W0080519

Drug Regulatory Affairs

Drug Regulatory Affairs

Papiya Bigoniya

BPharm MPharm PhD

Professor and Principal
DSKM College of Pharmacy
RKDF University, Bhopal

former faculty at Department of Pharmacy, Barkatullah University, and
Globus College of Pharmacy, Bhopal, and

former Professor and Principal, Radharaman College of Pharmacy, Bhopal

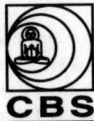

CBS

CBS Publishers & Distributors Pvt Ltd

New Delhi • Bengaluru • Chennai • Kochi • Kolkata • Mumbai
Bhopal • Bhubaneswar • Hyderabad • Jharkhand • Nagpur • Patna • Pune
Uttarakhand • Dhaka (Bangladesh) • Kathmandu (Nepal)

Disclaimer

Science and technology are constantly changing fields. New research and experience broaden the scope of information and knowledge. The author has tried her best in giving information available to her while preparing the material for this book. Although all efforts have been made to ensure optimum accuracy of the material, yet it is quite possible some errors might have been left uncorrected. The publisher, the printer and the author will not be held responsible for any inadvertent errors or inaccuracies.

Drug Regulatory Affairs

ISBN: 978-93-88902-96-0

Copyright © Author and Publisher

First Edition: 2020

Reprint: 2024

All rights reserved. No part of this book may be reproduced or transmitted in any form or by any means, electronic or mechanical, including photocopying, recording, or any information storage and retrieval system without permission, in writing, from the author and the publisher.

Published by Satish Kumar Jain and Produced by Varun Jain for

CBS Publishers & Distributors Pvt Ltd

4819/XI Prahlad Street, 24 Ansari Road, Daryaganj, New Delhi 110 002, India
Ph: 011-23289259, 23266861

Website: www.cbspd.com
e-mail: delhi@cbspd.com

Corporate Office: 204 FIE, Industrial Area, Patparganj, Delhi 110 092
Ph: 011-4934 4934   Fax: 011-4934 4935   e-mail: publishing@cbspd.com; publicity@cbspd.com

Branches

- **Bengaluru:** Seema House 2975, 17th Cross, K.R. Road, Banasankari 2nd Stage, Bengaluru 560 070, Karnataka, India
  Ph: +91-80-26771678/79   Fax: +91-80-26771680   e-mail: bangalore@cbspd.com
- **Chennai:** 7, Subbaraya Street, Shenoy Nagar, Chennai 600 030, Tamil Nadu, India
  Ph: +91-44-26680620, 26681266   Fax: +91-44-42032115   e-mail: chennai@cbspd.com
- **Kochi:** 42/1325, 1326, Power House Road, Opp KSEB, Power House, Ernakulam 682 018, Kerala, India
  Ph: +91-484-4059061-65   Fax: +91-484-4059065   e-mail: kochi@cbspd.com
- **Kolkata:** 147, Hind Ceramics Compound, 1st Floor, Nilgunj Road, Belghoria, Kolkata-700056
  West Bengal, India
  Ph: 033-25633055, 033-25633056   e-mail: kolkata@cbspd.com
- **Lucknow:** Basement, Khushnuma Complex, 7-Meerabai Marg (Behind Jawahar Bhawan), Lucknow 226001, India
  Ph: 0522-4000032   e-mail: tiwari.lucknow@cbspd.com
- **Mumbai:** PWD Shed. Gala no. 25/26, Ramchandra Bhatt Marg, Next to JJ Hospital Gate no. 2, Opp. Union Bank of India Noorbaug
  Mumbai-400009, Maharashtra, India
  Ph: 022-66661880/89   e-mail: mumbai@cbspd.com

Representatives

- **Hyderabad** 0-9885175004 • **Jharkhand** 0-9811541605 • **Nagpur**   0-8692091830
- **Patna**   0-9334159340 • **Pune**   0-9664372571 • **Uttarakhand** 0-9716462459

Printed at: Glorious Printers, Delhi, India

Preface

The regulatory affairs is a basic part of pharmaceutical science governing the ethical and legal issues that must be followed to safeguard public health. It implies with drug development, clinical trials, manufacturing, quality control, marketing authorization and sale of pharmaceutical products. Drug regulation is a multistep, multifunctional, interrelated practice that is to be adopted in three levels: Man, material, and method of a pharmaceutical organization. Understanding the impact of each level, proper coordinate functions are necessary to have an appreciable quality output, or it can result in dysfunctions with a quality defect. The overall aim of drug regulatory affairs is the integration of varieties of functions occurring at each level and to have a zero defect manufacturing mechanism. For example, when the quality of a vendor acquired material varies, the quality attributes of the final product will also vary despite the proper functioning of man and method.

In the current scenario, it is highly demanded to provide industry ready freshers who can quickly get a cohort in the assorted environment of a manufacturing firm. This requires the students to get exposed to theoretical concepts of drug regulation along with practical aspects of on-site implementation. As an author I have tried to make the content practical as much as possible, thus giving out this book with the abolition of the classical boundary between a textbook and a practical manual. Most of the pharmaceuticals, not all the personnel responsible for QC and QA related activities, belong to pharmacy background or had previous training. This was my endeavor to present this book in easily understandable verse that will be helpful for the persons of non-pharmacy background to relate with the subject comfortably and can effortlessly adopt in daily working. The book has been devised not only to give a detailed account of drug regulation but also has emphasized on the regulatory requirement of the agency like USFDA, WHO, EU, TGA, ICH, etc. The book contains information that I believe is essential to acquire a clear understanding of regulatory affairs and its practice in the industry.

This book contains tables, forms and lists apart from the text to provide with documentation and record keeping template that can be followed and further be adopted as per individual need. Concepts and processes are represented in the form of diagrammatic representations for easy understanding. As an integrated approach, the book is a step ahead by providing diagrammatic outlines and figures related to important drug regulatory concepts. Each chapter is provided with a chapter content list and key points to identify important subject matter and major issues covered. Basic terms in the text are displayed in bold or italic for easy recognition and memorization. The eight chapters contain information that is most relevant and applicable not only for students to gain knowledge but also for industries to apply in practice. The lists provide a list of important documents to be maintained by each section of the pharmaceutical manufacturing firm with a representative format that will serve as a template. The content of all the chapters has strong relevance to the implementation of cGMP quality practices in pharmaceutical manufacturing unit.

The content of this book has been designed to match the syllabus of drug regulatory affairs in BPharm and MPharm courses of various universities. The chapters are divided to accommodate subject content that is most commonly covered in the postgraduate syllabus and has updated and reviewed content in context to current global regulatory guidelines. I have integrated the subject matter in the particular chapters that are taught in the pharmacy institutions at undergraduate and postgraduate levels. The subject spectrum of drug regulatory affairs is very vast to accommodate in one book, so this is the first title in a line. Drug regulatory affairs is a subject of continuous evolution and change, the students and professionals should continue to study throughout their career. The bibliography has been incorporated at the end of each chapter that is suggested for further detailed study.

Papiya Bigoniya

Contents

Chapter 1

Drug Regulation in Nutshell

CHAPTER OVERVIEW

- Introduction
- Structure of drug regulatory organizations
- Major functions of drug regulatory authorities
- Drug regulation worldwide
  United States
    Federal Register and Code of Federal Regulations
    Orange Book
    Purple Book
- Canada
- Europe
  United Kingdom
  Norway
  Iceland
  Switzerland
- Japan
- China
- Brazil
- Australia
  Drug Regulation in India
- Central Drugs Standard Control Organization (CDSCO)
  The Drug Controller General of India (DCGI)
  Drug Technical Advisory Board (DTAB)
  Medical Devices Advisory Committee (MDAC)
  Medical Devices Technical Advisory Board (MDTAB)
  Subject Expert Committees (SEC)
  Drug Consultative Committee (DCC)
  Central Licences Approving Authority (CLAA)
  National Pharmaceutical Pricing Authority (NPPA)
  Indian Pharmacopoeial Commission (IPC)
- New Initiatives
  Central Drug Authority (CDA)
  Proposed Powers and Functions of CDA
- State Drug Control Organization
- International harmonization Initiative by regulatory bodies
- World Health Organization (WHO)
    Constitution of WHO
    Governance of WHO
    Functions of WHO
    Harmonization initiative
    Regulatory support activities
    Challenges for WHO
- European Union
- The International Council for Harmonisation (ICH)
- Harmonization in Africa
- Regional harmonization initiatives
    Pharmaceutical Inspection Convention and Pharmaceutical Inspection Co-operation Scheme (PIC/S)
    Global Harmonization Task Force (GHTF)
    Asia-Pacific Economic Cooperation (APEC; 21 member economies)
    Association of the Southeast Asian Nations (ASEAN; 10 economies)
    Gulf Cooperation Council (GCC 6 Gulf states)
    Pan American Network for Drug Regulatory Harmonization (PANDRH)
    Southern African Development Community (SADC 15 countries)
    East African Community (EAC 6 countries)
- Regulatory affairs personnel
- Qualification and experience required in regulatory professional
- Roles and responsibilities of pharma regulatory affairs personnel
- Bibliography

KEY POINTS

- The chapter compiles an overview of the purpose, applicability, relevance, history, and services of the regulatory authorities worldwide with major functions of the drug regulatory authorities in global perspective.
- Evolution, structure, legal frame, acts, and rules of various regulatory authorities like Indian, USA, Canada, Europe, China, Japan, Brazil and Australia, and their fundamental variability in the foundation of drug laws and scope of implementation.
- Organization and functional mechanism of Indian Drug Regulation with special focus to CDSCO, DCGI, and different committees along with an overview of the State Drug Control Organization.
- Looking into the differing level of control, astringency and complexity of the regulatory authorities worldwide, harmonization of technical requirements for medicines regulation is a need of the time. International harmonization initiatives have been adopted by different groups of countries to make uniform technical requirements for medicines regulation, viz. legislation, guidelines, procedures, quality, safety, and efficacy-related requirements.
- Regulatory Affairs is a fast developing department in pharmaceuticals with the expansion of business having broad scope. The roles and responsibilities of regulatory professionals cover not only to handle regulatory approval of drugs but also in research and development, clinical trials, manufacturing, advertising and post-marketing surveillance.

INTRODUCTION

Pharmaceuticals play a vital role in saving our lives, restoring health, preventing diseases and epidemics. In the period between 1930–50s, many pharmaceutical companies have flourished, and trade in the pharmaceutical industry has taken international dimensions. At the same time, circulation of toxic, substandard and counterfeit drugs on the national and international market has increased due to ineffective regulation of production and trade in pharmaceutical products. These substandard drugs have taken the lives of many as sulfanilamide incident in the United States of America in the mid-1930s led to deaths of 107 children and thalidomide disaster of the 1960s which caused congenital disabilities in children. Diethylene glycol contamination in paracetamol has led to multiple tragedies in Haiti and India. Safety and quality issues arise with the use of drugs containing toxic substances, impurities, unverified efficacy, substandard, outright fake and counterfeit drugs with the potential to cause unknown and severe adverse reactions. The problems of drug safety and efficacy

related severe adverse reactions can effectively be tackled by establishing robust drug regulatory system.

The therapeutically used drugs and other devices are strictly regulated by the jurisdiction in most of the countries worldwide to protect the public from harmful and dubious medicines. The primary aim of therapeutic goods regulation is to protect the health and safety of the population. Regulation ensures the safety, quality, and efficacy of the therapeutic products covered under the scope of the regulation. Drug regulation provides legal guidelines for manufacturing and marketing and trade-related activities of all types of products made available with medicinal claims by the public and private sectors. Development, production, importation, exportation, and distribution of therapeutic products are astringently regulated to ensure compliance with the prescribed standards. Therapeutic products are registered before they are allowed for distribution and marketing. The critical functions of drug regulatory bodies are the inspection of manufacturing facilities, product safety assessment and registration (marketing authorization), control of quality, adverse drug reaction monitoring, and control of drug promotion and advertising. Though each of these functions targets a different aspect of pharmaceutical activities, all of them are under taken simultaneously to ensure adequate consumer protection. Highly developed drug regulation framework is currently implemented in countries like the United Kingdom, the United States of America, Australia, Canada, Japan, and China. Well-formulated and strictly implemented drug regulation in these countries was possible with overwhelmed participation of consumers, and other stakeholders with enhanced political support that promoted transparency, accountability and protection from external influence.

STRUCTURE OF DRUG REGULATORY ORGANIZATIONS

Medicines regulation requires collective input of medical, scientific and technical knowledge and operates within a legal framework. Regulatory functions involve interactions with stakeholders, e.g. manufacturers, traders, consumers, health professionals, researchers and governments making implementation a real challenging job. Drug regulation is generously needed to be updated to match up with changes and new challenges in the scientific knowledge. The current scenario of drug regulation has evolved to its present status over a long time evolution. Along with this, the scope of legislative and regulatory powers has gradually expanded, to keep pace with the ever-increasing complexity of the sophisticated pharmaceutical sector. In most of the instances, the enactment of comprehensive drug laws was a result of public demand that led to the adoption of more restrictive legislation to provide stronger safeguards for the public following some significant public hazards due to adverse effects.

Worldwide legal structures of the regulatory authorities are considerably variable from the foundation of drug laws to their scope of implementation resulting in a regulatory gap between countries. For instance, in some countries, registration of herbal and homeopathic drugs are not required while, in others, legal mandates are not imposed on the exportation of drugs. Drug laws should be comprehensive enough to cover all areas of pharmaceutical activity in the respective country itself along with covering aspects of drugs which are exported to other countries. Regulatory guidelines describing the procedures and standards provide practical means to the regulatory authorities to implement laws. Whereas most of the drug regulatory organizations in developed countries have very well-defined and well-documented guidelines, but some drug regulatory authorities in underdeveloped countries do not have documented standard procedures for registration and inspection. WHO and other international agencies are providing support to countries in developing drug regulation structure, despite that less than 20% of WHO Member States have a well-developed system. Nowadays export and import of drugs and pharmaceuticals are flourishing as a growing market. The discrepancy in regulatory tools leads to variations in the implementation of the law and transparency of law enforcement.

In India, drug regulation is enforced both at state and national levels by various bodies. Some countries, such as the United States, drugs are regulated at the national level by a single agency, but in some other jurisdictions as in Australia, it is regulated at the state level only. In some countries, a single agency controls all functions related to drug regulation and jurisdiction having full command authority. In some other countries, like India, drug regulatory functions are assigned to more than one agency, at different levels of government control making the exercise of drug regulation fragmented. Under this type of organizational structure, command, coordination, and control of multitude regulatory functions to ensure adequate drug regulation is an enormous task. India, with a federal system of government, some drug regulatory activities are delegated to the State. Implementing public health policy through multiple levels of regulation concerning independent authorities requires a concerted effort between the agencies, and on the other side this type of system decentralize the activities and increases the effectiveness of the policy, but in a divided system, there can be a problem with the unity of command over drug regulatory functions. Indian drug regulatory structure is designed in a way that there is a central coordinating body (i.e. Drug Controller General of India) with overall responsibility and accountability for all aspects of drug regulation. The DCGI has an established official route for coordination and information flow at the national level covering entire country to support decision-making in all aspects of drug regulation. Drug regulation is not the sole mission of all the drug regulatory authorities, regulatory agencies in some countries are given non-regulatory functions due to political considerations or shortage of resources. This may lead to shift of focus from one function to another compromising performance and ineffective drug regulation.

Safety and quality issues are the main reasons that the authorities assess the medicines before they are placed on the market. Before placing a new Medicinal Product in the market, the applicant must perform extensive quality, toxicology, and clinical studies. The results of such studies are submitted to regulatory authorities for a review of conformance to the quality and safety standards of medicine, only then the medicines can be released in the market for consumers use. Regulatory agencies also work with custom and police department for inspecting medicinal products at ports and other points of entry, and distribution outlets. The regulatory authority helps in the detection and investigation of crimes involved in the illegal trade of medicines for apprehending and prosecuting criminals. The requirements made for veterinary medicines also same as that are intended for human consumption. Currently, the drug regulatory organizations, clinical evaluation boards, quality control laboratories, and pharmacovigilance information center have developed gradually to a level of excellence. Still though several areas in drug regulation *viz.* post-marketing surveillance, ADR reporting, control of drug information, etc. receive relatively little attention in the implementation process. Unlicensed manufacturers, importers, wholesalers, retailers and even individual persons engaged in the pharmaceutical business pose severe challenges to drug regulation. There is a big challenge in front of the regulatory agencies to control and monitor activities in the informal pharmaceutical sector. Informal sector mainly involves counterfeit products and products of dubious quality. Faulty exaggerated claims of efficacy especially related to herbal products are widespread in the informal sector. Increased globalization of the pharmaceutical trade has lead to the proliferation of harmful substandard and counterfeit medicines circulating in national and international markets. Pre-marketing safety and efficacy testing and documentation are primarily given more importance than post-marketing activities. Post-marketing surveillance, ADR monitoring and re-evaluation of registered products should also be given equal priority in drug regulation. Drug information received from the consumers and manufacturer has a significant influence on rational drug use. Monitoring of the post marketing safety along with accuracy and appropriateness of drug information provided to the public is generally inadequate which is now actively controlled by WHO with international pharmacovigilance networking system.

Regulatory, organizational structure and the working process need to have routine monitoring to identify problems in implementation and to determine loopholes in the system. Performance review by the supervisory body and peer analysis of guidelines implementation system should be implemented strictly by the regulatory bodies for performance appraisal and identification of areas requiring improvement. Drug regulation system in every country has some strength and weaknesses. Implementation of appropriate functional structure and continuous up gradation of guidelines ensures enforcement and enactment of policies. In many third world countries, medicine legislation and regulatory guidelines are 'copied' from other countries that do not reflect national realities and are not regularly updated. Every country should have drug regulation guidelines suitable to the national legislative framework. Regular updating of the medicine legislation and regulations must address new pharmaceutical issues arising as a result of continuous scientific and technological changes occurring in the field. Competent human resource, freedom from political and commercial influence, well defined standards and procedures, outcome-oriented systematic monitoring, comprehensive and up-to-date laws will contribute to regular and effective updating of drug regulation system in a country.

MAJOR FUNCTIONS OF DRUG REGULATORY AUTHORITIES

- Controlling and monitoring the quality of marketed medicines
- Ensure adequate supply of quality medicines at affordable prices
- Control the supply and pricing of essential and life saving medicines
- Define the medicinal products categories and activities to be regulated
- Provide legislation, Acts and Rules related to all the activities of medicines trade
- Define the roles, responsibilities, rights, and functions of all individuals/agencies involved in the manufacturing and trade of medicines
- Publish medicines regulation guidelines for better understanding of regulatory aspects and facilitate their implementation
- Define the norms, standards, and specifications applied for assessing the safety, efficacy, and quality of medicines
- Set the qualifications and standards required for all those handling medicines
- Licensing for the manufacturing, distribution, and sale of medicines
- Define the terms and conditions for suspending, revoking or canceling activity and product licenses related to manufacturing and sale of medicines
- Define prohibitions, offenses, penalties, and legal actions
- Marketing authorization for import and export of medicines
- Inspecting manufacture premises, wholesale and retail outlet of medicines
- Controlling promotion and advertisement of medicines
- Work with Pharmacopoeial commission that sets standards for all drugs manufactured, sold and consumed in India
- Work with Central Drug Testing Laboratory which is the appellate laboratory for testing of drugs
- Inspection and controlling of blood banks
- Inspecting and controlling clinical trials centers in respective states
- Monitoring adverse reactions of medicines
- Providing appropriate information on medicines to professionals and the public
- Train staff to carry out regulatory related functions
- Create mechanisms to ensure transparency and accountability in regulatory function

- Establish mechanisms to deal with public/consumer complaints
- Participate in state and central schemes, harmonization of regulatory processes and standards, mutual recognition of regulatory decisions with an aim to prevent duplication of effort to reduce workloads and save resources.
- Networking and exchange of information with other regulatory authorities

Many developing and underdeveloped countries are unable to ensure the safety, efficacy, and quality of medicines available on their markets because of limitations in standard regulatory systems. Countries with limited resources for regulatory implementation should primarily focus on encouraging the development of the pharmaceutical industry by controlling the sale and distribution of drugs. Drug regulation is perceived as an obstacle to the availability of low cost medicines in the markets of such countries. Drug regulation though in many instances may delay and prolongs the availability of new and potent molecules in the market for diseases of high lethality rate like cancer and AIDS.

On the other hand, the political environment in some countries favors the demand for new medicines for local patients without fully understanding the importance of effective guideline implementation that ensures the availability of effective and safe medicines. Balancing these two sides of the swift availability of new molecule and comprehensive assessment of safety is indeed a difficult task and can only be possible with a strict time line based regulatory system. Drug regulatory bodies must ensure both the viability of pharmaceutical industries as well as the availability of high standard medicines at a low cost. Harmonized or centralized regulation system in particular speeds up the reviews and evaluations in a fixed timeline so that new medicines can be approved in the shortest possible time.

DRUG REGULATION WORLDWIDE

UNITED STATES

In the United States, the US Food and Drug Administration (USFDA) regulates therapeutic goods. Under the joint jurisdiction of the FDA and the Drug Enforcement Administration (DEA) possession of some substances are prohibited as per schedule of the Controlled Substances Act. *Tea Importation Act* came into force on 1897 was possibly first consumer protection law in the USA. At that time, there were no Federal laws governing use or distribution of any drug. Heroin, morphine, and cocaine-like substances were readily available and sold as part of "patent" medicines to cure wide categories of pain from menstrual cramps to toothaches in children. In *1906, the Pure Food and Drug Act* was enacted strictly implementing a 'labeling law' for foods and drugs. The first comprehensive federal consumer protection law was implemented in 1906. *The Pure Food and Drug Act*, which prohibited misbranded and adulterated food and drugs in interstate commerce. The passage of the 1906 Act was due in large part to the untiring scientific and political efforts of Harvey Washington Wiley, who at that time was a chief chemist of the Bureau of Chemistry of the U.S. Department of Agriculture, FDA's predecessor. Previous to 1914, restrictions were on the State or local level only, and those restrictions were few and far between and commonly targeted to use by certain *groups*.

Up till the early 1930s, some egregious examples of consumer products that poisoned, maimed and killed many people spurred national outrage. The requirement of toxicity testing before marketing drugs or cosmetics was enacted in 1938 following a lethal toxic effect of sulfanilamide dissolved in diethylene glycol which unfortunately caused kidney poisoning and killed 107 people. This amendment also implemented directions needed to be used on the package and made the first mention of "use by an instruction from a physician only" in other words, prescription vs. non-prescription medicines. The enactment of the *1938 Federal Food, Drug, and Cosmetic Act* (FFDCA), replaced the earlier *Pure Food and Drug Act of* 1906. This has given authority to USFDA, to tighten controls over drugs and food. It includes protection of consumer from unlawful cosmetics and medical devices, and enhanced the government's ability to enforce the law. The amendment states that a drug had to be effective for what it was intended and approval had to be obtained before conduction human trial, which was introduced in 1962. Comprehensive *Drug Abuse Prevention and Control Act* (*Controlled Substance Act of 1970*) bought the drugs under the act and also under Federal jurisdiction that dealt with both narcotics and other "dangerous" drugs. The *Comprehensive Methamphetamine Control Act, 1996* restricted access to chemicals and equipment used in the manufacture of methamphetamine and increased penalties for possession of these plus the manufacture and sale of the drug. The act has been amended many times, till most recently to add requirements about preparations that can be used in bioterrorism. In the year 2009, President Obama signed the Family Smoking Prevention and Tobacco Control Act along with the formation of the FDA center for tobacco products.

The USFDA is an agency within the U.S. Department of Health and Human Services consisting of the Office of the Commissioner and four directorates overseeing the core functions of the agency. USFDA is responsible for protecting the public health by assuring the safety, effectiveness, and quality of human and veterinary drugs, vaccines and other biological products, medical devices, food, cosmetics, dietary supplements, tobacco products and products that give off radiation.

Some of the USFDA's specific responsibilities include control of:

- Product and manufacturing establishment licensing

- Establishing safety standards for blood transfusions
- Conduct research to establish product related standards and to develop improved testing methods
- Product approvals
- Drug manufacturing standards
- Quality and safety of biologics
- Quality and safety of drugs
- Quality and safety of cosmetics
- OTC and prescription drug labeling
- Quality and safety of all food products (except meat and poultry)
- Quality and safety of bottled water
- Quality and safety of medical devices
- Premarket approval of new devices
- Tracking reports of device malfunctioning and serious adverse reaction
- Quality and safety of radiation emitting electronic products
- Quality and safety of veterinary drugs and devices
- Quality and safety of livestock feeds
- Quality and safety of pet foods

Federal Register and Code of Federal Regulations

As required by law, the Food and Drug Administration publishes regulations in the *Federal Register* before issuing a final rule, in the federal government's official publication for notifying the public. All approved rules, proposed rules, notices, executive orders and other presidential documents of Federal agencies and organizations are officially published daily in the Federal Register that is published by the Office of the Federal Register, National Archives and Records Administration (NARA). The Federal Register is updated daily and is published on Monday through Friday, except Federal holidays.

The final rules promulgated by a federal agency are published in the Federal Register and ultimately reorganized by topic or subject matter as 'codified' in the Code of Federal

Regulations (CFR). The CFR is annually published in the Federal Register and in addition to this CFR is also published in an unofficial format online on the Electronic CFR website, which is updated daily. The CFR is divided into 50 titles that represent broad subject areas of federal regulation. The rule explaining the regulatory requirements of drugs are published under *Title 21 of Code of Federal Regulations*. The 21 CFR governs USFDA, the Drug Enforcement Administration (DEA) and the Office of National Drug Control Policy (ONDCP). The 21 CFR is divided into three chapters:

- Chapter I: Food and Drug Administration (The Federal Food, Drug, and Cosmetic Act.)
- Chapter II: Drug Enforcement Administration (for controlled substances)
- Chapter III: Office of National Drug Control Policy

Chapter I is divided into 12 subchapters that are concerned with drugs, cosmetics, biologicals, medical devices, tobacco products controlled by the Food and Drug Administration under the Department of Health and Human Services.

Orange Book (Approved Drug Products with Therapeutic Equivalence Evaluations)

The USFDA publishes a list of prescription drugs in 'Approved Drug Products with Therapeutic Equivalence Evaluations' that is commonly known as the Orange Book, identifying the drug products approved on the basis of safety and efficacy under the Federal Food, Drug, and Cosmetic Act. The Drug Price and Competition Act (Hatch-Waxman Act) requires FDA to publish the Orange Book.

The criterion for inclusion of any product in Orange Book is that the product has an effective approval and has not been withdrawn for safety or efficacy reasons. The publication does not include drugs on the market approved only on the basis of safety. The Orange Book contains therapeutic equivalence evaluations of approved multisource prescription generic drug products approved under Section 505 of the Federal Food, Drug, and Cosmetic Act to provide public information for state health agencies, prescribers and pharmacists. The Orange Book also lists patents and use codes provided by the drug application owner. The generic drug manufacturer can get the approval of a drug under the Hatch-Waxman Act only after expiration of the Orange Book listed patent or in case the patent is invalid or unenforceable. Orange Book was first published in 1980, and each subsequent edition has included new approvals and made appropriate changes in data. Orange Book is composed of four sections:

- Approved prescription drug products with therapeutic equivalence evaluations.
- Approved over-the-counter (OTC) drug products not covered under existing OTC monographs.
- Drug products approved under Section 505 of the Federal Food, Drug, and Cosmetic Act administered by the Center for Biologics Evaluation and Research.
- A cumulative list of approved products that have never been marketed, for exportation, for military use, have been discontinued from marketing or approvals other than safety or efficacy reasons after being discontinued.

This book index the prescription and OTC drug products by trade name (proprietary name) or established name (if no trade name exists) and by applicant name (holder of the approved application, who may not necessarily be the manufacturer of the product). Established names for active ingredients usually conform to official compendia names or the United States Adopted Names (USAN) as described in 21 CFR 2994e. The Addendum contains patent and exclusivity information of the prescription, OTC, approved drug products and the discontinued drug product. The Orange Book does not include drug products with tentative approvals, but it lists the drug product and the date of approval in the appropriate approved drug product list when the tentative approval becomes a final approval.

The multisource drug products are assigned a therapeutic equivalence code. The user can determine the approval status of the product following the coding system for therapeutic equivalence evaluations (e.g. a particular strength of an approved drug) as therapeutically equivalent to other pharmaceutically equivalent products (first letter) and to provide additional information on the basis of FDA's evaluations (second letter).

Multisource drugs are placed into two basic categories, indicated by the first letter of the relevant therapeutic equivalence code as follows:

a. Drug products that FDA considers to be therapeutically equivalent to other pharmaceutically equivalent products, i.e. drug products for which there is no known or suspected bioequivalence problems. These products are designated AA, AN, AO, AP, or AT, depending on the dosage form. The products are designated as AB, in case the actual or potential bioequivalence problems have been resolved with adequate *in vivo* and/or *in vitro* evidence supporting bioequivalence.

b. Drug products that FDA considers not to be therapeutically equivalent to other pharmaceutically equivalent products, i.e. drug products are designated as BC, BD, BE, BN, BP, BR, BS, BT, BX when the actual or potential bioequivalence problems have not been resolved by adequate evidence of bioequivalence.

Every product in the Orange Book is a subject to regulatory action at all times. Thus the approved products may be found in violation of one or more provisions of the Act. FDA believes that the retention of a violative product in the Orange Book will not have any significant adverse health consequences, as other legal mechanisms are available to prevent the product from marketing. FDA may, however, change a product's therapeutic equivalence rating or call for assessment as of whether the product meets the criteria for therapeutic equivalence. Efforts are made to ensure that the annual edition of the current Orange Book is accurate. Applicants are requested to inform the FDA about any changes or corrections, related to the product's marketing status that can result in the product being moved to the discontinued drug product list in writing within 180 days.

Purple Book (Lists of Licensed Biological Products with Reference Product Exclusivity and Biosimilarity or Interchangeability Evaluations)

The Patient Protection and Affordable Care Act (Affordable Care Act), 2010 authorize amendment of the PHS Act to include an abbreviated licensure pathway for biological products demonstrated to be biosimilar to or interchangeable with an FDA licensed biological product. A single biological product licensed by FDA under Section 351(a) of the Public Health Service Act (PHS Act) against which a proposed biological product is evaluated in an application submitted under Section 351(k) is considered as a reference product. Healthcare providers are allowed to prescribe biosimilar and interchangeable biological products similarly as they prescribe other medications. The Biologics Price Competition and Innovation (BPCI) Act of 2009 permits that an interchangeable product can be substituted for the reference product without the intervention of the healthcare provider who prescribed the reference product. In contrast, a biosimilar product should be specifically prescribed by the healthcare provider and cannot be substituted for a reference product at the pharmacy level.

The Purple Book lists biological products like biosimilar and interchangeable biological products licensed by FDA under the PHS Act. The Purple Book includes FDA evaluation status of a biological product licensed under Section 351(k) of the PHS Act as to be biosimilar to or interchangeable with a reference biological product already licensed as FDA biological product. Along with the evaluation status of the biological product for reference product exclusivity, the Purple Book also includes the date for licensing approval of the biological products under Section 351(a) of the PHS Act. Biosimilar and interchangeable biological products licensed under Section 351(k) of the PHS Act are listed under the reference product to which similarity or interchangeability was demonstrated. The resource lists all reference biological products licensed under Section 351(a), side-by-side with all corresponding biosimilars and interchangeable products licensed under Section 351(k) that is the primary purpose of Purple Book along with providing information on any existing reference product exclusivity protecting a reference biological product.

This book is designed to enable the user to verify whether a particular biological product has been determined by the Food and Drug Administration (FDA) to be a biosimilar or interchangeable with a reference biological product. The lists cross-reference the names of biological products licensed under Section 351(a) with the names of biosimilar or interchangeable biological products licensed under Section 351(k). A separate list is provided for the biological products regulated by the Center for Drug Evaluation and Research (CDER) and the Center for Biologics Evaluation and Research (CBER). The list will identify the date of the first licensure if a biological product is protected by a period of reference product exclusivity and will also mention the date for exclusivity expiry. The list does not identify periods of orphan exclusivity and their expiration dates for biological products. The Purple book lists are updated periodically to include the biological

products licensed under Section 351(a) or Section 351(k) and/or it determines the date of the first licensure for a biological product licensed under Section 351(a) of the PHS Act.

CANADA

In Canada, Food and Drugs Regulations are governed by the *"Food and Drug Act"* and associated regulations. The Therapeutic Products Directorate (TPD) implements the Food and Drug Regulations and the Medical Devices Regulations as per the authority of the *Food and Drugs Act*, to ensure safety, efficacy, and quality of pharmaceutical drugs and medical devices offered for sale in Canada. Under the authority of the Financial Administration Act, the TPD also administers fee regulations for drugs and medical devices. Food and drugs regulation have seven parts along with schedules defining different categories of drugs in list and tables:

• Part A: Administration
• Part B: Foods
• Part C: Drugs
• Part D: Vitamins, minerals, and amino acids
• Part E: Cyclamate and saccharin sweeteners
• Part G: Controlled drugs
• Part J: Restricted drugs

Part B contains regulation guiding safety and quality of alcoholic beverages, soft drinks, milk products, spice, fruits and vegetables, poultry products and food packaging details. Part C is for manufacturing licensing of drugs, GMP, radiopharmaceuticals, biologicals, clinical trials, drug categories like a new drug, non-prescription drugs, steroidal drugs, and sales regulation. Health Canada believes that disease prevention and health promotion can cut down the health care costs and improve the quality of life in the long term. Drug policy of Canada has traditionally favored punishment of even the smallest of offenders, until it was partially broken in 1996 with the passing of the *Controlled Drugs and Substances Act*. *Controlled Drugs and Substances Act* defines eight different schedules of drugs and describes new penalties enforced for the possession, trafficking, exportation, and production of controlled substances. This law replaced the *Narcotic Control Act* and Parts III and IV of the *Food and Drugs Act* which deal with the advertisement of controlled substances. Canada was the first country in the world to legalize the use of cannabis for the terminally ill patients in 2001. The Canadian Food Inspection Agency (CFIA) is assigned to the mission of safeguarding food, animals, and plants to enhance the health and well being of Canada's people, environment and economy.

EUROPE

United Kingdom

A comprehensive regulatory system was introduced in the United Kingdom in 1968 though there was some regulation previously imposed since the time of King Henry VIII. The first comprehensive licensing system for medicines in the UK was the *Medicines Act of 1968*. The new *Medicines Act* brought legislation on medicines with the introduction of many other legal provisions for the control of medicines. The Act provided a system of licensing of manufacturing, sale, supply, and importation of medicinal products into the UK. Safety monitoring is achieved by ensuring that product labels, leaflets, prescribing information and advertising meets the required standards lay down by the Regulations. A three-tiered classification system is enforced in the United Kingdom:

- General Sale List (GSL)
- Pharmacy Medicines (PM)
- Prescription Only Medicines (POM)

Controlled Drugs (CD) are some commonly known substances having high abuse/addiction liability separately scheduled under the *Misuse of Drugs Act 1971* within the POM and the *Misuse of Drugs Regulations 2001*.

Following the introduction of Medicines Act, 1968, many amendments were made, and the government consolidated medicines legislation, into one set of new regulations, the *Human Medicines Regulations 2012*. A comprehensive regime for the marketing authorization, manufacture, import, distribution, sale, supply, labeling, advertising and for pharmacovigilance of products were introduced. This regulations introduced some limited policy changes related to statutory warnings for over the counter products, membership of review panels, health professionals' exemptions, provisions for Patient Group Directions, pharmacist-instigated changes to prescriptions and repeal in some sections of the *Medicines Act 1968* with 349 regulations in 17 parts, followed by 35 schedules. Some of the other vital regulations are: The Medicines (Sale or Supply) Regulations 1980 (Miscellaneous Provisions), The Medicines (Pharmacy and General Sale—Exemption) Order 1980 and The Medicines (Products Other Than Veterinary Drugs) Order 1984 (General Sale List), that was consolidated by the Human Medicines Regulations 2001. The Medicines (Advertising) Regulations 1994 was revoked and consolidated by the Human Medicine Regulations 2001. The Medicines (Responsible Pharmacist) Regulations 2008 describes the duties of responsible pharmacists for safe and effective running of a pharmacy business at the outlets. The Medicines for Human Use (Marketing Authorisations, etc.) Regulations 1994, The Prescription Only Medicines (Human Use) Order 1997, The Medicines for Human Use (Manufacturing, Wholesale Dealing, and Miscellaneous Amendments) Regulations 2005 and The Medicines for Human Use (Prescribing by EEA Practitioners) Regulations 2008 was also revoked and consolidated.

Medicines and Healthcare products Regulatory Agency (MHRA) regulates the medicines for human use in the United Kingdom that is an executive agency of the Department of Health. The MHRA was formed in 2003 with the merger of the Medicines Control Agency (MCA) and the Medical Devices Agency (MDA). The MHRAs primary objective is to ensure that all medicines on the UK market meet appropriate standards of safety, quality, and efficacy to safeguard public health. The agency achieves its objective through a system of licensing before the marketing of medicines, and monitoring of medicines and acting on safety concerns after they have been placed on the market.

MHRA has three centers:
- The Clinical Practice Research Datalink (CPRD) aimed to improve public health by using anonymized NHS clinical data
- The National Institute for Biological Standards and Control (NIBSC) is a global leader in the standardization and control of biological medicines
- The MHRA responsible for safety, quality and effectiveness of medicines, medical devices, and blood components

The MHRA classifies drugs and regulates marketing authorization of the drug products. MHRAs prime objectives are:
- Inspection of the pharmaceutical manufacturing facility,
- Enforcement of requirements in manufacturing, sales, and distribution,
- Implementing medicines control policy,
- Representing UK pharmaceutical regulatory interests internationally and publishing quality standards for drugs,
- Promoting international standardization and harmonization to assure the efficacy and safety of biological medicines,
- Ensuring the adoption of a safe and secure supply chain for medicines, medical devices, and blood components,
- Supporting innovation and research beneficial for the development of public health,

- Educating the public and healthcare professionals about the risks and benefits of medicines, medical devices and blood components for safe and effective use.

Medicines must meet the standards of safety, quality and efficacy standards before granting marketing authorization for market release. This authorization covers all the main activities associated with the marketing of medicinal products and reviewing all the research and test results in detail. MHRA along with the expert advisory bodies set up by the Medicines Act ensures safety, quality, and efficacy as the primary criteria on which legislative control of human medicines functions. MHRA experts assess applications seeking approval for new medicines to ensure they meet the required standards. In April 2013, MHRA merged with the National Institute for Biological Standards and Controls (NIBSC). The MHRA also works closely with other health promotion bodies like National Patient Safety Agency (NPSA), Care Quality Commission (CQC), Health Protection Agency (HPA) and National Institute for Clinical Excellence (NICE) providing guidance on the promotion of good health and the prevention of ill health in national level.

Following the Brexit (British exit) pole, UK has decided in June 2016, a referendum to leave the European Union (EU) by March 2019. Following the event of the EU referendum, MHRA is analyzing for the best options and opportunities concerning effective regulation of medicines and medical devices in the UK. While negotiations continue, the UK remains a full and active member of the EU, with all the rights and obligations of EU membership firmly in place. UK Government gave a clear, public statement of its desire to retain a close working partnership in respect of medicines regulation after the UK leaves the EU in the interests of public health and safety. UK's current regulatory relationship with the European network remains unchanged until the exit negotiations are concluded. MHRA uploaded a link to update pharmaceutical companies on exit preparations in January 2018.

Norway

Norwegian Medicines Agency (NoMA) established in 2001 has united different branches of public administration of pharmaceuticals in Norway in one single agency. NoMA is subordinate to the *Ministry of Health and Care Services Act* as the legislative authority. NoMA supervises production, clinical trials, and marketing of pharmaceuticals. The Mission of the NoMA is to safeguard public and animal health by ensuring the efficacy, quality, and safety of medicines. NoMA is in charge of marketing authorization, classification, vigilance, pricing, supply chain, reimbursement and providing information on medicines to prescribers and the public.

The European Economic Area (EEA) comprises 28 EU member states, and the three EFTA (European Free Trade Association) states Iceland, Liechtenstein, and Norway. Through the EEA Agreement and the EEA Joint Committee Decisions Norway complies to implement EU regulations and directives though it is directly not a member country in EU, Norwegian regulation for pharmaceuticals is harmonized with EU regulation. These regulations and directives concern the marketing authorizations for manufacturing and distribution of pharmaceuticals, supervision of use and clinical trials. Norway, as part of the European Economic Area, adheres to EU-regulations regarding marketing authorizations. The NoMA contributes to the work of the European Medicines Agency (EMA), alongside agencies from the EU-member states. Ministry of Health and Care Services of the Norwegian government participates in binding work with the EU under The European Medicines Agency (EMEA) in various committees and working groups.

Medicines in Norway are divided into five separate groups:
- Class A: Narcotics, sedative-hypnotics and amphetamines in this class require a special prescription form
- Class B: Restricted substances which can easily lead to addiction
- Class C: All prescription-only substances
- Class F: Substances and package sizes not requiring a prescription
- Unclassified: Brands and packages not actively marketed in Norway

Iceland

Medicines in Iceland are regulated by the Icelandic Medicines Control Agency (IMA), a governmental Agency under the Ministry of Welfare. IMA's responsibilities are an assessment of quality and safety of medicinal products, medical devices, conduct inspections to confirm regulatory requirements and to guarantee consumer protection. The Agency issues permission for clinical trials, classifies natural products and food supplements, controls ads on medicines and publishes a catalog of Medicinal Products. IMA is an independent regulatory authority, functions under the Ministry of Welfare. One of its primary functions is to issue marketing authorizations for medicines in Iceland and also works in close collaboration with regulatory authorities in the European Economic Area (EEA). IMA controls surveillance of the pharmaceutical industry in Iceland and contribute to the availability of unbiased information on medicines to the health professionals and consumers.

Medicinal product is defined as 'Any substance or compound claimed to have properties which can be used for treating diseases in humans or animals or preventing diseases or any substance or compound which can be used by humans or in animals or given to them either for the purpose of restoring, rectifying or amending a physiological function through pharmaceutical or immuno-logical action or influencing the metabolism or for confirming a diagnosis of a disease' as per the amended *Medicines Act No 93/1994*. IMA issues list with the classification of substances and compounds concerning the pharmaceutical activity and/or harmfulness, including substances/compounds banned/permitted as consumer products, i.e. any substance independent of origin:

- Humans, e.g. blood or blood products
- Animals, e.g. microorganisms, animals, tissues, serum, toxic chemicals, extracts, substances processed from the blood.
- Herbs, e.g. plants or plants parts and extracts.
- Other substances, e.g. elements, substances from natural resources, substances formed by chemical reactions or combinations.

The IMA build up a formal quality management system in 2001 about other regulatory agencies in the field of medicinal products as well as guidelines from international agencies were foreseen at that time, and constant regulatory changes were also taken into account. Strengthening of quality management has been done at IMA by increasing the number of active procedures, establishing specific Procedures Teams to oversees implementation of quality related issues and the progress there off. Under the auspice of the Heads of Medicines Agencies (HMA), self-assessments helped in assessing the status of the quality management system in the agency. Benchmarking of European Medicines Agencies (BEMA) and internal audits initiated has benefited the management for reviewing essential functions of the agency. The advisory committee of the Agency, named Pharma-ceutical Committee comprises five members with broad expertise in medicine. The Chairman is appointed by Minister and other members are appointed in consultation with the Chairman for a four-year term. For dealing veterinary medicinal products the Chief

Veterinary Officer and a veterinarian appointed by the Ministry controls the regulation procedure. The IMA is responsible for regulatory surveillance of medical devices as per the *Act on Medical Devices, No. 16/2001*. Manufacturers should ensure that their devices are safe and fit for intended purpose before they are CE marked. In concern to pharmacovigilance, all adverse reactions should be reported to IMA by the healthcare professionals, veterinarians and members of the public. IMA is a Web trader in the EMA database, Eudra Vigilance, and reports all adverse reactions received to that database.

Switzerland

Swiss Agency for Therapeutic Products called SwissMedic is the central Swiss supervisory authority for therapeutic products. Medicines in Switzerland are regulated by Swissmedic public service organization of the federal government with headquarters in Bern. The country is not a member of the European Union and thus regarded as one of the easiest places to conduct clinical trials of new drug compounds. Swissmedic is linked to the Federal Department of Home Affairs (FDHA) which connects Swissmedic to the Federal Council (the Swiss government).

Five categories to cover different types of Delivery as per Swissmedic are:

a. Single delivery on medical prescription
b. Repeated delivery on medical prescription
c. Prescription free delivery after consulta-tion of a specialist, restricted to pharmacy/chemist
d. Prescription free delivery after con-sultation of a specialist restricted to pharmacy, chemist, and drug store
e. Prescription free delivery without consultation in all shops/stores

Switzerland's Federal Drug Policy aims at harmonization of the various drug strategies of the cantons (states) and the 1951 *Narcotics Act*. The history of Switzerland's drug policy began towards the end of the 1960s when there was an increase in psychoactive drug use. Like many other countries, at the beginning of the 1980s, HIV-AIDS epidemic hit Switzerland as a consequence of the miserable state of drug addicts. In the 1990s, Switzerland introduced new measures to reduce the problems associated with drug use and adopted a new national drug strategy. Currently known as "ProMeDro,"the Swiss government adopted a federal program to reduce the problems related to drug use on February 20, 1991, which was based on the concept of 'harm reduction.' These measures mark the beginning of Switzerland's drug policy, based on a fourfold approach: Prevention, law enforcement, treatment, and harm reduction. The Federal Council passed the *Ordinance Governing the Medical Prescription of Heroin* authorizing heroin-assisted treatment, setting objectives, eligibility criteria and administrative measures for providing such treatment on 1999.

The *Federal Act on Medicinal Products and Medical Devices (Therapeutic Products Act, TPA) 2000*, issued by the Federal Assembly of the Swiss Confederation, is to protect human and animal health and to guarantee that high quality, safe and effective therapeutic products are placed on the market.

The Medical devices ordinance along with the TPA forms the legal basis of regulation of medical devices in Switzerland which classify the medical device as

·Classical medical devices: corresponding to European directive 93/42/EEC

- *In vitro* diagnostic medical devices: Corresponding to European Directive 98/79/EC.

- Active implantable medical devices: Corresponding to European Directive 90/385/EEC.

- Devices produced using devitalized human tissue: Within Switzerland, these devices are counted as classical or active implantable medical devices.

In September 2003, USFDA and SwissMedic signed a memorandum of understanding (MOU) to enhance and strengthen communication and public health promotion, cooperative activities related to the regulation of human or animal pharmaceutical products and human medical devices in Switzerland and the United States. Information exchanged under the MOU also includes non-public information exempt from public disclosure under the laws and regulations of Switzerland or the United States. As per the mandate of the Federal Council in 2013, Swissmedic implements Marketing Authorisation for Global Health Products (MAGHP) procedure with the National Medicines Regulatory Authorities (NMRAs) of the East African Community (EAC) to accelerate and increase access to high-quality, essential medicines for populations living in low-income countries. This was aimed to increase the efficiency of the regulatory registration and review process focusing on stakeholders value-added activities and strengthening the regulatory authorities ability to protect citizens health. The WHO Pre-Qualification Team (WHO PQT) can also be involved in this marketing authorization procedure with Swissmedic.

In 2017 Swissmedic authorizes electronic application format for submission of documents (eDok) for authorization and variation requests regarding both human medicinal products. It does not replace the electronic Common Technical Document (eCTD) and is more straightforward, in technical respects, as the eCTD format. The electronic data replaces the necessary paper copies required with a paper submission. Swissmedic carries out the review based on the documentation submitted electronically and archives the paper original as a legally binding document. When submitted via the portal, the eDok format is considered to be a purely electronic format without the need for any paper documents. When submitted by post, the eDok format is considered to be a paper format requiring the submission of a complete paper copy as the original paper version. When eDok application is submitted via the Swissmedic eGov Portal, the uploads completely replace paper documents submission and data carriers. Even documents with signatures are no longer necessary since authentication takes place via the Portal log-in corresponding to a fully electronic application format.

JAPAN

The pharmaceutical regulatory authority of Japan is the Pharmaceutical and Food Safety Bureau (PFSB) of the Ministry of Health, Labor, and Welfare (MHLW), government organization similar in function to the FDA of other countries. The MHLW was originally established in 1938 aimed at improvement and promotion of social welfare, social security, and public health. The MHLW was merged with the Ministry of Health and Welfare (MHW) and the Ministry of Labour in 2001 as part of the government program. Japanese MHLW is a complex organization as its ancestor, the MHW which has implemented many current regulations and decisions. Consolidation of the services of the Pharmaceuticals and Medical Devices Evaluation Center of the National Institute of Health Sciences (PMDEC), formed the Pharmaceuticals and Medical Devices Agency (PMDA), established in 2004. In conjunction with the MHLW, the PMDA is responsible for reviewing drug and medical device applications. The PMDA works with the MHLW to assess new product safety, develop comprehensive regulations and monitor post-market safety. The PMDEC, usually known as 'The Center', is the actual decision maker for approval of new drug applications (NDAs).

The PMDA reviews new drugs, generic drugs, OTC drugs/behind-the-counter (BTC) drugs, and quasi-drugs, and conducts re-evaluations of previously approved drugs. Orphan drugs and other priority drugs are given priority reviews following their clinical significance. The Pharmaceutical Safety and Environmental Health Bureau (PSEHB) is one of the 11 bureaus of the MHLW. In addition to policies to assure the efficacy and safety of drugs, quasi-drugs, cosmetics, and medical devices, and safety in medical institutions, the PFSB also ensures the health of the general public including policies related to blood supplies and blood products, and narcotics and stimulant drugs. The PMDA evaluates new drugs for approval based on the reliability of the studies conducted, efficacy outcome based on properly designed clinical studies, the clinical significance of the results, any unacceptable risks overwhelming the benefits and ensures continuity in efficacy and safety of the drug from quality assurance standpoint. The essential tasks of the agency are:

- Scientific review of market authorization applications for drug and medical device as per Japanese pharmaceutical law.
- Review and approval of NDAs for drug and medical device.
- Advice on clinical trials and dossiers for the registration procedure.
- Inspection and conformity assessment as per Good Clinical Practice (GCP), Good Laboratory Practice (GLP), and Good Practice Systems and Programs (GPSP).
- Auditing and inspection of marketing authorization holder manufacturers ensuring conformance with GMP, and Quality Management System (QMS) as per product family.
- Collection, analysis, and distribution of data on post-marketing quality, efficacy, and safety of medicines and medical devices.
- Regulation of medical software
- Advising consumers on the safety issues of approved drug products.
- Research on the development of standards for post-marketing drug safety.
- Payment towards compensation for medical costs and lost wages for the

sufferers of injury or disability resulting from the use of medical products.

- Disbursement of compensation funds to the HIV infection victims due to blood transfusions.

Modern pharmaceutical legislation in Japan was originated with the enactment of the Regulations on Handling and Sales of Medicines in 1889. The Pharmaceutical Affairs Law (PAL) was enacted in 1943 and revised several times. The current PAL is the result of complete revisions in 1948 and 1960. In 2002, the PAL was revised for safety assurance of biotechnology, genomics and post-marketing surveillance policies. After that, the provisions on the enhancement of safety measures for biological products came into effect in 2003 and control on medical devices and regenerative medicine products in 2013. The current Japanese regulations laid out in the *Pharmaceuticals and Medical Devices Act* (PMD Act), came into force on 2014 replacing the Pharmaceutical Affairs Law (PAL) that consists of 17 chapters and 91 articles. The PMD Act secures the quality, efficacy, and safety of pharmaceuticals, medical devices, regenerative and cellular therapy products, gene therapy products and cosmetics. This act affects all aspects of Japanese medical product registration, including in-country representation, certification processes, licensing, and quality assurance systems. The PMDA defines cellular and tissue-based (regenerative medicine) products that are intended to be used for reconstruction, repair, or formation of structures or functions of the human body, treatment or prevention of diseases and gene therapy. To ensure early access to regenerative medical products, the PMD Act significantly shortens clinical trial phase period to approve on a conditional authorization basis.

PMDA classifies medical devices depending on the risk level:
- The general medical device (Class I)
- Controlled medical device (Class II)
- Specially controlled device (Class III and Class IV)

General medical devices do not need to undergo the approval process of MHLW and PMDA but only require notification/self-declaration on the product. Controlled medical devices can be certified by an authorized third-party or reviewed by the PMDA. Specially controlled medical devices must be reviewed and approved by the PMDA and MHLW.

CHINA

The pharmaceutical industry in the People's Republic of China covers synthetic chemicals and drugs, prepared traditional Chinese medicines, medical devices, apparatus and instruments, hygiene materials, packing materials and machinery. Impending growth of Chinese pharmaceutical market has persuaded the government to realize the importance of strict supervision of pharmaceutical market. The government has put forward several regulations and reform measures over the past couple of years. The Department of Drug Administration under the Ministry of Health, merged with the "State Pharmaceutical Administration of China" (SPAC) in March 1998, to become the State Drug Administration (SDA) to oversee all drug manufacturing, trade, and registration.

The current *Drug Administration Law* of the People's Republic of China came into effect on 2001 after several revisions. All institutions and individuals associated with research, production, distribution, use or administration of the drug in the People's Republic of China has to abide this Law. This Law was enacted to strengthen drug administration to ensure drug quality and safety for human subjects, protect the public health interest and legitimate rights of the drug users. It contains ten chapters covering drug manufacturing, distribution, quality and efficacy, packaging, pricing, advertising, hospitals, and legal liabilities.

Chapter I: General Provisions

Chapter II: Control over Drug Manufacturers

Chapter III: Control over Drug Distributors

Chapter IV: Control over Pharmaceuticals in Medical Institutions

Chapter V: Control over Drugs

Chapter VI: Control over Drug Packaging

Chapter VII: Control over Drug Pricing and Advertising

Chapter VIII: Inspection of Drugs

Chapter IX: Legal Liabilities

Chapter X: Supplementary Provisions

The SDA was restructured and become the State Food and Drug Administration (SFDA) in 2003. Formation of SFDA was an important step as with this the Chinese government established a single drug regulatory authority eliminating the diverge standards that prevailed among provincial government agencies centralizing the Chinese healthcare regulatory system. The current drug regulation law controls all the aspects of pharmaceutical manufacturing, drug distribution and sell, drug registration, requirements for manufacturing of Traditional Chinese Medicines (TCM), medicine packaging and medical device manufacturing. SFDA also overlooked advertising of all medications of both Western and TCM originated. SFDA implemented mandatory compliance with new GMP certification by all pharmaceutical companies in China in 2004 to sell drug products in China. In 2005, SFDA enforced GLP to investigative drugs, TCM injections and biotechnology products.

In March 2013, the SFDA was rebranded and restructured as the China Food and Drug Administration (CFDA), elevating to a ministerial-level agency directly under the State Council of the People's Republic of China. The CFDA has replaced the overlapping regulators with an entity similar to the FDA of the United States, streamlining regulation processes for food and drug safety.

The CFDA comprehensively supervises the safety of food, health food, and cosmetics also with authority of drug regulation in mainland China. CFDA is charged with the registration, testing, and administration of pharmaceuticals, over-the-counter drugs, traditional Chinese medicine, and medical devices.

CFDA categories for drug registration:

- Category I: New drugs not yet approved in any country.
- Category II: Drugs seeking approval for a new route of administration that is not approved in any country.
- Category III: Drugs approved in other countries but not in China.
- Category IV: Drugs made by changing the acidic or alkaline radicals or metallic elements of the salt of a drug approved in China without changing the original pharmacological effects.
- Category V: Changed dosage form of a drug approved in China without changing the route of administration.
- Category VI: Generic form of a drug with existing national standards in China.

The CFDA considers drugs approved and marketed in other countries as new drugs in China, and previously approved therapies are designated as category III import drugs that require clinical data from trials conducted in China to support an application. Full clinical development in China is required for drugs that have not been approved anywhere yet to submit a category I new drug application for market approval. Regulations for the Supervision and Administration of Medical Devices come into force in 2000. 'Medical devices' as defined by these regulations refer to any instrument, apparatus, appliance, material, or other articles that are being used alone or in combination, including the software necessary for its proper application. Rules for classification of medical devices were adopted at the executive meeting of CFDA in 2015, that became effective as on 2016.

According to the factors which may influence the degree of risk of medical devices, medical devices are divided as:

- Non-active and active medical devices, according to structural characteristics.
- Body-contacting and non-body-contacting devices, according to whether they are in contact with the human body.

According to the use pattern, structural characteristics are divided as:

- Non-active body-contacting devices
- Non-active non-body-contacting devices
- Active body-contacting devices
- Active non-body-contacting devices

According to the degree of risk (from low to high), the medical devices are divided into class I, class II and class III.

BRAZIL

The National Health Surveillance Agency, named the "Agência Nacional de Vigilância Sanitária" (ANVISA) enforced in 1999 regulates therapeutic goods in Brazil under the Brazilian Health Ministry. The autarchy is connected to the Ministry of Health and functions by a Board of Directors made up of five members under a special regime, with administrative independence, stability, and financial autonomy. ANVISA open spaces for society to give its opinion on critical health-related issues and to ensure transparency in regulatory actions. The basic regulation structure and the medical device classification schemes in Brazil are similar to those found in the European Medical Devices Directives (MDD) 93/42/EEC. For registration process of a medical device in Brazil the first step is to determine the device classification. This is critical for ensuring a smooth registration process. There are five main categories:

1. **Normal Medicines:** Cough, cold and fever medicines, antiseptics, vitamins and others which are sold freely in pharmacies and some supermarkets.

2. **Red Stripe Medicines:** These medicines are to be sold only with a medical prescription like antibiotic, antiallergenic, anti-inflammatory, etc. medicines. In Brazil, it is not uncommon to get this type of prescription medicine over the counter without a prescription, as governmental control is loose.

3. **Red Stripe Psychoactive Medicines:** These medicines are sold only with a "Special Control" white medical prescription with carbon copy, which is valid for 30 days. The pharmacist must retain the original after the sale, and the patient keeps the carbon copy. Drugs include anti-depressants, anti-convulsants, some sleep aids, antipsychotics, anabolic steroids, and other non-habit-inducing controlled medicines.

4. **Black Stripe Medicines:** These medicines are to be sold only with the "Blue B Form" medical prescription, which is valid for 30 days and must be retained by the pharmacist after the sale. This category includes sedatives (benzodiazepines), anorexia inducers and other habit inducing controlled medicines.

5. **"Yellow A Form" prescription medicines:** These medicines are sold only with the "Yellow A Form" medical prescription that is the most tightly controlled, which is valid for 30 days and must be retained by the pharmacist after the sale. This includes amphetamines and other stimulants (such as methylphenidate), opioids (such as morphine and oxycodone) and other strong habit-forming controlled medicines.

ANVISA is empowered to establish technical regulations, control and inspection procedures for drugs, medical devices, food, cosmetics, sanitizing products, pesticides, tobacco products, blood and blood products. The agency is also responsible for coordinating the National Health Surveillance System (SNVS), the National Program of Blood and

Blood Products and the National Program of Prevention and Control of Hospital Infections, monitoring of drug prices and performing pharmacovigilance activities.

The USFDA and the ANVISA have come under Statement of Cooperation (SOC) recognizing the importance of timely and effective communication and collaboration to enhance the activities of mutual interest in scientific and regulatory areas. This SOC is intended to strengthen existing structures and develop new opportunities for cooperative engagement in regulatory and scientific matters, and public health protection that is related to the products that both agencies regulate. This collaboration is intended to facilitate the effective exchange of information, develop new or strengthen existing cooperative efforts/initiatives, and coordinate with other countries and with stakeholder groups relevant to product regulation within their respective countries or a broader global context.

AUSTRALIA

The Therapeutic Goods Administration (TGA) regulates therapeutic goods in Australia. Drugs and poisons are regulated through scheduling under individual state legislation under the guidance of the national Standard with Uniform Scheduling of Drugs and Poisons (SUSDP). Under the SUSDP, medicinal agents generally belong to one of the five categories:

• Unscheduled/exempt
• Schedule 2 (S2): Pharmacy Medicines
• Schedule 3 (S3): Pharmacist Only Medicines
• Schedule 4 (S4): Prescription Only Medicines
• Schedule 8 (S8): Controlled Drugs

The legislation governing medicines in Australia is the *Therapeutic Goods Act 1989* which establishes a national system of controls for medicines. The Therapeutic Goods Advertising Code and the Australian Code of Manufacturing Practice for Therapeutic Goods are the two main codes that govern the advertising and manufacturing of medicines in Australia. The *Therapeutic Goods Act 1989*, that came into effect on 15 February 1991, provides a national framework for the regulation of therapeutic goods in Australia and ensure their quality, safety, and efficacy. The TGA regulates therapeutic goods via pre-market assessment, enforcement of standards, licensing of Australian manufacturers, post-market monitoring and verifying overseas manufacturer's compliance with the same standards as their Australian counterparts. TGA regulates medicines, medical devices, chemicals, gene technology, blood, blood and tissues products. Medicines are classified as registered medicines or listed medicines, depending on their ingredients and claims made. Registered medicines are further classified as non-prescription (low risk) registered medicines and as prescription (high risk) registered medicines. The degree of control imposed on registered medicines is higher than that of listed medicines as they are evaluated for safety, quality, and efficacy while listed medicines are evaluated for safety and quality only. The regulatory framework is based on a risk management approach designed to ensure public health and safety, but at the same time also endeavor to relax the industries from the unnecessary regulatory burden.

Necessarily, any product for which therapeutic claims are made must be entered in the Australian Register of Therapeutic Goods (ARTG) before the product can be supplied in Australia. The ARTG is a computerized database of information about therapeutic goods for human use approved for supply in/or exported from Australia. *The Therapeutic Goods Act* (1989), regulations and orders set out the requirements for inclusion of therapeutic goods in the ARTG including advertising, labeling, product appearance and appeal guidelines. The relevant state or territory legislation covers some provision such as the scheduling of substances and the safe storage of therapeutic goods.

TGA exercise overall control on the supply of therapeutic goods by three main processes:

Pre-market assessment: Prescription medicines, some non-prescription medicines and medical devices assessed to have a higher level of risk are evaluated for quality, safety, and efficacy. Once approved for marketing in Australia these products are included as 'registered' products and are identified by a number. Products assessed having a lower risk like many non-prescription medicines including most complementary medicines and low risk medical devices are also evaluated for quality and safety. Once approved for marketing in Australia, these products are included as 'listed' products and are identified by a number. Product strength, side effects, potential harm caused after prolonged use, toxicity and the seriousness of the medical condition for which the product is intended to be used are the factors taken into account while assessing the level of risk.

Licensing of pharmaceutical manufacturers: All Australian manufactures of therapeutic goods should be licensed with TGA. The manufacturing processes must comply with the principle of good manufacturing practice (GMP). The aim is to protect public health by ensuring that medicines and medical devices meet pre-defined standards of quality assurance and are manufactured in a clean and free of contaminants condition.

Postmarketing vigilance: Postmarketing activities include investigating reports of ADR related problems. Laboratory testing of products available in the market and monitoring of products is done to ensure compliance with the legislation.

The TGA is the leading government agency responsible for enforcing the regulations of medicines in Australia, as part of the Health Products Regulation Group (HPRG) in the Australian Government Department of Health. The TGA is responsible for administering the provisions of the legislation. The TGA carries out assessment and monitoring activities to ensure that the therapeutic goods available in Australia are of an acceptable standard. The TGA ensures that the Australian community has access to therapeutic advances within a reasonable time. TGA has three major divisions:

- Medicines Regulation Division: This division evaluates applications to approve new medicines for supply in Australia and monitoring of medicines approved for supply in Australia.
- Medical Devices and Product Quality Division: This division monitors medical devices approved for supply in Australia and works to ensure Australian and international therapeutic goods manufacturers meet specified standards.
- Regulatory Practice and Support Division: This division provides operational, regulatory, policy advice and specific support services that ensure efficient, best practice administrative operations in the Health Products Regulation Group.

The TGA has seven statutory expert committees it may call upon to obtain independent advice on scientific and technical matters. The TGA is focusing on implementing changes to ensure greater emphasis on transparency of regulatory decision-making processes, business process reform and a more strategic approach to the use of information technology to support regulatory operations. In 2009, the TGA commenced a significant program of business process reforms (BPR program) for the regulation of prescription medicines in Australia. An advertising regulatory framework was released in 2011, for therapeutic goods other than prescription medicines. In concern to medicines and medical devices regulation, some changes have now been implemented under the Government's Response to the Review of Medicines and Medical Devices Regulation in 2016, with further reforms in progress or upcoming. The first set of legislative changes were passed in 2017 focusing on new assessment pathways for medicines and medical devices. The second tranche of legislative review is underway.

DRUG REGULATION IN INDIA

The Indian pharmaceutical industry sector is one of the largest, most advanced and rapidly growing among the developing countries with a wide range of products. Keeping in pace with this fast growth, the Indian pharmaceutical industry, the regulatory bodies are also coming out with major inclusions, amendments and revisions in guidelines to be in equivalence with international regulatory perspective. Indian pharmaceutical industry is having an advanced infrastructure, technological capability and qualified work force. India regulatory system is implementing and adopting the changes in guidelines, i.e. Good Manufacturing Practices (GMP), Good Clinical Practices (GCP) and Good Laboratory Practices (GLP) to be at peer with global standards to ensure supply of quality drugs at affordable prices to the Indian population.

Manufacturing, sale and distribution of medicines in India are regulated by Central Drugs Standard Control Organization (CDSCO) under Ministry of Health and Family Welfare and respective states licensing authorities headed by Directorate General of Health Services. CDSCO regulate the pharmaceutical products through Drug Controller General of India (DCGI) of India. CDSCO is India's prime regulatory body for pharmaceuticals and medical devices.

CENTRAL DRUGS STANDARD CONTROL ORGANIZATION (CDSCO)

The CDSCO is the Central Drug Authority for discharging functions assigned to the Central Government under the Drugs and Cosmetics Act. CDSCO regulates the manufacturing of large volume parenteral (LVPs), blood bank, new drugs, clinical trials, class III, and IV diagnostic kits. Under the *Drug and Cosmetics Act*, manufacture, sale, and distribution of drugs is the primary concern of the State authorities while the Central Authorities are responsible for approval of new drugs, clinical trials, developing standards for drugs, control the quality of imported drugs, coordination of the activities of State Drug Control Organisations. CDSCO provides expert advice encouraging uniformity in the enforcement of the Drugs and Cosmetics Act. CDSCO headquarter is located at FDA Bhawan, New Delhi. CDSCO has six zonal offices (Mumbai, Kolkata, Chennai, Ghaziabad, Hyderabad, and Ahmedabad), five sub-zonal offices, 13 port offices and seven central laboratories under its control. The Zonal Offices work in close collaboration with the State Drug Control Administration and assist them in securing uniform enforcement of the Drug Act and other related legislation. The zonal offices do pre-licensing and post-licensing inspections, post-market surveillance and recall when necessary.

The CDSCO establishes safety, efficacy and quality standards for pharmaceuticals and medical devices. The primary functions of CDSCO are:

- Laying down standard and approval of new drugs
- Approval and licensing to manufacture LVPs, vaccines, sera and biotechnological products as Central Licence Approving Authority
- Licensing of blood banks and setting standards for blood products
- Licensing of medical devices and class III and IV diagnostic agents
- Grant of test license and NOCs for export of drugs
- Grant of license for the export of drugs for personal use
- Import registration and licensing and regulation of standards of imported drugs

- Regulation and approval of clinical trials and clinical research
- Amendment of Drug and Cosmetics Act and Rules
- Participation in WHO GMP certification scheme
- Publishing and updating the Indian Pharmacopeia
- Publishing and updating the list of drugs approved for marketing
- Publishing and updating the list of regulated pharmaceuticals and devices
- Publishing and updating the list of banned drugs and cosmetics
- Publishing and updating the list of drugs prohibited for manufacture and sale
- Publishing and updating the list of banned medical devices and diagnostics
- Laying down standard and publication of guidance documents registration requirements of LPVs, vaccines, sera, biological, medical devices and diagnostics
- Testing of drugs by central laboratories
- Monitoring adverse drug reactions
- Conducting training programmes for regulatory officials and government analysts
- Quota distribution of narcotic drugs for use in medicinal formulations.
- Developing regulatory measures, amendments to Acts and Rules and guidance on all technical matters concerned to drug regulation.
- Coordinating the State Drugs Control Organizations to achieve uniform administration of the Act and policies.

For all drug and device licensing applications CDSCO appoints notified bodies to perform conformity assessment and testing to ensure compliance with their standards. CDSCO safeguards public health by ensuring the quality, safety, and efficacy of drugs, cosmetics and medical devices as the Central Drug Authority. For fulfilling functions allocated by the Central Government under the Drugs and Cosmetics Act, CDSCO formatted different committees with eligible members to review clinical trials of new drugs, and medical devices. CDSCO endorses experts of 25 panels from various therapeutic areas. Experts are selected and approved by the government from various therapeutic fields of medicine all over the country. The names of experts from various Govt. Medical Colleges and hospitals are added as deemed necessary by the government.

In addition to its regulatory functions, the CDSCO also offers technical guidance, training to the regulatory officials and analysts, and monitors adverse events. The CDSCO works with the WHO to promote Good Manufacturing Practice (GMP) and international regulatory harmony in India. CDSCO has adopted the Common Technical Document (CTD) format for technical requirements for registration of pharmaceutical products for human use since 2008. The adoption of Drug Master File (DMF) and drug product dossier concepts as in CTD format in tune with the global requirements are helping the Indian pharmaceutical industry for quick entry to the global markets, and simultaneously patients are assured to receive good quality and safe medicines.

The Drug Controller General of India (DCGI)

DCGI is responsible for licensing of specified categories of drugs such as blood and blood products, IV Fluids, vaccine and sera. Within the working structure of CDSCO, the Drug Controller General of India (DCGI) is responsible for approval of new drugs, medical devices and clinical trials in India. DCGI is appointed by central Govt., Directorate General of Health Services, all the state drug control organization named Food and Drug Administration (FDA) function under this umbrella. The Drug Technical Advisory Board (DTAB) and the Drug Consultative Committee (DCC) advise the DCGI on related issues. Central Licensing Approval Authority (CLAA) handles the licensing and classification of medical devices. DCGI headquarter deals with new drugs, import of drugs and medical devices, whereas the six zonal offices (Mumbai, Kolkata, Chennai, Ghaziabad, Ahmedabad, and Hyderabad) perform GMP audit, inspection of manufacturing units of LVPs, sera, vaccines, and blood products, and maintain coordination with state authorities. Six Central Drug Testing Laboratories (Mumbai, Kolkata, Chennai, Kasauli, Guwahati, Chandigarh) function under the DCGI overseeing quality control of drugs and cosmetics, and validation of test protocols.

Drug Technical Advisory Board (DTAB)

DTAB is a statutory body under the provision of *Drugs and Cosmetics Act* to advise the Central Govt. on the technical matter related to implementation of *Drugs and Cosmetics Act* and Rules and to carry out other assigned duties by this Act. DTAB counsels Central and State government on drug control related technical issues. The DTAB consists of the following members as per the current Drugs and Cosmetics Act, 1940 and Rules, 1945 amended up to the 31st Dec 2016:

1. The Director General of Health Services *ex officio, as* Chairman
2. The Drugs Controller, India, *ex officio*
3. The Director of the Central Drugs Laboratory, Calcutta, *ex officio*
4. The Director of the Central Research Institute, Kasauli, *ex officio*
5. The Director of the Indian Veterinary Research Institute, Izatnagar, *ex officio*
6. The President of the Medical Council of India, *ex officio*
7. The President of the Pharmacy Council of India, *ex officio*
8. The Director of the Central Drug Research Institute, Lucknow, *ex officio*
9. Two persons nominated by the Central Government from states drugs control office

10. One person elected by the Executive Committee of the Pharmacy Council of India (teaching faculty of Pharmacy from an Indian university or an affiliated college)
11. One person elected by the Executive Committee of the Medical Council of India (teaching faculty in medicine from an Indian university or an affiliated college)
12. One person nominated by the Central Government from the pharmaceutical industry
13. One pharmacologist elected by the Governing Body of the Indian Council of Medical Research
14. One person elected by the Central Council of the Indian Medical Association
15. One person elected by the Council of the Indian Pharmaceutical Association
16. Two persons appointed as Government Analyst nominated by the Central Government

All the nominated and elected members of the Board hold office for three years but also eligible for re-nomination and re-election. The Board subject to the previous approval of the Central Government, make bye-laws fixing a quorum and regulating its procedure to conduct all functions. The Board can constitute sub-committees for a period not exceeding three years or in a case as decided temporarily for the consideration of particular matters with persons who are not members of the Board. The Central Government appoints a person to act as Secretary of the Board and also provide clerical and other staff as considered necessary as per the Drugs and Cosmetics Act 1940 and Rules 1945 (amended up to 31st Dec 2016).

Medical Devices Advisory Committee (MDAC)

MDAC is to advise the CDSCO in making decisions on approval of new medical devices, import registration and marketing authorization of devices. The importer/manufacturer of the new medical device is required to furnish clinical data to satisfy the MDAC. The Committee members review and assess the safety and efficacy data submitted with the application, where industry representatives require to present the data about concerned projects. Based on the recommendations of MDAC decision on the product approval is taken by CDSCO. Seven MDAC is now functioning under CDSCO, namely:

1. MDAC: Cardiovascular
2. MDAC: Dental
3. MDAC: Reproductive and Urology
4. MDAC: Orthopedics
5. MDAC: Ophthalmic
6. MDAC: General
7. MDAC: Miscellaneous

Medical Devices Technical Advisory Board (MDTAB)

The Drugs and Cosmetics (Amendment) Bill, 2013, recommends insertion of new Section 5A. As per this section, the Central Government shall, by notification, constitute a Board to be called the Medical Devices Technical Advisory Board. This board is deemed to advise the Central Government and State Governments on technical matters pertaining to medical devices, arising out of the administration of this Act and other functions as assigned by or under this Act. The Board shall consist of the following members, namely:

1. The Director-General, Indian Council of Medical Research, who shall be the Chairperson, *ex officio*;
2. The Drugs Controller General of India, *ex officio*;
3. One expert each with qualifications and experience in the field of medical devices, to be nominated:
   a. The Department of Science and Technology;
   b. The Department of Atomic Energy;
   c. The Department of Electronic and Information Technology;
   d. The Central Government from the Government testing laboratories connected with the testing of medical devices;
   e. The Indian Council of Medical Research;
   f. The Bureau of Indian Standard;
   g. The Defence Research and Development Organisation;
4. One expert from the field of biomedical technology from recognized technical educational institutions, to be nominated by the Central Government;
5. One expert from the field of biomaterial or polymer technology from recognized technical educational institutions, to be nominated by the Central Government;
6. One person representing recognized consumer associations to be nominated by the Ministry of Consumer Affairs;
7. One pharmacologist to be nominated by the Central Government from recognized medical or research institute in the field of medical devices;
8. One expert to be nominated by the Central Government from recognized medical or research institute from amongst persons involved in the conduct of clinical trials;
9. One person to be nominated by the Central Government from the medical device industry.

The nominated members of the Board shall hold office for three years, and shall be eligible for re-nomination for not more than two consecutive terms. The Board may, in consultation with the Central Drugs Authority, and subject to previous Central Government approval can make bye-laws fixing quorum and regulating the procedure for the conduct of all business transacted to it. The Board may constitute sub-committees and may appoint to such sub-committees, the persons who are not a member of the Board for a period not exceeding three years, as it may decide, for the consideration of particular matters. The Central Drugs Authority shall appoint a person to be the Secretary of the Board and shall provide the Board with such staff as the Central Drugs Authority considers necessary.

Subject Expert Committee (SEC)

SEC is formed by CDSCO comprising of 8 experts from medical specialties out of which one has to be a pharmacologist. In case of absence of an expert in a meeting, another member from the approved panel, having requisite specialization and experience, can be invited to attend the meeting. The experts comprehensively review and assess the non-clinical data, toxicology data, preclinical data, clinical trial phase I, II, III data and make essential statements advising Drug Controller General of India (DCGI) on the approval recommendations. The panel held high standards and follow the national regulations and specific rules that need to adhere for approval and licensing of drugs. Each member evaluates individually and gives written expert comments within a time frame of 6 weeks of receiving the proposal. SEC give its final opinion after the evaluation of the proposal within the regulatory framework and practical utility of the products. In case of a suggestion or revision is required in the initial proposal, the committee can deliberate meeting considering the initial decision. The experts are required to be nondiscriminatory in the recommendations and maintain utmost discretion of the documents submitted by the applicants. SEC works on approval of the following categories:

- To evaluate applications of potential new substances or new drugs of chemical and biological origin
- To evaluate applications of biological product vaccines and r-DNA derived products

- To evaluate applications of fixed dose combinations of two or more drugs that are to be presented for the first time in the country
- To assess the status of global clinical trials happening all across the world for the new drug applied for approval in the country
- To evaluate the applications of global clinical trials filled by manufacturer outside India
- Procedural matters like safety or root cause analysis when needed or asked by the Ministry or Government requiring expert opinion
- To counsel and assist in the planning and preparation of guidelines for clinical research industry and for developing the acceptance/rejection criteria for marketing of new drugs belonging to different therapeutic categories.
- To recommend a road map of research to the pharmaceutical companies to manufacture new medications that cater to the Indian population
- To examine the utility and anticipated nature of new drugs that include assessment of risk versus benefits for patients for the innovated new drug compared to existing drugs and the unmet need in the country.
- To assist in any other matters that CDSCO needs advice.

SEC currently in function are:
1. Ophthalmology
2. Oncology and hematology
3. Nephrology
4. Pulmonary
5. Antimicrobial, antiparasitic, antifungal and antiviral
6. Cardiology and renal
7. Metabolism and endocrinology
8. Neurology and psychiatry
9. Analgesics, anesthetics and rheumatology
10. Gastroenterology and hepatology

11. Reproductive and urology
12. Dermatology and allergy
13. Orthopedics
14. Vaccine section
15. Endocrinology
16. Radio-diagnostic
17. Dentistry

New Drugs Advisory Committee (NDAC)

NDAC was formally assigned by CDSCO to take decisions on approval of new drugs, new formulations, fixed dosage combination(s), modified dosage forms, a formulation with additional indication/formulation with additional strength. Twelve New Drug Advisory Committee's (NDAC) were in function previously before DCGI renames new drug advisory committee as subject expert committee in 2014.

Drug Consultative Committee (DCC)

It is a statutory body under Section 7, Chapter II of the Drugs and Cosmetics Act with all State Drugs Controllers as its members to advise the central government, the state government and the DTAB on matters relating to the uniform administrative implementation of the Drugs and Cosmetics Act and Rules throughout the country. DCC consists of two representatives of the central government and one nominated representative from each state government. DCC enforces drug control measures in all the states and forms rules for national level implementation. DCC issues license for import of biological, biotechnological and other related unique products. The Drugs Consultative Committee consists of two nominated representatives of the Central Government and one nominated representative from each state government. The Drug and Cosmetics Amendment Bill 2013 and 2015, recommends substitution of Section 7 to constitute a consultative committee to be called the "Drugs, Cosmetics and Medical Devices Consultative Committee." This committee will advise the central government, the state governments, the Drugs Technical Advisory Board and the Medical Device Technical Advisory Board on any matter tending to secure uniformity throughout India regarding administration of this Act. The Drugs, Cosmetics and Medical Devices Consultative Committee shall consist of the following members, namely:

a. The Drugs Controller General of India, who shall be the chairperson, *ex officio*;
b. Two representatives of the Central Drugs Authority nominated by it;
c. The Secretary-cum-Scientific Director of the Indian Pharmacopoeia Commission;
d. One representative of the Pharmaceuticals Export Promotion Council nominated by it;
e. One representative of the Department of Revenue, Ministry of Finance, Government of India dealing with the administration of the Narcotic Drugs and Psychotropic Substances Act, 1985; and
f. One representative of each state government who is incharge of the matters relating to the regulation of drugs, cosmetics and medical devices in that state.

The DCMDCC must meet at least twice in a year or when required by the central government or, as the case may be. The Central Drugs Authority have the power to regulate its procedure. Though proposed, this has not been implemented in The Drugs And Cosmetics Act, 1940 and Rules, 1945 amended up to 31st Dec 2016.

Central Licences Approving Authority (CLAA)

CLAA issues license for blood banks, blood components, manufacturing of LVPs, medical devices manufacturing and approval for the commercial laboratory. The CLAA is responsible for classification of medical devices, publishing and updating guideline, enforcing safety standards, appointing notified bodies to oversee conformity assessment, conducting post-market surveillance, and issuing warnings and recalls for adverse events of the related products. The CLAA acts as the chief regulatory authority for medical devices. The Third Schedule proposed for inclusion after the Second Schedule in the Drugs and Cosmetics (Amendment Bill) 2013 was to empower the CLAA to issue the license for the following categories of drugs, though not been implemented in The Drugs and Cosmetics Act, 1940 and Rules, 1945 amended up to the 31st Dec 2016:

1. RNA interference based products
2. Monoclonal antibodies
3. Cellular products and stem cells
4. Gene therapeutic products
5. Xenografts
6. Modified living organisms

National Pharmaceutical Pricing Authority (NPPA)

NPPA was formed by the Government of India under the *Drugs (Prices Control) Order, 1995*, to fix/revise the prices of controlled bulk drugs and formulations towards enforcing price regulation and availability of the medicines in the country. The organization is also entrusted with the task of recovering any overcharged amounts to the consumer by the manufacturers for the controlled drugs. It also monitors the prices of decontrolled drugs as an effort to keep them at reasonable levels. The functions of NPPA are:

1. To implement and enforce the provisions of the Drugs (Prices Control) Order.
2. To advice the central government on changes/revisions required in the pharmaceutical policy.
3. Monitor the availability of drugs, identify shortages and take remedial steps
4. Collect and maintain data of production, exports, and imports, the market share of individual companies, and the profitability of companies for bulk drugs and formulations.

5. Undertake, sponsor studies relevant to the pricing of drugs and pharmaceuticals.
6. Recruit the officers and other staff members of the Authority.
7. Deals with all legal matters arising out of the decisions of the Authority.
8. Assist the Central Government in the parliamentary matters relating to the drug pricing.

One of the major responsibilities of NPPA is to formulate, revise and implement national 'Pharmaceutical Policy' to ensure abundant availability of good quality essential pharmaceuticals at reasonable prices within the country. The 'Pharmaceutical Policy' formulates Government approach relating to drugs and pharmaceutical sector, covering all aspects of pharmaceutical business, i.e. quality control over drug and pharmaceutical production, distribution, encouraging research and development in the pharmaceutical sector, cost effectiveness, exports promotion of pharmaceuticals by reducing barriers to trade, promoting rational use of pharmaceuticals, import promotion and encouraging pharmacy education. This policy reflects the approach of the government for the overall growth of the pharmaceutical sector compatible with the country's needs and with a particular focus on endemic diseases relevant to India by creating an environment conducive to channelizing a higher level of investment into research and development and education in pharmaceuticals in India. The objective of this policy is to create an incentive framework for the pharmaceutical industry which can promote new investment in the pharmaceutical industry and encourages the introduction of new technologies and new drugs.

Indian Pharmacopoeial Commission (IPC)

IPC is an autonomous institution that acts under the Ministry of Health and Family Welfare, Government of India dedicated for the setting of standards for drugs, pharmaceuticals and healthcare devices. It also provides Reference Standard substances and training for the professionals. The IPC is a registered Society since 9th December 2004, under the provisions of the Societies Registration Act, 1860, under Act No. 21 (1860) related to registration of Literary, Scientific and Charitable Societies. The primary functions and working areas are:

- Develop comprehensive monographs for drugs, active pharmaceutical ingredients, excipients, dosage forms and medical devices for inclusion in the Indian Pharmacopoeia. IPC also revise and update Indian Pharmacopoeia on a regular basis.
- Prepare monographs of drugs like national essential drugs list and their dosage forms.
- Prepare monographs for products in the market for not less than two years except for particular categories of new drugs like antiretrovirals, antitubercular and anti-cancer drugs and their formulations introduced recently requiring priority attention.
- Develop Pharmacopoeial tests methods with special attention to the manufacturing methods used by the indigenous industry for monitoring the toxic impurities of the concerned drugs.
- Upgrade the levels of testing methods as per the sophistication in analytical testing/instrumentation available while framing the monographs.
- Preparation, certification, and distribution of Indian Pharmacopoeial Reference Substances including the impurities and degradation related products.
- Collaborate to at peer with the standards of international pharmacopoeias like the European Pharmacopoeia, British Pharmacopoeia, United States Pharmacopoeia, Japanese Pharmacopoeia, harmonizing with global standards.
- Organize educational programs and research activities for spreading and

establishing awareness on the need and scope of quality standards for drugs and related materials.

NEW INITIATIVES

The Indian pharmaceutical regulatory bodies are coming out with significant changes to keep pace with the international regulatory scenario. In pursuance of the same, the Amendment Bill of Drugs and Cosmetics Act 2013 have proposed new implementations to bring about revolutionary changes in the Indian pharmaceutical industry. Some of the initiatives are the revision of DTAB and DCC constitution along with the revision of CLAA powers.

Drugs defined as New Drugs under the Drugs and Cosmetics Act are subjected to bioavailability/bioequivalence (BA/BE) evaluations through clinical trials, which are reviewed by the DCGI. A drug has a New Drug status for four years from the date of first permission. After four years, the State Licensing Authority grants the license, but they do not insist for BA/BE and clinical trial studies which are essential to establish the efficacy of the drugs. Central Drugs Standard Control Organisation (CDSCO) has come out with new draft guidelines on the approval of clinical trials and new drugs.

Central Drug Authority (CDA)

The CDA is an initiative to centralize the drug licensing in respect of 17 categories of very critical drugs. The central licensing authority is empowered to issue licenses for categories of drugs as of sera, serum proteins intended for injection, vaccines (including DNA vaccines and vaccines containing living genetically engineered organisms), toxins, antigens, and anti-toxins, antibiotics (beta-lactams and cephalosporins), preparations meant for parenteral administration, hormones and preparations containing hormones. The other drugs like r-DNA derived drugs, RNA interference based products, monoclonal antibodies, cellular products, and stem cells, therapeutic gene-products, xenografts, cytotoxic substances (anti-cancer drugs), blood products and modified living organisms are included in the list as per the bill. The bill introduced in the Rajya Sabha on 29th August, 2013 for Drugs and Cosmetics (Amendment) Act, 2013 proposed insertion of new chapter, namely Chapter IA after the Chapter I of the Principal Act proposing formation of a new body called CDA though not been Implemented in The Drugs And Cosmetics Act, 1940 and Rules, 1945 amended up to 31st Dec 2016.

Proposed Constitution of CDA

The Central Government shall constitute an Authority to be known as the CDA to exercise the powers conferred on, and perform the functions assigned to it by or under this Act by notification in the Official Gazette.

The CDA shall be a body corporate by the name aforesaid, having perpetual succession and a common seal, with the power to acquire, hold and dispose of property, movable and immovable both and to contract by the said name, sue or be sued. The head office of the CDA shall be in the National Capital Region. The CDA may, with the prior approval of the Central Government, by notification in the Official Gazette, can establish its offices at places considers necessary in India.

Proposed Composition of CDA

The CDA shall consist of the following:

a. Secretary to the Government of India, Ministry of Health and Family Welfare, Department of Health and Family Welfare—*Chairperson, ex officio*

b. Secretary to the Government of India, Ministry of Health and Family Welfare, Department of Ayurveda, Yoga and Naturopathy, Unani, Siddha and Homoeopathy—*Member, ex officio*

c. Secretary, Department of AIDS Control and Director General, National AIDS Control Organisation, Ministry of Health and Family Welfare—*Member, ex officio*

d. Secretary to the Government of India, Ministry of Commerce and Industry, Department of Commerce—*Member, ex officio*

e. Secretary to the Government of India, Ministry of Chemicals and Fertilisers, Department of Pharmaceuticals—*Member, ex officio*

f. Secretary, Department of Health Research and Director General, Indian Council of Medical Research, Ministry of Health and Family Welfare—*Member, ex officio*

g. Secretary to the Government of India, Ministry of Science and Technology, Department of Biotechnology—*Member, ex officio*

h. Director General Health Services, Directorate General of Health Services, New Delhi—*Member, ex officio*

i. Additional Secretary or Joint Secretary and Legislative Counsel in the Legislative Department, Ministry of Law and Justice, incharge of the Group dealing with the work relating to the Ministry of Health and Family Welfare—*Member, ex officio*

j. Additional Secretary or Joint Secretary in charge of the Drugs Quality Control Division in the Ministry of Health and Family Welfare—*Member, ex officio*

k. Four experts having such qualifications and experience to be nominated by the Central Government in such manner as may be prescribed—Member (shall hold office for three years from the date of their nomination, and shall be eligible for re-nomination)

l. Four State Licensing Authorities to be nominated by the Central Government in such manner as may be prescribed—Member

m. Drugs Controller General of India—Member-Secretary, *ex officio*

Proposed Powers and Functions of CDA

a. As specified by regulations, the guidelines, norms, structures, and requirements for the effective functioning of the Central and State Licensing Authorities

b. Assess the functioning of the Central and State Licensing Authority periodically

c. Issue directions to the Central Licensing Authority and the State Licensing Authorities to ensure compliance with the guidelines, norms, structures, and requirements specified

d. Review, suspend or cancel a permission, license or certificate issued by the Central Licensing Authority or the State Licensing Authorities

e. As specified by regulations, collect the fees or charges for issue or renewal of licenses, certificates, approvals and permissions by the Central Licensing Authority and the State Licensing authorities

f. Coordinate, mediate and decide upon the disputes arising out of the implementation of the provisions of the Act and rules and regulations made thereunder between two or more States Licensing Authorities

g. Constitute such committees or sub-committees as it considers necessary for the efficient discharge of functions and exercise of powers under this Act

h. Recommend to the Central Government the measures as regard to the standards of drugs, cosmetics and medical devices for effective implementation of the provisions of this Act

i. Perform such other functions as may be prescribed by the Central Government.

The powers of the CDA is going to be with the Central Drugs Standard Control Organisation (CDSCO), as per specifications by regulations, the guidelines, norms, structures, and requirements for the effective functioning of the Central and State Licensing Authority. The DCGI shall act as the Central Licensing Authority and shall have powers to:

a. Issue, renew, suspend or cancel licenses or certificates or permission, as the case may be, for import, export or manufacture of drugs, cosmetics or medical devices or permission for conducting clinical trials;

b. Recall or direct to recall any drug, cosmetic or medical device;

c. Collect the fees or charges for issue or renewal of licenses, certificates, approvals and permissions issued by the Central Licensing Authority under this Act.

Formation and implementation of CDA have not been materialized in The Drugs And Cosmetics Act, 1940 and Rules, 1945 amended up to 31st Dec 2016.

STATE DRUG CONTROL ORGANIZATION

Every State and Union territory in India has its individual setup of food and drug control administration headed by Drugs Controller/Commissioner under the State Health Ministry. Deputy Drugs Controller, State Licensing Authorities and Drugs Inspectors work under the administrative powers of Drugs Controller. The state drug testing laboratory functioning under the FDA is involved in testing the quality of drugs sampled by the regulatory personnel. Functions of the state FDAs are:

- Administrative regulation of medicinal product retailers, wholesalers, and manufacturers
- Inspection and licensing of pharmaceutical manufacturing units in the respective state
- Licensing of commercial drug testing laboratories
- Approval of drug formulation for manufacturing
- Monitoring quality of drugs and cosmetics manufactured in the respective state
- Monitoring quality of drugs marketed in the respective state
- Pre and Post licensing inspections
- Recall of substandard drugs

- Investigation and prosecution in respect of the contravention of legal provisions
- Inspection and licensing of wholesale and retail medical shops

INTERNATIONAL HARMONIZATION INITIATIVE BY REGULATORY BODIES

The term "regulatory harmonization" has different definitions depending on the context of its usage. The virtual interpretation can be "the process by which the interpretation and/or application of technical guidelines can be made to be uniform or mutually compatible between the participating agencies". Harmonization of drug regulation signifies harmonization of technical requirements for medicines regulation, viz. legislation, guidelines, procedures and all quality, safety, and related efficacy requirements of the medicinal products. Worldwide from country to country these requirements differ in the level of control, astringency, and complexity in different types of marketing authorization applications. Harmonization of technical requirements for medicines regulation is a need of the time looking into the fast growing and expanding business scenario of multinational companies. Globalization of medicinal product related activities, i.e. research and development, manufacturing and distribution increasingly demand regulatory cooperation across borders, which inevitably affects the initiatives driven by a group of countries having a similar economic interest. Identification of the particular "harmonization" requirements that each harmonization initiative aims is indispensable in determining future directions. The driven benefits of any harmonization initiative are:

- Companies can apply for marketing authorization to all the collaborating countries of a particular harmonization umbrella with only one data set for all regions, and consequently, the amount of human and animal experimentation is reduced as the scientific study parameters applicable are same.
- Fast regulatory communication and information sharing are possible due to common regulatory standards for scientific evaluation and inspection of premises which facilitate quick processing.
- Local products are likely to be easily acceptable for export to other countries under universal harmonization treaty as quality related aspects will be trustable to the general public.
- The cost of regulatory documentation development for both new and multi-source/generic medicines are reduced due to exemption from multiple regulatory licensing application submission with saving of the application fee and working hour requirements, which can lead to lower prices.
- Faster access and availability of medicines with high public health value (pediatric medicines, medicines for commonly occurring diseases or emergencies in public settings) and for rare diseases (orphan drugs) are assured.
- Harmonization, in turn, increases competitiveness not only between the pharmaceuticals of national level but also international level between the member countries resulting from the availability of shared markets.
- The most important benefit of drug regulation harmonization is the equality in quality of medicines available to the population of underdeveloped, developing and developed countries assuring the equal right of everybody to have quality medicine irrespective of the physical and economic barrier.

Harmonization policy works on the successful collaboration of the regulatory organization of all the member countries' under the treaty. It could not be effective if all significant aspects of regulation are not addressed. All these benefits of drug regulatory harmonization can be achieved when harmonization policy development aims at the real goal of:

- True harmonization is not just development of common standard documentation, it requires continuous communication, effective collaboration, information sharing, mutual recognition and shared working cultures aimed at building capacity and trust between member countries.
- Harmonization can be adopted for similar or collaborative approaches in drug registration paving the way for mutual recognition and/or centralized registration in the longer-term future.
- Harmonization does not require the loss of national sovereignty/autonomy, but the similarity in policy adoption and execution is expected.
- Common documentation should be developed stipulating the requirements for registration and marketing authorization. Joint scheduling and drug product classification can be adopted between member countries with specific legislation applicable to a particular country.
- Regular effective and meaningful communication enables member countries to choose what information they will use and why.
- Collaborative mechanisms, such as joint assessments of applications or inspections of facilities, does not always imply collaborative decision-making, which will help safeguard the individual legal interest of the member countries.
- Harmonization of technical requirements can create a "common technical language" for collaborating regulators. Continuous training, effective communication, and collaboration are needed to build mutual trust and avoidance of duplication.
- Political will and support by member country governments are required for defining and achieving clear long-term objectives like creating a common market and faster market access.

- Strong commitment from major concerned stakeholders (regulators), effective governance structure, well-resourced secretariat, support of authorities, adequate human and financial resources, clearly defined processes and procedures, continuous updating and follow-up, transparent and effective communication between stakeholders is mandatory to brought forward a highly effective harmonization program resulting implementation of all objective driven guidelines.
- The primary factors responsible for futile harmonization effort are: Lack of political support and transparency with poor communication, ambiguously defined objectives with no 'reality check' for implementation, ineffective governance, inefficient functioning secretariat, absence of mechanisms to ensure timely update implementation, lack of experience, human resource and financial allocation.

The Nordic Council on Medicines (NLN) was formed in 1975 with the five European Nordic Countries (Denmark, Norway, Sweden, Finland, and Iceland) as members. NLN was a successful cooperation and supported in the development of modern medicines regulations in these countries. The Nordic Council was closed down in 2002, as all member countries inclined for participation in the EU procedures coordinated by the European Medicines Agency in London. The European Community (EC now the European Union) started harmonization of regulatory requirements of healthcare products in the member states in the 1980s.

World Health Organization (WHO) initiated its harmonization process in 1980 with the organization of International Conference of Drug Regulatory Authorities (ICDRA), which is now biennially convened by the WHO. In the same period of 1980s bilateral discussions between Europe, Japan, and the US started on possibilities for harmonization. Specific action plans began to materialize in 1989 at WHO

International Conference of Drug Regulatory Authorities (ICDRA) in Paris. Soon afterward, the authorities of Europe, Japan and US approached the International Federation of Pharmaceutical Manufacturers and Associations (IFPMA) to discuss a joint regulatory international harmonization initiative. The International Conference on Harmonization (ICH) came into existence in a meeting in April 1990, hosted by the European Federation of Pharmaceutical Industries and Associations (EFPIA) in Brussels conceptualizing a unique harmonization initiative involving the regulators and research-based industries of US, EU, and Japan.

WORLD HEALTH ORGANIZATION (WHO)

The "United Nations," was conceptualized by the United States President Franklin D. Roosevelt in the Declaration by League of Nations in 1942, during the Second World War with representatives of 26 nations. The UN emerged as an international organization in Allied conferences of 1943. In 1944, representatives of the Republic of China, the United Kingdom, the United States, and the USSR represented proposal outlining the purposes of the United Nations organization, its membership, and organs, as well as initiatives to maintain international peace and security encouraging international economic and social cooperation. Brazil, Syria and some other countries qualified for membership by declarations of war of 1945.

In 1945, representatives of 50 countries met in United Nations Conference held in San Francisco to draw up the United Nations Charter and decided to set up a global health organization concerned with international public health. WHO headquarters in Geneva, Switzerland came into force on 7 April 1948, with (celebrated every year as World Health Day) constitution signed by all 61 countries of the UN in the first meeting of the World Health Assembly.

Constitution of WHO

The World Health Organization, objective is to attain the highest possible level of health by all people. As per WHO, health is a state of complete physical, mental and social well-being and not merely the absence of disease or infirmity. The enjoyment of the highest attainable standard of health is one of the fundamental rights of every human being without distinction of race, religion, political belief, economic or social condition. Healthy development of the child is of fundamental importance for the ability to live harmoniously in a coherent environment. Unequal development concerning to promotion of health and control of disease, especially communicable disease, is a common danger in different countries.

Governance of WHO

The World Health Assembly is the supreme decision making body for WHO. The WHO is headed by the director-general, appointed by the health assembly based on the nomination of the executive board. The general meeting of delegates of all the member state is held in Geneva every year in May. Its primary function is to determine the policies of the organization. The health assembly appoints the Director General, supervises the financial policies of the organization, reviews and approves the proposed programme budget.

Health assembly works considering the reports of the executive board, composed of 32 members technically qualified in the field of health. Executive board members are elected for the term of three years. The central board meeting decides the agreed agenda and resolutions for forwarding to the health assembly that adopts the administrative matters. The primary function of the board is to make the decisions and policies of the health assembly and to facilitate its work. The WHO secretariat has approximately 3500 health and other experts and support staff on fixed-term appointments, working at the headquarters of the six regional offices and countries all over the world.

Functions of WHO

Thriving to achieve its objectives, the WHO functions on:

- Act as the directing and coordinating authority of international health work.
- Establish and maintain effective collaboration with the United Nations, specialized health care agencies, governmental health administrations, professional groups, and other such organizations.
- Assist governments in strengthening health services.
- Furnish appropriate technical assistance in emergencies with necessary aids upon the request or acceptance of governments.
- Provide and also assist in providing health services and facilities to special groups, such as the peoples of trust territories.
- Establish and maintain administrative and technical services as may be required, including epidemiological and statistical services.
- Stimulate advance work for the eradication of epidemic and endemic diseases.
- Promote cooperative working with specialized agencies towards the prevention of accidental injuries, improvement of nutrition status, housing, sanitation, recreation, economic development, betterment of working conditions and other aspects of environmental hygiene.
- Promote cooperation among scientific and professional groups contributing to the advancement of health.
- Propose conventions, agreements, regulations, and make recommendations concerning international health matters.
- Promote maternal health and child welfare.
- Foster activities in the field of mental health promotion, especially those affecting the harmony of human relations.
- Promote and conduct research activities in the field of health services.
- Improve standards of teaching and training in the health, medical and related professions.
- Study and report on administrative and social techniques affecting public health and medical care from the point of view of preventive and curative care including hospital services and social security.
- Provide information, counsel, and assistance in the field of health.
- Assist in developing a system of informed public opinion among all people on matters of health.
- Establish and revise as necessary international nomenclatures of diseases, causes of death and public health practices.
- Standardize diagnostic procedures as necessary.
- Develop, establish and promote international standards for food, biological, pharmaceutical, and similar products.

WHO had played a leading role in the eradication of smallpox. WHO's priorities are:

- Control of communicable diseases particularly HIV/AIDS, malaria and tuberculosis
- The mitigation of non-communicable lifestyle related diseases
- Eradication of epidemic, endemic and other diseases
- Safeguard of sexual and reproductive health, development and aging
- Promotion of nutrition, food security, and healthy eating
- Promotion of environmental hygiene like housing, sanitation, recreation, economic, working conditions, and other aspects
- Awareness related to occupational health issues
- Prevention of drug abuse
- Development of networking reporting, health status related data collection, handling, and publication.

As of 2013, the WHO has 194 member states, two associate members, Puerto Rico, and Tokelau and several other countries with observer status. WHO fulfills its objectives of strengthening international health services acting as the directing and coordinating authority. The WHO maintains an active collaboration of the UN with the specialized agencies, governmental health administrations, professional groups and such other organizations working on promotion of health. WHO also furnish appropriate technical assistance to promote co-operation between specialized agencies, scientific and professional groups to establish and maintain administrative and technical services. WHO's significant contributions are the promotion of conventions, agreements, and regulations, and to make recommendations on harmonization of international drug regulatory organizations.

Harmonization Initiative

Currently, only about 20% of countries have a well-developed system for medicines regulation, about 50% have regulation of varying capacity and level and rest 30% have minimal drug regulation. The problems of weak drug regulation are not bound to the national borders but have global implications. Illegal manufacturing, distribution, sales and smuggling of medicines are widespread in some countries. Many lower-income countries are unable to ensure the safety, efficacy, and quality of medicines circulating on their markets and these medicines can get access to other surrounding countries also as often controls on exported medicines are less stringent than for those used domestically. Medicines are traded as several intermediaries in free-trade zones, repackaged and relabelled which can hide their true source or identity, leading to the circulation of counterfeit medicines.

The drug regulation guidelines worldwide are different, and assessment procedures in many countries are not up to international standards and are often of administrative rather than technical nature. Medicines regulation deals with the products, processes, and practices that involve rapid scientific and technological changes. The government department responsible for drug regulation must be empowered to formulate new regulations and to propose modifications in the existing ones as and when required. In some countries, drug regulation functions come under the jurisdiction of a single agency with full authority. While in some countries, the functions are distributed between different authorities, either horizontally (e.g. the ministry of health and family welfare, the ministry of chemical and fertilizer) or vertically (central, state and union territory governments) and to function effectively coherent coordination at the national level is required which is difficult to achieve. The countries like Australia (TGA) and the United Kingdom (MHRA) recover 100% of all regulation costs from fees levied for services, whereas in Canada and the United States recover around 50–70% of their costs. In the developing and underdeveloped countries, regulatory fees are less compared to the other counterparts where the government finds it exceptionally difficult to finance the regulatory functions adequately. The fees should somehow reflect the actual cost of services as in most instances the government resources alone are insufficient to ensure effective and sustainable medicine regulation in the developing countries. Inadequate resources in the third world countries severely limit the technical assessment of dossiers. Wide-ranging exemption clauses exist between country to country which should be compromised upon while justifying risk assessment and safety evaluation of drugs. Weak political will and commitment, lack of adequate human and financial resources, inappropriate facilities and absence of substantial enforcement power make the drug regulation inadequate.

Effective enforcement of drug legislation requires coherent work between regulatory agency, customs, police, and prosecutors, but in many countries cooperation is non-existent. In many developing countries, no written policy and guidance exist for staffs on the principles, practices, and methods to be followed. Monitoring and evaluation of guideline implementation are difficult because of the lack of information and weak data management.

Despite resource constraints, only a few countries rely on regulatory decisions made by other competent authorities (such as stringent MHRAs or by the WHO Prequalification Programme). Looking into the widespread conflicts and dissimilarities, WHO is promoting regulatory collaboration and harmonization worldwide. WHO provides technical assistance for developing evidence-based regulatory systems worldwide. Direct technical support (capacity building tools, and guidance) is provided to the collaborative agencies of various regions and countries to facilitate communication among national/regional regulatory systems facilitating relevant network meetings (e.g. WHO Annual Pharmacovigilance Centres meetings, and International Regulatory Cooperation for Herbal Medicines (IRCH). WHO also helps in forming global Regulators Networks like Blood Regulators Network and Paediatric Regulators Network.

The WHO has a dual role in medicines regulation and guideline development. The first aspect is to develop internationally recognized norms, standards, and guidelines. The second aspect is to provide guidance, technical assistance, and training in order to enable countries to implement global guidelines to meet their specific medicines regulatory environment and needs.

Regulatory Support Activities

The medicines regulatory support activities of WHO focus on supporting the work of national regulatory authorities by working on:

- Assessing national medicines regulatory systems
- Preparing regulatory information and practical manuals
- Providing training opportunities
- Preparing model website for medicines regulatory authorities
- Developing a model system for computer assisted medicines registration
- Quality certification of pharmaceutical products moving in international commerce
- Organizing international conferences of drug regulatory authorities
- Promoting international cooperation and harmonization

Successful harmonization initiative of technical requirements for medicines regulation is based on collaboration in the field of legislation, technical guidelines, and procedures. Implementation of the medicines regulation could not be effective without addressing all significant regulation aspects.

Harmonization of technical requirements for medicines regulation is advantageous for future development goals:

- Companies have to generate only one data set for all regions, and consequently, the amount of human and animal experimentation is reduced.
- The cost of development of regulatory documentation both for new drugs and multisource/generic medicines is reduced, which can lead to lower prices.
- Common regulatory standards for scientific evaluation and inspection facilitate regulatory communication and information sharing.
- Local products are more likely to be acceptable for export to other countries.
- Faster access to medicines of higher public health value (pediatric medicines, medi-

cines for common diseases or emergencies in national settings).

• Increase in competitiveness resulting from newly developed common markets.

Challenges for WHO

WHO is a highly recognized institution with its well-organized infrastructure reaching out to all countries through its regional and country offices, and has competitive advantages over other organizations. The future of quality pharmaceuticals depends on worldwide adoption of regulatory harmonization. Due to the sophistication of science, new amount of information and data is always to appraise as there is no alternative to efficient scientific communication and collaboration. The patients will always pay the price for the failure of regulators to act. WHO has promoted regulatory collaboration and harmonization since long time and bringing upon new ideas and changes. WHO is one of the most critical organizations giving help to less resourced regulators. WHO is still going through the reform process and this brought upon both opportunity and challenge.

EUROPEAN UNION

In order to ensure health protection and free movements of medicines across the European Economic Community (EEC), the European Union (EU) has harmonized requirements for research and testing among the Member States. Medicines control was an early activity area of the EEC. The first and primary EEC directive for control of medicines was introduced in 1965 (Directive 65/65/EEC) as requirement for the control of medicinal products by the *Medicines Act 1968*, matching with existing European Directives. European Community legislation then has taken precedence over the Medicines Act, its Instruments and Orders, which were amended from time to time to align with new EC requirements. The European Medicines Agency (EMA) located in London plays a central role in the network of close collaboration among the medicines authorities, concerning marketing authorizations and surveillance of medicines. EMA began operations in 1995 with the responsibility of scientific evaluation, supervision and safety monitoring of medicines in the EU. EMA is responsible for the centrally authorized medicines, but the individual Member States perform the assessments of application for National and Mutual recognition aspects. The most current relevant legislation of medicinal products for human use, given in Directive 2001/83/EC was amended by Directives 2002/98/EC, 2003/63/EC, 2004/24/EC, and 2004/27/EC. The regulations implemented in EU Directive 2010/84/EU, introduced a strengthened, clarified and more proportionate regime for pharmacovigilance in the EU market.

In the EU the two main routes for authorizing medicines are the centralized route and the national decentralized (route). For consideration under centralized authorization procedure pharmaceutical companies submit a single marketing authorization application to EMA. EMA's Committee for Medicinal Products for Human Use (CHMP) or Committee for Medicinal Products for Veterinary Use (CVMP) carry out scientific assessment of the application and give recommendation. Once approved, the centralized marketing authorization issued is valid in all EU Member States as well as in the European Economic Area (EEA) and countries like Iceland, Liechtenstein and Norway. After approval by a single marketing authorization, the license holder can market the medicine throughout the EU. The national route is based on the regulatory framework of each country of EU. The decentralized marketing authorization is valid for the respective country only.

The EU has mutual recognition agreements (MRAs) with third country authorities concerning the conformity assessment of regulated products, GMP inspections and batch certification of medicines. MRAs allow EU authorities and their counterparts to facilitate mutual market access and greater harmonization in the implementation of standards and compliance protecting consumer safety. These agreements benefit authorities by reducing duplication of inspections, facilitate trade by reducing costs for manufacturers and waiving re-testing of products upon importation.

The regulatory guideline of the European Community document with its explicit legal basis is referred to as legislative framework intended to provide advice to applicants or marketing authorization holders, competent authorities and/or other interested parties on the best and most appropriate ways to fulfil the legal obligations laid down by the pharmaceutical legislation of the EU. The basic EU legislation is thus supported by a series of guidelines published by the Commission, grouped broadly as regulatory or scientific. The concept of regulating medical device is well established in EU, whereas many countries did not have any significant medical device regulation. The EU has implemented the New Approach Directive for medical devices, making the first significant conceptual advance in healthcare regulation in last nearly 100 years. The New Approach Directive provides broad concepts on the law, and the bulk of the technological detail delegated to comply with recognized updateable standards. The Global Harmonization Task Force has mostly adopted the European Model of medical device regulation as a general template.

THE INTERNATIONAL COUNCIL FOR HARMONISATION (ICH)

The ICH, formerly known as the International Conference on Harmonisation (ICH) of Technical Requirements for Registration of Pharmaceuticals for Human Use, was launched in 1990. ICH has brought together the drug regulatory authorities of Europe, Japan, and the United States along with the pharmaceutical trade associations from these three regions, to discuss scientific and technical aspects of drug product registration. Well-defined objectives of ICH is to improve the efficiency of new drug development and registration process, promotion of public health, prevention of duplication of clinical trials in humans and to minimize the use of animal for preclinical testing without compromising safety and efficacy. ICH's mission is to reduce duplication of testing and reporting required for the research and development of new medicines. This was achieved by harmonization in the interpretation and application of technical guidelines and requirements for product registration implementing universal single application and approval system.

In the first ten years, ICH has created and developed procedures and guideline in the areas of safety, efficacy, and quality of medicinal products. In the year 2003, ICH introduced Common Technical Document (CTD) which has revolutionized the submission procedures for industry's regulatory staff. CTD has offered benefit to industry far higher than any other harmonization initiative by significantly saving time and resources. CTD greatly reduces the requirement of the huge work force and financial burdens of assembling regulatory submission to a particular drug regulatory agency and then having it reformatted for another agency. CTD replaced complex multiple submissions by a single technical dossier, which is submitted for consideration simultaneously in the three ICH regions facilitating fast approval and launch of new drugs. The CTD has also made the possible easier exchange of information among drug regulatory authorities. Earlier, USFDA and the EMA have had a confidentiality arrangement allowing the sharing of confidential information, significantly increasing interactions between the two agencies.

In recognition to the aspiring global face of drug development, ICH updated its logo in 2010 emphasizing the benefits of harmonization for better global health. The electronic CTD (eCTD) was implemented, disseminating guideline information to non-ICH countries, yielding additional benefits to both regulators and industry. The eCTD has significantly improved the application submission efficiency and reviewer efficiency, besides delivering submission material to the reviewer in an expedited manner. In the eCTD format, it is easier to develop standardized reviewer e-templates and review tools. The CTD has rapidly become the marketing application technique of choice, and regulators are now using the principles of the CTD as a springboard to incorporate newer and better ideas in regulatory review practices.

The globalization of industry in the field of both innovative and generic medicines drove a need for common standards, which has spurred the interest of non-ICH countries also promoting earlier access to new therapies. The ICH guidelines are now recognized as reference documents due to science-based principles and defined approaches having broad utility, not limited to new drugs, giving them broader relevance. In March 1999, ICH created the Global Cooperation Group (GCG) to facilitate open communication and fluid dissemination of information with a desire to establish global linkages that extend beyond the three ICH regions. The crucial operating principal of GCG is precise that, ICH will never impose its views on any country or region and it will work closely with WHO and other international organizations to achieve its goals. The mission statement "to promote mutual understanding of regional harmonization initiatives to facilitate the harmonization process related to ICH guidelines regionally and globally and to facilitate the capacity of drug regulatory authorities and

industry to utilize them" was recognized for GCG's in November 2003, to achieve the overall goal of partnership with Regional Harmonization Initiatives (RHI).

The representatives from five RHIs actively participate in GCG discussions for harmonization for better health are Asia-Pacific Economic Cooperation (APEC), the Association of the Southeast Asian Nations (ASEAN), the Gulf Cooperation Council (GCC), the Pan American Network for Drug Regulatory Harmonisation (PANDRH), and the Southern African Development Community (SADC). GCG was expanded in 2007, with the creation of a Regulators Forum including Chinese Taipei, Singapore, South Korea, Brazil, China, India and Russia. This is to authorize the representation of individual countries drug regulatory authorities (DRAs) as they were a major source of active pharmaceutical ingredients (APIs), clinical trial data, and had adopted ICH guidelines. The representatives from five RHIs and the newly established Regulators Forum promoted participation of non-ICH countries interested in implementing ICH's strategies. This initiative has created a common regulatory language promoting faster access to life-saving treatments to patients beyond ICH regions. GCG efforts have evolved from mere information sharing to active dialogue between ICH and non-ICH member countries. GCG has fostered a spirit of trust and cooperation between ICH representatives and colleagues from RHIs and DRAs perhaps the most important key to future success of ICH.

HARMONIZATION IN AFRICA

Africa is a continent of many small countries having huge diversity and complex unity, with numerous Regional Economic Communities (REC) and politically complicated environment.

Potential benefits of harmonizing medicines registration have encouraged WHO to develop a concept paper describing the proposed approaches supporting drug registration harmonization within and across the African region (WHO Drug Information, Volume 22, Number 3, 2008). After further discussions and orientation, African Medicines Regulatory Harmonization Initiative (AMRHI) was established in 2009. AMRHI is intented to improve health in the African Region by increasing access to safe, effective and right quality medicines with strengthening of the technical and administrative capacity of participating national medicines regulatory authorities. WHO support the RECs, for necessary actions related to national implementation, strengthen national regulatory agencies and promote the inter-REC and continental exchange of information, coordination and technical consistency. WHO invited summary project proposals from committed RECs seeking financial and technical support.

The collaborative mechanism was aimed at improving the regulatory approval process and operational efficiencies at the national/regional/sub-regional levels for medicines regulatory systems and processes. AMRHI focuses on medicine registration specifically of essential medicines (mostly generic pharmaceuticals) in order to maximize near-patient benefit and impact the critical disease burden that Africa is facing. The initiative works for increasing the capacity of national medicines regulatory authorities, harmonize technical requirements for the regulation of medical products, strengthening the administration, structural and technical elements of medicines regulation. AMRHI helps the member countries to enhance and facilitate decision making processes regarding the registration of medicines, establishment of a framework for joint evaluations of application dossiers and inspections of medicine manufacturing sites, information exchange as well as exercise more control over medicines circulating on the market. WHO provided technical assistance to develop harmonized approaches for medicinal product registration, GMP inspection, quality management, and information management systems development and support capacity building and training. In 2010 World Bank joined the process as a Multi-Donor Trust Fund Holder and provided advocacy for resource mobilization, fiduciary oversight, and dissemination of lessons.

REGIONAL HARMONIZATION INITIATIVES

Pharmaceutical Inspection Convention and Pharmaceutical Inspection Co-operation Scheme (PIC/S)

The PIC and PIC/S are two international conventions between countries and pharmaceutical inspection authorities providing constructive co-operation in the implementation and maintenance of harmonized GMP standards of inspectorates in the field of medicinal products. The PIC/S based in Geneva is an instrument to improve co-operation in the field of GMP implementation between regulatory authorities and the pharmaceutical industry. The PIC was founded in 1970 by the European Free Trade Association (EFTA), initially comprising Participating Authorities of 10 member countries. The inclusion of new member countries in PIC was not possible due to incompatibility between the Convention and European law. European law did not permit individual EU countries having a membership of PIC to sign agreements with other countries seeking to join PIC.

Pharmaceutical Inspection Co-operation Scheme was formed in 1995 as an informal agreement between health authorities instead of a formal treaty between countries to formalize inclusion of new members. PIC and the PIC Scheme, which operate together in parallel, are jointly referred to as PIC/S. PIC/S works on developing and promoting harmonized GMP standards and guidance documents, training of GMP inspectors, exchange of inspectional information, continuous assessing of inspectorates and facilitating networking of competent authorities with international organizations. Currently, there are 52 Participating Authorities in PIC/S which include most EU Member States, Switzerland, South Africa, Australia, Canada, Singapore, and others. PIC/S Expert Circles facilitates discussions, and the exchange of information among Inspectors specialized in a specific area of GMP such as blood, Computerised Systems, Active Pharmaceutical Ingredients, and Quality Risk Management. Expert Circles meet regularly to develop draft guidance, recommendations, and offer training in their respective fields of specialization.

PIC/S Committee setup the Sub-Committee on Strategic Development (SCSD) in 2009 to discuss issues related to the improvement of the operation of the Scheme. Following suggestion of the Irish Medicines Boards more Sub-Committees were established, which was successfully implemented in 2014, with the mandate to define PIC/S' strategy, future policy and make proposals for improvement of structure and operation of PIC/S. PIC/S activities are now shared by 7 Sub-Committees that report back to the PIC/S Committee on the activities covered by their respective Sub-Committees in fields of:

1. Training (SCT)
2. Expert Circles (SCEC)
3. Strategic Development (SCSD)
4. Compliance (SCC)
5. GM(D)P Harmonisation (SCH)
6. Budget, Risk, and Audit (SCB)
7. Communication (SC COM)

The SCSD is also responsible for making proposals on the possible expansion of PIC/S' mandate to other areas, discuss new projects, funding options and issues related to the improvement of co-operation with PIC/S Partner Organisations. In 2010, USFDA

became a member of the PIC/S network. Centre for Biologics Evaluation and Research (CBER) of USFDA has a representative on the FDA Steering Committee managing the Agency's interactions with PIC/S and actively participates in the technical group known as the PIC/S Expert Circle on Human Blood, Tissues and Cells. Australia is a member of PIC/S since 1993 while Japan got membership in 2014. Indonesia and Thailand are the only two Asian countries having a formal association with PIC/S. Mexico, Iran, and Turkey became the new member of PIC/S effective from Jan 2018.

Global Harmonization Task Force (GHTF)

The Global Harmonization Task Force (GHTF) fosters international harmonization in the regulation of medical devices. The GHTF was founded in 1992 in an endeavor to fulfil the growing needs for international harmonization in the regulation of medical devices. The GHTF was a voluntary group of representatives from regulatory, and industry authorities of Europe, Asia-Pacific, and North America collaborated to encourage the harmonization of regulatory practices to ensure the safety, effectiveness, and quality of medical devices. A Harmonization and Multilateral Relations representative serves on the GHTF Steering Committee. It has members from different national medical device regulatory authorities and members of the medical device industry whose goal was to standardize medical device regulation across the world. The representatives from five founding members, the EU, the US, Canada, Japan, and Australia actively regulates medical devices using their unique regulatory framework. The GHTF also serves as an information exchange forum for countries with underdeveloped medical device regulatory systems where thay are benefited by sharing experiences with GHTF Founding Members. The GHTF disbanded late in 2012 as the mission has been taken over by the

International Medical Device Regulatory Forum (IMDRF), a successor organization composed of officials from regulatory agencies around the world but not industry.

Asia-Pacific Economic Cooperation (APEC: 21-member economies)

The APEC forum was established in 1989 aiming to facilitate economic growth and prosperity in the 21 members of Pacific Rim countries; secretariat is based in Singapore. APEC seeks to promote free trade and economic cooperation throughout the Asia-Pacific region. APEC forum operates by non-binding commitments, open dialogue and equal respect for views of all participants. It takes decisions by consensus and commit-ments are undertaken on a voluntary basis. It provides coordination, technical and advisory support as well as information management, communications, and public outreach services between the member countries. APEC aims to strengthen regional economic integration by removing trade and investment impediments 'at the border', enhancing supply chain connectivity 'across the border', and improv-ing the business environment 'behind the border'. APEC supports the multilateral trade negotiations of WTO and complements the goals of the G-20 Framework for healthy, sustainable and balanced growth in the Asia-Pacific region.

APEC leaders have recognized the impor-tance of good regulatory performance in contributing to life sciences innovation and supported the initiative, Life Sciences Innova-tion Forum (LSIF) in 2002 as an 'enabler of regulatory harmonization.' APEC has adopted existing international standards and best practices for medical products and served as a vehicle to promote prospective harmoni-zation dialogue in the area of advanced therapies. LSIF is unique as it does not work on formulating new harmonized guidelines, instead promotes the use of existing inter-national guidelines. It encourages linkages of

Asia-Pacific rim countries with the inter-national harmonization initiatives having complementary roles in government, industry, and academia. The LSIF supports a strategic, coordinated approach to harmoni-zation activities, and strives to complement rather than duplicate. The LSIF has endorsed the establishment of the APEC Harmonization Center and Regulatory Harmonization Steering Committee (RHSC), inaugurated in June 2009 leveraging resources and efforts towards effective medicine harmonization.

The APEC has developed and implemented a five-year plan cutting across GMPs, Good Distribution Practices (GDPs), Good Import/Export Practices, Good Pharmacy Practices and Internet sales that have a powerful influence on global regulatory harmonization scenario in the pharmaceutical supply chain realm. Besides the Pacific Rim Member countries, regulatory and standards organi-zations, including FDA, EMA, U.S. Pharmacopeial Convention (USP), Health Canada, European Directorate for the Quality of Medicines (EDQM), WHO and the Nigerian government are participating in the plan. FDA and Health Canada were instrumental among the other participants in convincing this multi-national body about the benefits of pharma-ceutical supply chain regulation harmoni-zation as an essential component in achieving its goals. APEC has addressed eight 'choke-points' from regulatory impediments to customs procedures and infrastructure bottlenecks with improvement in supply chain performance regarding time, cost and uncertainty. The delivery time to import goods dropped by an average 25% while the preparation period for export fell by 21% in the region. APEC economies have centralized making the export-import processes online at the border. This widely known Single Window virtual system links all government agencies involved in the export-import process, allowing companies to submit documents electronically. Fourteen APEC economies had already adopted various stages of the Single Window system, and this also aims to link all 21 members coming on board by 2020. The member economies are committed to reducing energy intensity in the region near 45% by 2030.

Association of the Southeast Asian Nations (ASEAN: 10 economies)

The Association of Southeast Asian Nations (ASEAN) formed in 1967, is a geopolitical and economic organization of ten countries located in Southeast Asia. The members are Indonesia, Malaysia, the Philippines, Singapore, Thailand, Brunei, Myanmar, Cambodia, Laos, and Vietnam. ASEAN aims to accelerate economic growth, social progress, cultural development, protection of regional peace, stability and providing opportunities for peaceful open discussion between members. ASEAN celebrated its 40th anniversary in 2007, with an aspire to carry out free trade agreements with China, Japan, South Korea, India, Australia, and New Zealand by 2013. This Regional Comprehensive Economic Partnership (RCEP) was formed in 2018, in line with this ASEAN Economic Community (AEC) establishment in 2015 forming a more integrated group. The AEC intent to espouse industrial production capacity, encourage competitiveness, support growth and regional integration as a single market presenting for the global economy. The pharmaceutical market in South East Asia is relatively small, but the region remains attractive to the global pharmaceutical industry due to its growth potentials.

The regulatory environment in the ASEAN countries is similar in certain features but there are differences in systems and practices, and have problems of lack of consistency and transparency in the review procedure. Many of the regulatory agencies in these countries suffer from having rather weak infrastructures primarily due to limited human resources. Although a few scientific guidelines have been established in the region, the ICH guidelines are well adapted in most countries. The requirement of CPP (Certificate of Pharmaceutical Product) from the country of origin (COO) remains a crucial barrier to the registration of new drugs in the region. Among the ten ASEAN members, the five founding member countries (Singapore, Malaysia, Thailand, Philippines, and Indonesia) are more progressive with drug registration and drug development clinical trial activities. The different drug regulatory agencies in South East Asia are National Agency of Drug and Food Control in Indonesia; Drug Control Authority in Malaysia; BFAD, DoH in Philippines; ThaiFDA, Drug Control Division in Thailand; Health Sciences Authority (HSA), Centre for Pharmaceutical Administration (CPA) and Centre for Drug Evaluation (CDE) in Singapore.

Efforts toward harmonization of ASEAN pharmaceutical regulations were initiated in 1992 through the formation of ASEAN Consultative Committee for Standards and Quality (ACCSQ). ASEAN has started a harmonization initiative given many regulatory barriers and diversity in requirements hindering simultaneous regulatory submission in ASEAN countries. In this direction, a Product Working Group on Pharmaceutical (CCCSQ-PPWG) was initiated in 1998 aimed at establishing common technical requirements and quality guidelines for product registrations, and it started functioning in 1999. PPWG's objective is to develop harmonization scheme for pharmaceuticals regulations in the ASEAN member countries, to complement and facilitate elimination of technical barriers to trade posed by the regulations without compromising on quality, efficacy, and safety of drugs.

PPWG has developed and harmonized ASEAN product guidelines, i.e. ACTR (ASEAN Common Technical Requirement), ACTD (ASEAN Common Technical Dossier) and Technical "Quality, Safety, Efficacy" guidelines. PPWG has adopted guidelines from WHO, ICH, and International pharmacopeia and developed ASEAN Quality guidelines:

- Analytical Validation guideline
- BA/BE Studies guideline
- Process Validation guideline
- Stability Study guideline

ACCSQ-PPWG in cooperation with international organizations and dialogue partners has developed projects like:

- WHO-ASEAN Harmonization project,
- ACCSQ-US Cooperation project—with three PPWG project proposals (i) Developing the Guidelines on Quality, (ii) Training on Clinical Data and (iii) Developing and Implementing the "Guideline & Implementation SOP."

ACCSQ-PPWG was also expanded for implementation of the harmonized ASEAN documents into the possible "Sectoral MRA (Mutual Recognition Agreement)." The ACCSQ-PPWG has made considerable progress, despite limitations in the existing capability and capacity of the Regulatory Authorities of ASEAN member countries. The Singapore agency HSA has progressed in the direction of harmonization by making international cooperation, signing a pact with the health authority of Australia, TGA. The cooperation is aimed at a better sharing of experiences, and this has bought an improved reviewing process to Singapore. ASEAN's drug regulatory authorities are working in very close partnership with one another and with the pharmaceutical industry to ensure the smooth functioning of implemented initiatives.

Gulf Cooperation Council (GCC: 6 Gulf states)

The Cooperation Council for the Arab States of the Gulf is a political and economic union of Arab states established in 1981, known as the Gulf Cooperation Council (GCC). The members are Bahrain, Kuwait, Oman, Qatar, Saudi Arabia, and the United Arab Emirates. The Gulf Cooperation Council states are similar in language, geography, values, traditions, economic resources, in social and cultural factors. The pharmaceutical market in the GCC has witnessed considerable progress over the years as a result of favorable demographic and economic growth and strong government support for healthcare sector. The pharmaceutical market in these countries has reached up to 5.6 billion dollars in 2010 and predicted that sales would reach 10.8 billion dollars by 2020.

The GCC regulatory authorities have formed the Gulf Central Committee for Drug Registration (GCC-DR) including Bahrain, Kuwait, Oman, Qatar, Saudi Arabia, United Arab Emirates, and Yemen in 1999. GCC-DR headquarter is located in the executive office for Health Ministers Riyadh, Saudi Arabia. The responsibilities of GCC-DR include:

- Registration of pharmaceutical companies.
- Registration of pharmaceutical preparations.
- Inspection of pharmaceutical companies for GMP compliance.
- Review of technical and post-marketing surveillance reports.

The company registration must be approved before the product registration, and the model used by the Gulf central registration system for all major application is an abridged assessment. GCC-DR has adopted two processes for drug registration, the Centralized registration procedure, and Decentralized registration procedure. For centralized registration, the manufacturer should fill companies registration form and pharmaceutical chemical entity/preparation registration form separately. Filled registration form and samples of chemical entity should be submitted to the executive office along with dispatching of the form and sample for the respective countries. Every concerned country forward the file to committee after study with the recommendation. The executive office analyses the sample by a reference accredited laboratory. Following submission of prescribed fee for centralized registration GCC-DR executive office approve the registration of the company and/or chemical entity and issues a registration certificate. The remaining authentication, documentation, and fees are finalized on the country basis as per their prescribed and approved policies. Though centralization registration of drugs is not mandatory in GCC, for special classes, as follows registration through the centralized process is necessary:

- Generic drugs for which bioequivalence studies cannot be done, e.g. inhalable medicines and some nasal inhalers.
- Drugs supported by biotechnology for which bioequivalence studies cannot be done and which require clinical or pharmacodynamic studies.
- Orally administered drugs with narrow therapeutic spectrum.

In the decentralized registration process, the drug registration is regulated separately by main countries of GCC. Although there is a centralized and harmonized process for drug registration in GCC countries, the regulatory requirements for a few big countries like Saudi Arabia, UAE, Bahrain, and Kuwait are separate with well-established regulatory systems and enforcement. The GCC countries adopted the Common Technical Document (CTD) framework in 2009 and had since progressively moved towards to its implementation. Saudi Food and Drug Authority is the main regulatory body in Saudi Arabia. SFDA has a system for online application form submission followed by hard copy submission within 12 weeks. SFDA prefers drug dossier submission in eCTD format along with stability study data submission following GCC guideline for three initial batches. Ministry of Health, Bahrain, requires all necessary documents similar to other GCC countries for drug registration in the Kingdom of Bahrain but also focus on the details of company profiles and business mergers.

Medicines in Kuwait are regulated by quality, safety, efficacy standards, price control, and patent protection. Kuwait Food and Drug Authority (KuFDA) is the head regulatory agency to register pharmaceutical products. The GCC pharmaceutical market is dominated by patented drugs, whereas generics have only about 5–6% market share. Foreign drug manufacturers can only market drug products in a GCC country through local importing and distribution companies registered with the health ministry. Foreign investors are restricted to work in the pharmaceutical wholesale and distribution segment. Apart from regulating investments and drug registration, the health ministry and other government agencies also control the price of pharmaceutical products.

Pan American Network for Drug Regulatory Harmonization (PANDRH)

The Pan American Network for Drug Regulatory Harmonization (PANDRH) is a continental forum on drug regulatory harmonization established in November 1999. It is an initiative of the national regulatory authorities within the Pan American Health Organization (PAHO) region. PANDRH supports the pharmaceutical regulatory harmonization process in the America, within the framework of national and sub-regional health policies abolishing the pre-existing asymmetries.

The Components of PANDRH are:
- The Pan American Conference on Drug Regulatory Harmonization (PANDHR)
- The Steering Committee (SC)
- The Technical Working Groups (WGs)
- Secretariat

These constitute a continental forum ensuring the presence of regulatory authorities of all PAHO member states, representatives from the regional pharmaceutical industry associations, representatives of organisms for economic integration (like Latin American Association for Integration, the Andean Community), academics, consumer groups, representatives of regional professional associations and other groups interested from all the continents sub-regions. This forum also facilitates the integration of the countries from the continent that do not belong to the sub-region blocks as Cuba, Dominican Republic and Chile. The conference disseminates the decisions of global initiatives on drug regulatory harmonization. The PANDRH is a member of the Global Cooperation Group of the ICH. Its primary objective is to support the harmonization processes through the analysis of specific regulatory aspects, the adoption of recommendations on priority subjects and harmonization of guidelines proposed by the working groups.

The PANDRH Steering Committee is the decision-making body for the strategic and operational management of the network, guiding progress on projects and activities, and making recommendations for evaluation and discussion at the Conference. The Steering Committee is composed of the Secretariat and members officially designated to represent each sub-region as North America, Central America, Cuba, the Dominican Republic, the Caribbean, the Andean Region, and the Southern Cone. Steering Committee Members are appointed for four years, ensuring rotation among the countries in each subregion. The Pan American Health Organization serves as Secretariat providing technical and administrative support to PANDRH.

PANDRH has working groups on bioequivalence, biotechnological products, combat counterfeit medicines, good clinical practices, good laboratory practices, good manufacturing practices, medical plants, medicines classification, medicines promotion, medicines registration, pharmacopoeia, pharmaco-

vigilance, and vaccines. PANDRH regular activities are to support the countries for implementation of approved guidelines, external quality control programs, organizing national seminars and running educational programs. The PANDRH's mission is to promote drug regulatory harmonization covering all aspects of quality, safety, and efficacy of pharmaceutical products with a pursuit for the betterment of quality of life and healthcare of the citizens of the American Member Countries. PANDRH's scope of harmonization/cooperative activities includes updating technical guidelines, standards, and regulatory processes, and strengthening of national regulatory agencies to improve drug quality assurance.

Southern African Development Community (SADC: 15 countries)

The Southern African Development Community (SADC) is an inter-governmental organization supporting socio-economic cooperation and integration along with political and security cooperation among 15 southern African states. The Southern African Development Coordination Conference (SADCC), the forerunner of SADC, was formed as a liberate alliance of nine majorities ruled states in Southern Africa with the aim of coordinating development projects to lessen economic dependence in 1980. The founding member states were Angola, Botswana, Lesotho, Malawi, Mozambique, Swaziland, United Republic of Tanzania, Zambia and Zimbabwe.

The encouraging transformation of the organization from a Coordinating Conference to a Development Community (SADC) took place on 1992 in Windhoek, Namibia when the Declaration and Treaty were signed at the Summit of Heads of State and Government giving the organization a legal status. The Member States are the Democratic Republic of Congo, Madagascar, Mauritius, Namibia, Seychelles, and South Africa. SADC headquarters is located in Gaborone, Botswana. On 2001, the SADC treaty was amended with an overall impact on the structures, policies, and procedures.

All SADC Member States have an official or draft national medicines policy, as well as medicines legislation and regulations framework, who function under a shared regulatory network. All countries in the SADC region are members of the World Trade Organisation (WTO) and signatory in the Agreement on Trade Related Aspects of Intellectual Property Rights (TRIPS). *Medicines Registration Harmonisation Project* has been developed in the interests of regional integration of regulatory authorities in the SADC to register and control medicines using the common set of regional minimum standards. The SADC region has developed guidelines for medicines regulation and other pharmaceutical strategies focusing to improve access to medicines. SADC has strategic policy documents such as the SADC Health Policy Framework, SADC Protocol on Health, SADC Trade Protocol developed for SADC *Pharmaceutical Programme*. SADC *Pharmaceutical Programme* has these priority areas in medicine regulation:

- Strengthen capacity to review and monitor ethical clinical trials
- Strengthen the region's training centers
- Facilitate information exchange on the safety, quality. and efficacy of medicines
- Ascertain laboratories capacitation and facilitate access for testing of essential medicines and African Traditional Medicines

The SADC *Pharmaceutical Business Plan* was then developed and approved for 2007–2013 in order to operationalize the SADC Health Programme and plan. The goal of the Pharmaceutical Business Plan is to ensure availability of essential medicines along with African Traditional Medicines to reduce disease burden in the region, and to improve sustainable availability and access to essential medicines. In order to achieve the overall goal and objective the following strategies were pursued:

1. Facilitate trade of pharmaceuticals within SADC.
2. Harmonization of standard treatment guidelines and essential medicine lists
3. Developing and retaining competent human resources
4. Maximizing research and production capacity of the local and regional pharmaceutical industry
5. Strengthening regulatory capacity, supply, and distribution of pharmaceutical products
6. Promoting joint procurement of medicines of acceptable safety, proven efficacy moreover, quality at affordable prices
7. Establishing regional data bank of traditional medicine, medicinal plants, and procedures to ensure their protection following regimes and related intellectual property rights preservation
8. Developing mechanisms to respond in cases of emergency pharmaceutical needs

Development of regulatory policy and legislative framework for regulation and validation of the African Traditional medicines safety, quality, and efficacy is equally essential. Populations throughout the SADC region extensively use traditional medicines to cater their primary healthcare needs. Medicinal plants contain a vast wealth of active ingredients that can be used in the production of herbal medicines. SADC medicine registration harmonization project and business plan have actively included the African Traditional Medicines in their harmonization and quality assurance system. The SADC Free Trade Area was achieved in 2008. The SADC Secretariat was officially recognized in 2012 as having international standards in accounting, audit, internal controls and procurement.

East African Community (EAC: 6 countries)

The EAC is the regional intergovernmental organization of five countries, the Republic of Kenya, Republic of Uganda, the United Republic of Tanzania, Republic of Rwanda and Republic of Burundi. The EAC Secretariat headquarters is in Arusha, Tanzania. South Sudan is the newest member, joined the EAC in 2016. It is also referred to as the youngest nation in Africa after gaining independence in 2011. The vision of EAC is to have a stable and politically united East Africa with a deep economic, political, social and cultural integration that will improve the quality of life through value added production, trade, and investments.

The EAC has implemented a harmonized medicines regulatory system by the 1999 Treaty engaging various stakeholders in facilitating implementation of the initiative. In 2000, the Health Committee of EAC Council established working groups and medicines were placed under research, policy and health systems working group. This working group drafted a common drug policy to harmonize drug registration procedures for the partner states. EAC National Medicines Regulatory Authorities (NMRAs) has been tasked to assure the quality, efficacy, and safety of medicines by subjecting pre-marketing evaluation and authorization/registration of pharmaceutical products. Formation of EAC Customs Union in January 2005 established common external tariffs on medicines.

The main Organs of the EAC are the Summit, the Council of Ministers, the Co-ordinating Committee, the Sectoral Committees, the East African Court of Justice, the East African Legislative Assembly and the Secretariat. The Summit comprises heads of government of partner states. The Council is the central decision-making, and governing organ of the EAC constitutes with Ministers or Cabinet Secretaries from the partner states. The Co-ordinating Committee is responsible for regional co-operation and co-ordinates the activities of the Sectoral Committees. It also recommends the establishment, composition, and functions of such Sectoral Committees. The Coordinating Committee meets twice a year preceding the meetings of the Council. Sectoral Committees conceptualize programmes and monitor their implementation. The East African Court of Justice is the major judicial organ of the community which ensures adherence to the law in the interpretation and application of compliance with the EAC Treaty. The Legislative Assembly has members comprising of 45 elected members (nine from each partner state), and seven ex-officio members consisting of the minister or cabinet secretary responsible for EAC affairs from each partner state. Currently, it has 6 Standing Committees to execute the mandates:

- The accounts committee
- The committee on legal, rules, and privileges;
- The committee on agriculture, tourism, and natural resources;
- The committee on regional affairs and conflict resolution;
- The committee on communication, trade, and investment, and
- The committee on general purpose.

The Secretariat is the executive organ of the community ensuring the adoption of regulations and proper implementation of directives by the Council.

In line with the AMRHI Programme, Situation Analysis on Medicines Registration Harmonization (MRH) for the East African Community has been carried out to develop a strategy for regional medicines registration harmonization as a precursor to broader medicines regulatory harmonization initiatives on the continent in 2012. The report recommended proposal development for the EAC MRH project. The project proposal development process has been completed through collaborative consultations by stakeholders. This includes proposal writing workshop held in Entebbe, Uganda in September 2009 and consultation and project finalization meeting held in Zanzibar, Tanzania in May 2010. The progress of the EAC Union is encouraging, with establishment of the Common Market in 2010 and the implementation of the East African Monetary Union Protocol in 2013. An appraisal of the EAC partner states before the implementation of the MRH project was held in October 2011. This appraisal aimed at sensitizing the Ministers of Health, Finance and the National Medicines Regulatory Authority on the project governance and project management structures to get their support during the implementation. Members on the appraisal team included representatives of the EAC Secretariat, The World Bank, the WHO, and the NEPAD Agency. The project proposal whose goal is to have a harmonized and efficient functioning medicines registration system within the EAC by following national and internationally recognized policies and standards, have received approval for funding. The EAC MRH project was successfully launched on 30th March 2012 in Arusha, Tanzania.

REGULATORY AFFAIRS PERSONNEL

The functions of the regulatory personnel in healthcare industries are vital in making safe and effective healthcare products. Regulatory professionals ensure compliance of guidelines in manufacturing, preparing documents for regulatory approval submissions, coordinate functions of clinical affairs and quality assurance. Regulatory professionals are employed by private sector pharma industry, government, academia, consultancy service providers involved with a wide range of products and services, including:

• Pharmaceuticals
• Medical devices
• *In vivo* and *in vitro* diagnostics
• Biologics and biotechnological products
• Nutritional products
• Cosmetics
• Veterinary products

QUALIFICATION AND EXPERIENCE REQUIRED IN REGULATORY PROFESSIONAL

In a pharmaceutical industry involvement of the regulatory professionals begin with the research and development phase of medicinal product development, moving into clinical trials and extending through premarket approvals, manufacturing, labeling, and advertising up to postmarketing surveillance.

Regulatory Affairs departments are nowadays growing in a breakneck pace with the expansion of pharmaceutical business having scope to work outside as well as within companies. As the guidelines and resources necessary to fulfil the regulatory requirements are changing and evolving, some companies also choose to outsource or outtask regulatory affairs related documentary work to external service providers. So there are many service provider entrepreneurship agencies providing free launch regulatory services for the pharmaceutical companies. Regulatory Affairs department is continually evolving and growing and is the one which is least impacted during recession, acquisition and mergers phase from 2006 to 2013. Global harmonization approaches implemented by ICH and WHO has considerably raised the standards of guidelines which has led to consistent upgradation approach in regulatory submissions and reviews, expanding the scope and work possibilities of regulatory personnel. Regulatory affairs professionals have opportunities to work in such fields which require high knowledge level involving multiple activities.

Regulatory personnel should have a proficient knowledge of the scientific background of the pharmaceutical field from preclinical to marketing authorization and formulation development to liaising.

1. Regulatory personnel should be well aware of the latest developments within the pharmaceutical industry. Exhaustive knowledge of CFDA, GMP, cGMP, WHO and other international guidelines, *viz.* USFDA, MHRA, TGA, etc is a must have.

2. Thorough knowledge of Indian, US, Australian, Canadian, Nordic and African countries Acts, laws and legislation enforced on food, drug, cosmetics, and herbals are necessarily required.

3. Scope and aspects of current harmonization guidelines like ICH, OECD, and other mutual recognition policies, between a group of countries, export and import laws and documentary requirements related updated knowledge is must for the persons working in the regulatory field.

4. Thorough knowledge of free or reduced tariff areas with the mutual recognition treaties like WTO (World Trade Organization), ASEAN (Association of South East Asian Nations), TRIPS (Trade-Related Aspects of Intellectual Property Rights), Doha Declaration on TRIPS and Public Health, South Asian Association for Regional Cooperation (SAARC) and North Atlantic Treaty Organization (NATO) between the group of countries is required. Regulatory personnel must keep abreast with policy changes and approval process related to trade and marketing of drugs and cosmetics.

5. Thorough knowledge of national and international drug laws and legislation controlling legal aspects of drugs and medicines, *viz.* Indian Penal Code, Drugs and Cosmetics Act 1940, 21 Code of Federal regulation, Federal Food, Drug, and Cosmetics Act 1938, Australian Therapeutic Goods Act 1989, etc.

6. Jobs in pharma regulatory affairs eventually require a firm background of working in the relevant industry, business knowledge, excellent oral and written communication skill, good leadership capability and team work. To be an effective negotiator, good organizational and interpersonal communication, and coordination skill is required.

7. Strong IT skill is required along with knowledge of several computer application used for data preparation, statistical analysis, interpretation, and representation.

8. The international scope of most of the companies working in the field of pharmaceuticals essentially requires knowledge of a second/third language. It is also generally desirable to know one/two foreign languages expending the possibilities of work area helping in the proper understanding of legal and social requirement of a country.

9. In depth knowledge of different steps and stages involved in drug development, beginning from research and development to finally the new drug approval.

10. Thorough knowledge of pharmacovigilance activities.

11. Information of electronic representation and submission of data and forms, like the Common Technical Document (CTD) and Drug Master File (DMF).

12. Ability to innovatively search for solutions for complex technical and procedural problems related to drug manufacturing, marketing, and legislation.

13. Work experience with clinical or pharma organizations is desirable for working in giant multinational pharmaceuticals having diverse customer groups all over the world.

14. Regulatory personnel is involved in writing product labels and patent

information, so knowledge of all legal requirements related to copyright, trademark and patent registration is required.

The current new approach to drug regulation adopted by the regulatory bodies of developed countries will eventually become essential for all healthcare organizations of underdeveloped and developing countries as it represents the best model for delivering new healthcare advances in a reasonable time with acceptable safety. These astringent guideline implementations will, in turn, increase the job opportunities for regulatory personnel.

ROLES AND RESPONSIBILITIES OF PHARMA REGULATORY AFFAIRS PERSONNEL

Regulatory personnel has an essential role in every phase of formulation and process development. They also plan regulatory approval strategy of a new drug formulation along with planning for the post-marketing activities. Drug regulation is multidimensional profession having an international scope. Professionals working in pharmaceutical regulatory affairs handle many different tasks:

1. Active participation in discussions with Quality Assurance (QA) team and coordination of team activities.
2. Assess the completeness and accuracy of all the documentation and records maintained by the QA team.
3. Managing and collaborating regulatory inspections within the company and reviewing practices when required to meet with new or updated regulatory requirements and maintenance of regulatory approval status of all the already approved marketed drugs.
4. Collaboration between multidisciplinary team to collect and collate large amounts of information and documents required for preparing drug product licensing submissions.

5. Supervise preparation of Marketing Authorization Application for new pharmaceuticals and diagnostics including report on quality, safety, efficacy, indication, adverse reaction, and side effects and packaging specifications. Address all issues related to a product review, managing reports, and tracking post-marketing activities.
6. Ensure regulatory compliance of ND/AND application submission and tracking with FDA approval.
7. Liaising with doctors and scientists for conducting clinical trials and negotiating with regulatory authorities for ND or AND. Supervision and auditing of clinical trial sites for adherence and compliance with all regulatory guidelines and coordination between multisite clinical trials.
8. Filling application with all relevant documents for marketing authorization of drugs with new dose, new indication or a new formulation called an Investigational New Drug (IND).
9. Provisional documentation clearance from FDA for pilot scale production, manufacturing in small quantity for conduction of trials, export of drugs for testing and clinical trials, import of drug for an investigational purpose.
10. Provide advice and guidance to the international clinical research teams on drug development related issues. Supervise all steps in drug development for preparation of documentary submission required for regulatory authority approval of clinical trials from phase I to III.
11. Preparation, and monitoring of all types of documentary submissions to regulatory bodies.
12. Ensure prompt and satisfactory answers to comment or requests generated during the submission review process.

13. Facilitate data/report collection, analysis, and communication about risk and benefit of health products to regulatory agencies, medical care systems, and the general public.
14. Review of labeling, insert, information sheets and advertisement materials especially for the overseas market.
15. Negotiate most favorable labeling and product monograph insert design as per sponsors business activities while still consistent with the legal requirements of regulatory bodies. Supervise editing of labeling text in the local language, packaging leaflets, product profile and other relevant documents designed for promotion of a particular product in the market. Regulatory approval of all promotional materials and drug information leaflets before market launch.
16. Planning and monitoring of product launch activities.
17. Responsible for assuring government obligations and market driven demands.
18. Responsible for maintaining and securing approval or authorization status of the existing authorized drug products by continually fulfilling regulatory documentation requirement needed to be submitted periodically (*viz.* stability data or post-marketing safety data/pharmacovigilance data) and renewal of authorization on due time course.
19. Report state/national regulatory authorities about an adverse drug reaction or side effect.
20. Manage patent and trademark registration status of all the relevant products and procedures in the company. Maintaining and negotiating in-licensing and out-licensing agreements for most favorable conditions.
21. Keep company management up to date on the status of specific product registration, problems encountered and solutions provided there in. Inputs regarding legislation and policies changes or new guideline amendments related to scientific as well as political influences on the national and international drug regulatory scenario are also to be provided to the management.
22. For being updated with current events in drug regulation attending the seminar, conferences and meeting at the national and international platform are expected to be a part of the responsibility.
23. To serve as a representative of the company in the international platform while being a member of the global drug regulatory affairs team. Coordinate regulatory affair activities worldwide and also responsible for performing all the assigned actions required for multi-country Marketing Authorizations.

The principal objective of drug regulation for every government regulatory agency is the promotion and protection of public health. Harmonization of registration requirement initiatives supported by the international community is successfully delivering the target object as measurable public health gains. Substantial improvement in drug regulation was observed over the last several decades as the pharmaceutical manufacturers are following the business strategies required for the fulfilment of global marketplace demands. Value addition is a relatively new phrase in science and business which is equally applicable to pharmaceuticals also. The core asset of the harmonized drug regulation is its significant contribution towards public health advances that have been realized as direct benefits of harmonization, improving quality, safety, and efficacy of marketed products. These initiatives mitigate the risks of medicines related harm, greater transparency of review and approval processes, and decreased costs for the industry as a harmonized application format reduces the expense of preparing registration dossiers eliminating duplication of activities. Increased public trust in approved medicines is the vital achievement of international harmonization apart from helping drug developers and regulatory authorities. The coming progressive future of harmonization directives will depend on:

- Strong commitment of major stakeholders, governments and pharma industries
- Allocation of necessary resources
- Information sharing to improve overall regulatory performance
- Involvement of expert knowledge base and resources
- Formation of active networks among national regulatory authorities
- Supporting cooperation, collaboration, and international understanding
- Enhancing public trust on regulatory authorities.

BIBLIOGRAPHY

1. A timeline of Canadian Cannabis Legalization. Ontario Cannabis Activist Network. https://ggs-greenhouse.com/marijuana/blog/a-timeline-of-canadian-cannabis-legalization. World Health Organization. Effective drug regulation: what can countries do?(Discussion paper). Geneva, WHO Essential Drugs and Medicines Programme, 1999(Document WHO/HTP/EDM/MAC(11)/99.6).

2. Ageel AM. Drug Registration in the Gulf States: Comparative Study. Application for registration of a medicinal product. DC/TA/F001.Ministry of Health-United Arab Emirates. http://www.moh.gov.ae/admincp/assetsmanager/Files/Pharmacusts/3.Application%20for%20 Registration% 20of%20a%20 Medicinal%20 Conventional%20Product.pdf.

3. Ageel AM. Drug Registration in the Gulf States: Application form for the registration of pharmaceutical product. Ministerial Decree 302/80. http://www.ccras.nic.in/country%20 wise%20compendium/kuwait%20207-210.pdf.

4. ASEAN good manufacturing practices guidelines. 2nd Ed. Jakarta, Association of SouthEast Asian Nations, 1988.

5. Center of Medicine Research International, CMR R&D Briefing No 37. December 2002. http://www.cmr.org.

6. Controlled Drugs and Substances Act 1996. Department of Justice, Government of Canada. Retrieved May 21, 2018.

7. Dukes G. The effects of drug regulation: a survey based on the European studies of drug regulation. Lancaster, MTP Press Ltd., 1985.http://www.moh.gov.bh/PDF/Publications/Guideline/Guide_drugs.pdf.

8. Fenn CF, Wong E, Zambrano D. The contemporary situation for the conduct of clinical trials in Asia. International Journal of Pharmaceutical Medicine 2001; 15: 169–173

9. Friedman MA, Woodcock J, Lumpkin MM, Shuren JE, Hass AE et al. The safety of newly approved medicines: do recent market removals mean there is a problem? Journal of the American Medical Association. 1999; 218(18): 1728–1734.

10. Geiling E, Cannon P. Pathogenic effects of elixir of sulfanilamide (diethylene glycol) poisoning. A clinical and experimental correlation. Journal of the American Medical Association 1938; 111: 919–926.

11. Good manufacturing practice for medicinal products in the European Community. Brussels, Commission of the European Communities, 1992.https://ec.europa.eu/health/documents/eudralex/vol-4_en.

12. Good manufacturing practices for pharmaceutical products. In: WHO Expert Committee on Specifications for Pharmaceutical Preparations. Thirty-second report. Geneva, World Health Organization, 1992 (WHO Technical Report Series, No. 823, Annex 1).

13. Guidance for submission. Version 2. Saudi Food and Drug Authority.http://colleges.ksu.edu.sa/CollegeofPharmacy/Documents/Conference 1989/10.pdf.

14. Guidance for submission. Version 2. Saudi Food and Drug Authority. http://www.sfda.gov.sa/NR/rdonlyres/F7CF9563-9DD8-4C64-B183-AEB487A00E26/0/GuidanceforSubmissionv 2.pdf.

15. Information on Japanese regulatory affairs. Regulatory Information Task Force. Japan Pharmaceutical Manufacturers Association. Pharmaceutical Administration and Regulations in Japan.http://www.jpma.or.jp/english/parj/pdf/2018.pdf.

16. Nagata R, Raflzadeh-Kabe JD. Japanese pharmaceutical and regulatory environment. Dialogues in Clinical Neuroscience 2002; 4(4): 470-474.

17. O'Brien KL, Selanikio JD, Hecdivert C, Placide MF, Louis M, Barr DB. et al. Epidemic of pediatric deaths from acute renal failure caused by diethylene glycol poisoning. Journal of the American Medical Association 1998; 279(15): 1175–1178.

18. Perspective on Canadian Drug Policy. Volume 1. John Howard Society. Retrieved on May 21, 2018.

19. Ratanawijitrasin S, Soumerai S, Weerasuriya K. Do national drug policies and essential drug programs improve drug use? A review of experiences in developing countries. Social science and medicine 2001; 53(7):831–844

20. Registration guidelines. Pharmacy and Drug Control Directorate, Kingdom of Bahrain. Available

21. Singh J, Dutta AK, Khare S, Dubey NK, Harit AK, Jain NK, et al. Diethylene glycol poisoning in Gurgaon, India, 1998. Bulletin of the World Health Organization 2001; 79(2):88–95.

22. The GCC Guidelines for Stability Testing of Drug Substances and Pharmaceutical Products. Edition Two. 1428 H–2007 G. http://www.sgh.org.sa/PDF/GCC_STABILITY .pdf.

23. Thompson FJ. The enduring challenges of health policy implementation. In: Litman TJ, Robins LS, eds. Health politics and policy.2nd Ed. New York, Delmar Publishers Inc.,1991.

24. World Health Organization. Global comparative pharmaceutical expenditures: with related reference information. (Health Economics and Drugs EDM Series No. 3). Geneva, 2000 (Document EDM/PAR/2000.2).

Chapter 2

International Organization for Standardization

CHAPTER OVERVIEW

- Significance of ISO
- ISO standard development process
  Conformity assessment
- Key principles in standard development
  ISO standards respond to a need in the market
  ISO standards are based on global expert opinion
- Popular categories of ISO standards

- ISO certification process
  Pre-requisite to ISO certification
  Process of certification
  Cost of the ISO certification process
  The time required in ISO certification
- Impact of ISO
- Benefits of ISO certification
- Bibliography

KEY POINTS

- Organization Internationale de Normalisation (ISO) is a network of national standards institutes of 161 different countries. ISO develops standards for all type of organizations, government bodies, trade officials, professional, suppliers, customers, and services. ISO standards ensure the quality and safety of products and services to consumers.

- ISO standard development process starts with conformity assessment of specific standard requirements that are usually communicated to the national member by any industry sector initiated by market-driven needs. The technical scope of the proposed future standard is defined by working groups comprising technical experts and following agreement on technical aspects the detailed specifications are negotiated on consensus. Finally, the resulting draft of the international standard is formally approved.

- Majority of ISO standards are specific to a particular product, material or process among those are the ISO 9000 for quality management, ISO 14000 for environmental management and ISO 31000 for risk management are most widely known and applicability in the pharmaceutical sector.

- ISO certification is done by external bodies or third party that are accreditation by ISO assuring the agencies authenticity. Applicant formulates the certification objectives, choose the type of standard, develop and implement the quality system, choose the certification agency to carry out quality document review, submit final quality manual for approval after assessment by registrar certificate is issued.

- As a benchmark of quality ISO certification of any industry or enterprise help in extending market potential with quality compliance, improved efficiency, cost savings, and higher customer satisfaction.

SIGNIFICANCE OF ISO

Organization Internationale de Normalisation is a network of national standards institutes of countries. In English it is adopted as an International Organization for Standardization (ISO) with principal activity as to develop technical standards. The word ISO is derived from the Greek ISOS meaning 'equal' International standardization began with the International Electrotechnical Commission in 1906, which led to the development of International Federation of the National Standardizing Associations (ISA) in 1926. ISO originated from the union of two organizations; the ISA and the UNSCC (United Nations Standard Coordinating Committee) in 1946 when over 25 countries met at the Institute of Civil Engineers in London to create a new international organization, with an objective to 'facilitate the international coordination and unification of industrial standards.' From this, the new organization ISO was established in 1947, as a non-government federation of national standards bodies of around 150 different countries. According to British Standards Institution (BSI), a standard is "specification that establishes a common language, and contains technical specification and other precise criteria designed to be used consistently, as a rule, a guideline, or a definition."

ISO officially began operations in February 1947. ISO is a network of the national standards institutes of 161 countries, 776 technical committees and subcommittees, 3117 published standards and 532 standards under development as on Jan 2018. The central secretariat of ISO is in Geneva, Switzerland that coordinates the whole system with 135 full time working staff, by one member per country. Though ISO is a non-governmental organization, it forms a bridge between the public and private sectors. ISO Standards cover a wide variety of items ranging from medical equipment to ship building, i.e. machinery, construction, aerospace, fuels, energy, transportation, information, technology, quality, measurements, safety, environment, medical, and consumer goods.

The ISO developed standards are useful to industrial and business organizations of all types, governments and other regulatory bodies, trade officials, conformity assessment professionals, product suppliers and customers, services in both public and private sectors, and ultimately, to people in general as end users. ISO is a network of national standards bodies of different countries, where these national standards bodies make up the ISO membership, and they represent ISO in their country. Since inception ISO has published more than 19500 International Standards covering almost all aspects of technology and manufacturing, food safety to computers and agriculture to healthcare. ISO provides a technical base to the governments for providing health, safety, and environmental legislation. ISO standards ensure the safety and quality of products and services to the consumers and other users, to safeguard from using the counterfeit and misbranded products.

ISO standards have essential economic and social consequences. First ISO standard was published in 1951. ISO standards are beneficial not only to the manufacturers but also to the whole society as they contribute in the development, manufacturing, and supply of products and services, which are more efficient, safer and cleaner. ISO provides news and information on standards and standard development. ISO give state-of-the-art specifications for products, services, and good practices, helping to make the industry more efficient and effective. ISO standards ensure that products and services are safe, reliable and of good quality. These strategic tools can reduce costs by minimizing waste and errors and increasing productivity. They help companies to expand business in new market places, maintain the quality standards of the products for developing countries and facilitate fair global trade. The ISO 9000 standards have a different impact across countries of different economic status.

ISO STANDARD DEVELOPMENT PROCESS

An ISO standard can be of few pages to several hundred pages long documents, now increasingly available in electronic format. It carries the ISO logo and the "international standard" designation. Published in A4 page format which is itself one of the ISO standard paper size.

Conformity Assessment

Conformity assessment process assures that a product, service or system meets its specified requirements. These requirements are likely to be contained in an ISO standard, but ISO itself does not perform conformity assessments.

The benefits of showing that a product, service or system meets certain requirements are:

• It provides the consumers with added quality.
• It gives the company a competitive edge.
• It helps to ensure the health, safety or environmental conditions are met.

The primary forms of conformity assessment are inspection, testing, and certification. ISO certification to any organization, product or service is given after assessing quality standards as per the specified requirements of ISO.

Experts from all over the world participate in standard development that is required by their sector. An ISO standard is developed by a panel of experts, within a **technical committee**, through a consensus process. When there is a need for a standard to be established, the experts meet to discuss and negotiate a draft standard. The developed draft is shared with ISO's members who put their comments and vote for it. The draft becomes an ISO standard if a consensus is reached, if not, it goes back to the technical committee for further editing.

International standardization is market-driven and therefore based on voluntary involvement of all interested in the marketplace. There are three main phases of the ISO standard development process, viz.

1. The need for a standard is usually expressed by any industry sector, which communicates this need to a national member. Once the need for an international standard has been recognized and formally agreed, the first phase involves defining the technical scope for the proposed future standard. Working groups comprising technical experts from countries interested in the subject matter carries this phase.

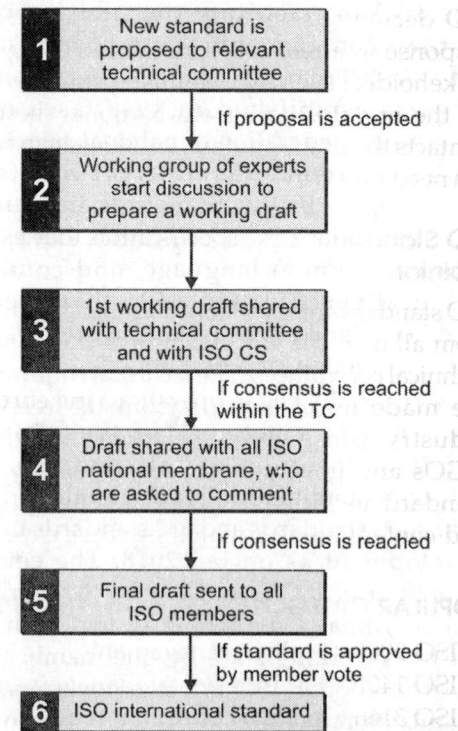

Source: http://www.iso.org/iso/home/standards_development

Fig. 2.1: Process of ISO standard development

2. Once an agreement has been reached on technical aspects, in the second phase countries negotiate the detailed specifications within the standard by consensus building.
3. The final phase comprises the formal approval of the resulting draft international standard. The acceptance criteria stipulated as the approval by two-thirds of the ISO members involved in the standards development process and approval by 75% of all members that vote. After which the agreed text is published as an ISO international standard.

KEY PRINCIPLES IN STANDARD DEVELOPMENT

ISO Standards Respond to a Need in the Market

ISO decides to develop a new standard in response to a request from industry or other stakeholders such as consumer groups but not by the organization itself. National member contacts the ISO for a standard whenever there is a need raised by an industry sector or group.

ISO Standards Based on Global Expert Opinion

ISO standards are developed by experts groups from all over the world acting as members of technical committees. The technical committees are made up of experts from the relevant industry, consumer associations, academia, NGOs and government. All aspects of the standard, including its scope, key definitions, and content are negotiated by these experts.

POPULAR CATEGORIES OF ISO STANDARD

- ISO 9000: Quality management
- ISO 14000: Environmental management
- ISO 3166: Country codes
- ISO 26000: Social responsibility
- ISO 50001: Energy management
- ISO 31000: Risk management

- ISO 22000: Food safety management
- ISO 4217: Currency codes
- ISO 639: Language codes

The majority of ISO standards are highly specific to a particular product, material or process. The ISO 9000, ISO 14000 and ISO 31000 families are among ISO's most widely known and successful standards applicable in the pharmaceutical sector. ISO 9000 has become an internationally acclaimed reference in quality requirements in business dealings. ISO 14000 helps organizations to meet their environmental challenges, and ISO 31000 focuses on risk assessment concepts, processes and the selection of risk assessment techniques. The standards of the ISO 9000 and ISO 14000 families has earned a worldwide reputation and are known as "generic management system standards." Generic signifies that these standards can be applied to any organization, large or small, whatever a product or a service, in any sector of activity, whether it is a business enterprise, public administration, or government department. "Management system" refers to what the organization does to manage its processes or activities. "Generic" also signifies that no matter what the organization deals with or works for when it wants to establish a quality management system or an environmental management system, it must comply with all the essential features, described in the relevant standards of the ISO 9000 or ISO 14000 families.

ISO 9000

ISO 9000 is concerned with 'quality management' that explains standards to be followed based upon the processes utilized. Introduced in 1987, the ISO 9000 family of standards is a 'generic quality management standard' that has a great impact on company performance. ISO 9000 standards help in creating consensus on requirements and standards all around the world. ISO 9000 specifies the necessary components of a quality management system in the structural framework of business in broad terms. ISO 9000 applies to all types of organization irrespective to its size or function. ISO 9000 does not describe product standards but the system standards. Certification under ISO 9000 is not mandatory by legislation but only voluntary. The ISO 9000 was convinced in 1987 and updated in 2000 which has three series 9001 for design and servicing, 9002 for production and installation and 9003 for final inspection and testing. Few of the ISO norms are enlisted below:

ISO 9000:1993: Quality management and quality assurance standards—part 4: A guide to dependability programme.

ISO 9000:1994: Quality systems—model for quality assurance in design, development, production, installation, and servicing.

ISO 9000:1997: Quality management and quality assurance standards—part 3: Guidelines for application of ISO 9001:1994 for the development, supply installation, and maintenance of computer software.

ISO 9000:2000: Quality management system—fundamentals and vocabulary.

ISO 9001:2000: Quality management systems—requirements.

ISO 9001:2008: Quality management system—requirements.

ISO 9002:1994: Quality systems—a model for quality assurance in production. Installation and servicing.

ISO 9003:1994: Quality systems—a model for quality assurance in final inspection and test.

ISO 9004:2000: Quality management systems—guidelines for performance.

ISO 9005:1994: Uranium dioxide powder and sintered pellets—determination of oxygen/uranium atomic ratio—amperometric method.

ISO 9006:1994: Uranium metal and uranium dioxide powder and pellets—determination of nitrogen content—a method using ammonia-sensing electrode.

ISO/TR 9007:1987: Information processing systems—concepts and terminology for the conceptual scheme and the information base.

ISO 9008:1991: Glass bottles—verticality—test method.

ISO 9009:1991: Glass containers—height and non-parallelism of finish concerning container base test methods.

ISO 9010:1997: Synchronous belt drives automotive belts.

Since introduction in 1987, the ISO 9000 has been revised and represented many updated versions. Names of standard reflect each version of it. Though most of the revisions were relatively minor, a significant change has been made in 2000. ISO 9001 standards are for companies and organizations who are engaged in the creation of new products that want to ensure quality assurance in design, development, production, installation, and service. ISO 9002 standards only differ with 9001 in requirements concerning new product development. ISO 9003 standards cover only final inspection of finished product, regardless of production procedure. ISO 9001: 2008 determine requirements for process implementation and their application in the organization. It monitors, measures and analyze action implementation and ensures continual improvement of processes. ISO 9000 is the most successful international management standard issued by the ISO as it integrates all the activities that have a direct or indirect effect on the quality of a product or service. ISO 9000 is considered as a benchmark for measuring quality. ISO 9000 certification offers a competitive edge to a company by improving efficiency thus minimizing repeated auditions and inspections and also helps to sell products in European countries.

ISO 14000

ISO 14000 is primarily concerned with "**environmental management.**" It is concerned with the standards of the functions of the organization to minimize harmful effects on the environments caused by its activities and continues to improve its environmental performance. It sets out the criteria for an environmental management system that can be certified. Any organization regardless of its activity or sector can use it. This assures company management and employees as well as external stakeholders that environmental impact is being measured and improved.

ISO 14001:2004: Environmental management systems—requirements with guidance for use.

ISO 14004:2004: Environmental management systems—general guidelines on principles, systems and support techniques.

ISO 14064:2006: Greenhouse gases—Part 1: Specification with guidance at the organization level for quantification and reporting of greenhouse gas emissions and removals.

ISO 14006:2011: Environmental management systems—guidelines for incorporating ecodesign.

ISO 31000

ISO 31000 is concerned with "**risk management.**" Risks affecting organizations can have consequences regarding economic performance and professional reputation, as well as environmental, safety and societal outcomes. Managing risk can effectively help the organizations to perform well in an environment full of uncertainty.

ISO 31000:2009: Risk management—principles and guidelines that provide a framework and process of managing risk. The ISO 31000 cannot be used for certification purposes but it is a guidance system for internal or external audit programmes. Organizations using it can compare their risk management practices with the internationally recognized benchmark for effective management and corporate governance.

ISO Guide 73:2009: Risk management—vocabulary complements is for providing a collection of terms and definitions relating to the management of risk.

ISO/IEC 31010:2009: Risk management—risk assessment techniques that help the decision makers to understand the risks that could affect the achievement of objectives as well as the adequacy of the control measures already in place.

ISO 13485 Medical Devices

A medical device is an instrument, machine, implant or an *in vitro* reagent that is used in the diagnosis, prevention, and treatment of diseases or other medical conditions. Medical devices range from simple tongue depressors to complex programmable pacemakers with micro-chip technology and laser surgical devices. In contrast to drugs medical devices are not intended to achieve their purposes through chemical action within and are not dependent upon being metabolized for the achievement of its primary intended purposes. For the medical devices, product conformity is as much as crucial and vital to that of a drug product concerning quality control of design and manufacturing. Implementation of ISO standard in the medical device manufacturing industry is a vital way for the safeguard of product conformity while simultaneously harmonizing requirements internationally. ISO 13485 publishes comprehensive requirements for quality management systems related to design and manufacturing of medical devices first time in 1996. Organizations involved in the design, production, installation, and servicing of medical devices and related services use ISO 13485 1996 guidelines. All ISO standards are reviewed once in every five years to scrutinize need of revision in order to keep it current and relevant for the marketplace.

ISO 13485 was revised for the first time in 2003. The primary objective of revised ISO 13485:2003 is to facilitate harmonized medical device regulatory requirements for quality management systems. The ISO 13485:2003 specifies requirements for the quality management system of the organizations demonstrating its ability to provide medical devices and related services that consistently meet customer and regulatory requirements. It includes particular requirements for medical devices and excludes some of the requirements of ISO 9001 that are not appropriate as regulatory requirements. The principal difference is that ISO 9001 requires the organization to demonstrate continual improvement, whereas ISO 13485 assures that the quality system is effectively implemented and maintained for product safety, risk management, design control, traceability of implantable devices, validation of sterile implants and effectiveness of corrective and preventive action.

The effective edition of current ISO 13485 was published on 1 March 2016. ISO 13485:2016 is designed to respond to the latest quality management system practices, including changes in technology and regulatory requirements and expectations. ISO 13485:2016 specifies requirements for the quality management system intending the organizations involved in one or more stages of medical device life-cycle, including design and development, production, storage and distribution, installation, or servicing. Along with design and development, the provisions of associated activities (e.g. technical support) are also included. ISO 13485:2016 can also be used by suppliers or external parties providing product along with quality management system-related services to such organizations. The new version has strong emphasis on risk management and risk-based decision making, also includes changes related to the enhanced regulatory requirements for organizations working in the supply chain management.

ISO 13485 is now considered to be inline with the standard and requirement for medical devices of the International Medical Device Regulatory Forum (IMDRF) that has become universal standards for design,

manufacture, export, and sales of various medical devices. The certification of ISO 13485 quality management system, specifically for medical devices, is advantageous, and in many cases essential, for companies which export their products to the global market.

ISO CERTIFICATION PROCESS

ISO itself does not provide any direct certification to the companies. Certification is done by the accredited external bodies or a third party. ISO certification is a written assurance in the form of a certificate that the product, service or system provided by the applicant meets specific requirements of ISO guidelines. Accreditation is the formal recognition of an external organization by ISO, assuring that the certification agency operates according to international ISO standards.

1. **Pre-requisite to ISO certification**
   a. *Formulating the ISO certification objectives:* Quality objectives are the primary requirements for the ISO certification. The quality objectives spotlight the key elements of the quality policy and find a focal point for the personnel efforts in the organization to work toward improvement. Improvement is the principal reason for a company to implement a Quality Management System.
   b. *Choosing the type of ISO certification standards:* The type of ISO certification required for a particular business is decided upon between the various types of ISO certification available such as:
   ISO 9001 2008: Quality Management
   ISO 14001: Environmental Management
   ISO 27001: Information security Management
   ISO 22008: Food Safety Management and so on.
   c. *Choosing an ISO certification agency:* It is imperative to choose a well reputed,

recognized and credible certification agency. While choosing the ISO registrar, these factors should be considered:

- Evaluate several ISO certification service providers before finalizing the external agency, which must meet the requirements of ISO accreditation bodies. An accredited certification agency can be found in the national accreditation body of the respective country or the International Accreditation Forum.
- ISO's Committee on Conformity Assessment (CASCO) released some standards related to the certification process, which are used by certification bodies. Confirm that the certification agency is following the CASCO standards. CASCO also works on issues relating to conformity assessment of the accredited certification agencies.
- Checking for accreditation status is also important as it confirms the competence of the agency.

d. *Development and implementation of a quality system:* Quality objectives are formulated focusing the main goals of the company as per the quality policy that is set forward and planned for further improvement. The quality policy should be created following the customer requirements and then quality objectives can be linked back to the customer requirements. Before finalization quality objectives are communicated to each level of the organization to achieve the overall planned goal. The quality objective can target product or process objectives, often referred to as key performance indicators.

2. **Process of certification:**

a. *Application contract with the certification agency:* The applicant and the registrar of the certification agency agree on a contract defining rights and obligations of both parties including liability issues, confidentiality, and access rights. Certification agency request the applicant organization to provide information regarding:

- The desired scope of the certification.
- The general features of the applicant organization: Name, address, location, aspects of the process, operations and other relevant legal obligations.
- The relevant standard and field of certification for which the applicant organization is seeking certification relates to the applicant organizations activities, human and technical resources and functions.
- Information of all outsourced processes that can affect conformity to requirements.
- Information of the consultancy services used relating to the management system.

The application is submitted in the prescribed format with a copy of the quality manual and necessary fee.

b. *Quality document review:* The ISO auditor views all quality manuals and documents related to various policies and procedures performed in the organization. Review of existing work is also done by ISO auditor to identify the possible gaps against the requirements stipulated in the ISO standards. ISO auditors work in contract to registrars to perform registration assessments and surveillance as a front line in the certification process. The registrars are responsible for ensuring that the auditors meet qualification requirements. Auditors must have training in auditing and ISO 9001 requirments. At least one member of the audit team must have experience in the industrial sector of the company being audited. Auditors collect the objective evidence demonstrating the effectiveness of the company's quality management system and make registration recommendations to the registrar.

c. *Development of an action plan:* Following the ISO auditors communication related to existing gaps in the quality objectives of the applicant organization, an action plan is prepared to eliminate these gaps. The list of the required tasks is prepared and performed to bring the desired changes in the procedures. Training to the employees is provided to work efficiently while adopting new procedures. The employees are made aware of the ISO standards required to maintain the quality standards.

d. *Initial certification audit for self analysis:* The initial certification audit has two categories: Stage 1 and Stage 2.

Stage 1: Stage 1 audit is conducted before the certification audit mostly following client desire. It provides a macro level assessment of the implementation status and identification of major deficiencies if any in documented quality system compliance as per requirements of the certification standards. It provides valuable inputs to the clients and saves time by taking necessary corrective action in advance of the certification audit. Stage 1 audit is must for all types of cases, and it is also ensured that the auditors sign the conflict of interest before every visit. Stage 1 audit findings are documented and communicated to the client by the team leader. It includes identification of any areas of concern that could be classified as nonconformity during the stage 2 audit. The non-conformities are divided into minor and significant non-conformities. The applicant care-

fully assesses all these non-conformities and do all required modification in the techniques and processes to get it aligned as per the desired quality standards.

Stage 2: Stage 2 audit is intended to ensure that the applicant's management system confirms the effectiveness to the requirements of the applicable standard/specification. The stage 2 audit evaluates the implementation, including the effectiveness of the applicant's management system. After the organization does all the required changes to rectify the non-conformities, the ISO auditor does the final auditing to check elimination of all the non-conformities. At the end of the assessment duly signed written report by the team leader are prepared and handed over to the applicant including non-conformities identified if any, and recommendation for certification. The recommendation is made for certification in the audit reports when the ISO auditor is satisfied, and the final audit report is forward to the registrar.

e. *Submission of the final quality manual for approval:* The final quality manual is submitted to the certification Committee to review the audit findings and agree on the audit conclusions after analyzing the information and audit evidence gathered during stage 1, and stage 2 audits.

f. *Pre-assessment by registrar:* The final audit report along with comments on the non-conformities and, where applicable, the correction and corrective actions taken by the applicant are provided to certification agency registrar to carry out the application review. If not recommended for certification due to improper implementation of corrective actions on non-conformities, it is reversed for further implementation of corrective action by the applicant.

g. *Implementation of corrective action if any:* The implementation of corrective actions on nonconformities observed if any by the assessment team is reviewed and verified. A minor nonconformance is a minor infraction of procedures or minor failures of the system in meeting the ISO requirements. A major nonconformance deals with issues where the nonconforming product is likely to reach the customer or possibility of a breakdown in the quality system resulting in systems inefficiency to meet the requirements of the standard. Registration cannot proceed until all major nonconformities are closed and verified by the registrar. This is the primary difference between a major and minor nonconformance. This usually involves a re-audit with associated costs. Minor nonconformities require a corrective action plan assuring closing at the first surveillance.

h. *Final assessment by the registrar:* After all, nonconformities are addressed, and all the findings are put in the ISO audit report, the registrar grant the ISO certification. The registrar recommends whether or not to grant certification, together with any conditions or observations. The registrar makes the certification decision by the evaluation of audit findings, conclusions, and other relevant information.

i. *Issue of certification:* Certification should always be mentioned or displayed along with the name of the standard, i.e. not 'ISO certified' but 'ISO 9001:2015 certified'.

j. *Surveillance audits:* Surveillance audit is primarily conducted from time to time to ensure that ISO quality standards are being maintained and continuously followed by the organization.

3. **Cost of the ISO certification process:** Cost for getting ISO certification is not fixed and varies from organization to organization. The ISO certification agencies mostly calculate the cost of certification for an organization after considering different parameters such as:
   - Number of employees
   - Processes complexities
   - Level of risk associated with the scope of services of the organization
   - The complexity of the management system
   - The working scope and spectrum of the organization

4. **The time required in ISO certification:** Time taken in completing the whole process of ISO certification again varies from organization to organization. The ISO certification agency can give a fair idea after assessing the size and scope of a company. Generally, the time required to complete the process of ISO certification is approximately 6–8 months for small organizations, 8–12 months for medium organizations and 12–15 months in case of a large organization.

IMPACT OF ISO

Standards are introduced as a common language as they reduce variability, confusion and help companies to take advantage of industrial scales by reducing labor and production costs, and consequently products price. The ISO series of standards acts as 'quality management standards', that it is intended to be applied to the quality management of any organization or business in particular regardless of the size of ownership, profit status, manufacturing or service provider. ISO standards emphasize adoption of 'manual' by companies to form the base for their quality benchmarks for self improvement. The standards are used to guide internal process development. ISO requires the organizations to build and develop their own "quality manual" in order to document procedures developed addressing the ISO 'elements' and to log any activities that affect the quality system. ISO itself does not provide ISO certification neither it is compulsory to pursue certification, however, without certification, companies cannot claim adherence to ISO standards. The ISO standards codify international management practices which act as a foundation for certification. Independent audit companies issue ISO certifications and once certified is not for the lifetime, as companies must be re-audited every three years to ensure that they still adhere to the ISO requirements.

Every year ISO performs a survey of certifications that shows the number of valid certificates to ISO management standards (ISO 9001 and ISO 14001) reported for each country. This survey counts the number of certificates issued by certification bodies that have been accredited by members of the International Accreditation Forum (IAF). A total of 1.6 million valid certificates were recorded across nine standards in 2016 compared to 1.5 million in 2015, with an increase of 8%. ISO 9000 certifications have a 'push' effect for exports from developing countries to developed countries leading to expanding the volumes of exports and also regarding the number of destination countries. The trade effect of ISO 9000 certifications also depends on the stringency and reputation of the certification body or agency. Itself the quality of ISO 9000 is questioned when there is doubt about the auditing competencies of the certification agency. To establish trust in the certification agency accreditation bodies have been created. Accreditation body confirms the competency and auditing conformity of the certification bodies. The accreditation body certifies the certifier. Monitoring and surveill-

ance of accreditation bodies are done through a series of peer evaluations to approve as signatories. The IAF is responsible for reliability of accreditors of certification bodies, and established regional accreditation groups (European Cooperation for Accreditation, Pacific Accreditation Cooperation, etc) under 'multilateral recognition arrangement' (MLA). Companies both from developed and developing countries get benefited from ISO certification. The international network of accreditation bodies has developed an agreement (the IAF-MLA) that verifies the implementation of equivalent accreditation programs leading to worldwide acceptance of certification.

BENEFITS OF ISO CERTIFICATION

Each ISO standard supports the management system that have scope within every organization. However, the collective benefits of the certifications include widened market potential, compliance with procurement tenders, improved efficiency and cost savings, higher customer service and satisfaction, and heightened staff morale and motivation. ISO 9001 certification provides maximum benefit to an organization when implemented practically. ISO 9001 certification is not only suitable for large organizations, but small organizations can also get benefited by adopting efficient Quality Management Systems that save time and cost, improve efficiency and ultimately improve customer relationships. Companies with ISO certification communicate commitment to quality for both customers and regulators. Proper implementation of ISO standards improves working efficiency and reduce chances or errors in the manufacturing process for future rejections and rework. The benefits of ISO certification are:

1. Adoption of ISO signifies continuous quality improvement by providing sustained assessment and improvement.

2. ISO encourages independent/third party audits demonstrating a commitment to quality.

3. ISO certification helps to improve overall performance, eliminate uncertainty and widen market opportunities locally and internationally.

4. ISO standard implementation increases operating efficiency, productivity, and profit by costs cutting and monitoring supply chain performance.

5. ISO certification upgrades companies credibility and improves public image, thus in turn level of customer satisfaction.

6. Adoption of ISO standards assures process evaluation and standardization.

7. Training new and old employees for a better and comprehensive understanding of process fundamentals and quality attributes.

8. ISO Quality Management System ensures clear organizational structures, tasks, and responsibilities distribution throughout the entire organization, which improves the working atmosphere and reduces the pressure of work.

9. ISO is a globally recognized standard providing the objective proof that a certified organization committed to the implementation of effective and robust ISO Quality Management System, is being checked regularly by an independent party.

Implementation of ISO standards is demanding for resources and time consuming, and also the document formulation requires administrative expenses. The assessment and registration process is also expensive for small and medium enterprises. ISO 9001 is currently in use by over one million organizations around the world. It is indeed a worldwide standard for quality. ISO is the world's largest developer and publisher of International Standards for the public and private sectors and serves over 50,000 new customers every year. Operationally, 18,000 ISO standards are available in multiple languages.

BIBLIOGRAPHY

1. Bizmanualz Policies, Procedures and Processes. https://www.bizmanualz.com/quality-manual/iso-9001-procedures-manual.

2. Docking DS, Dowen JR. Market Interpretation of ISO 9000 Registration. The Journal of Financial Research (1999); XXII(2): 147–160.

3. Hudson J, Jones P. 'International trade in Quality Goods?: Signaling Problems for Developing Countries. Journal of International Development 2003; 15 (8): 999–1013.

4. International Organization for Standardization. https://www.iso.org/iso-9001-quality-management.html, and https://www.iso.org/the-iso-survey.html.

5. ISO 13485:2016 Medical devices: Quality management systems—Requirements for regulatory purposes. Retrieved 2016-03-24. (www.iso.org). http://sic.com.ua/wp-content/uploads/2009/11/iso-13485-2003.pdf.

6. The Trade Impact of ISO 9000 Certifications and International Cooperation in Accreditation. https://www.researchgate.net/publication/267961486_The_Trade_Impact_of_ISO_9000_Certifications _and_International_Cooperation_in_ Accreditation.

7. World Trade Organization. Benefits of the ILAC & IAF Multilateral Mutual Recognition Arrangement. G/TBT/GEN/117. Committee on Technical Barriers to Trade. World Trade Organization, Geneva, Switzerland. 2011.

International Council for Harmonisation

KEY POINTS

- The International Council for Harmonisation (ICH), formerly known as International Conference was incepted in 1990 with focus on a mission to make recommendations towards achieving greater harmonization in interpretation and application of technical guidelines for pharmaceutical product registration. ICH facilitates the adoption of new technical research and development approaches resulting in more economical use of human, animal and material resources without compromising safety.
- In 2015, ICH became an international association with a legal entity under Swiss law. The governance structure of reformed ICH is made up of assembly, management committee, MedDRA, secretariat and coordinators, working groups and auditors.
- ICH harmonization activity is initiated with a concept paper having a short summary of the proposal and business plan outlining the costs and benefits of the proposed topic. The ICH assembly endorses the concept paper and business plan with the establishment of an expert working group, which pass it through the five step-wise procedure of implementation of the harmonized guideline in the ICH regions.
- v ICH implement harmonized tripartite guidelines under headings of 'Quality,' 'Safety,' 'Efficacy' and 'Multidisciplinary' technical document that is adopted by the regulatory agencies in the three ICH regions.
- v Till 2017, ICH has successfully developed 112 harmonized guidelines covering 51 major topics that are adopted and implemented by the regulatory agencies. WHO is playing a crucial role as observer coordinating liaising between ICH and non-ICH countries ensuring information exchange.

The International Council for Harmonisation (ICH), was previously known as the International Conference on Harmonisation. The ICH objective is to propose recommendations for the attainment of harmonization in the interpretation and application of technical guidelines and requirements for pharmaceutical product registration. Endeavors toward obviation of testing duplication carried out during research and development of new human medicines. Regulatory harmonization offers many direct benefits to both regulatory authorities and the pharmaceutical industries with a beneficial impact on public health protection. Key benefits include: Preventing duplication of clinical trials in humans and minimizing the use of animal testing without compromising safety and effectiveness; streamlining the regulatory assessment process for new drug applications; shortening of the drug development duration and rational use of resources for drug development. ICH Tripartite Guidelines development was initiated to achieve process harmonization between drug regulatory authorities.

HISTORY OF ICH

It is essential to have an independent evaluation of medicinal products before they are allowed to reach the market in different regions. However, the realization to perform detailed safety and efficacy study on new drugs was driven by tragedies like thalidomide disaster causing malformed limbs in babies occurred in the 1960s. Laws, regulations, and guidelines for reporting and evaluating data on the safety, quality, and efficacy of new medicinal products were implemented in many countries worldwide in the 1960s and 1970s. The pharmaceutical industries gradually became multinationals seeking approval of new drugs for global markets. However, huge technical requirements divergence was there from country to country. It was obvious to duplicate many time consuming and expensive test to market

new products, internationally repetitively for new territories. The over rising price of health care with the escalation of the R&D cost has rationalized the urgent need to harmonized drug regulation. The need was also impelled to meet the public expectation of minimizing delays in marketing safe and efficacious new treatments available to the patients in need.

Initiation of ICH

Harmonization of regulatory requirements was pioneered by the European Community (EC), in the 1980s, as the EC (now the European Union) moved towards the development of a single market for pharmaceuticals. The success achieved in Europe demonstrated future potential of harmonization initiatives. Bilateral discussions between Europe, Japan, and the US on possibilities for harmonization was started by that time. At 1989, WHO International Conference of Drug Regulatory Authorities (ICDRA), held in Paris, the specific plans for action began to materialize. Soon afterward, the authorities approached the International Federation of Pharmaceutical Manufacturers and Associations (IFPMA) to discuss a joint regulatory industry initiative on international harmonization, and ICH was conceived. The ICH was created at a meeting in 1990, hosted by the European Federation of Pharmaceutical Industries and Associations (EFPIA) in Brussels. Representatives from the regulatory authorities and industry associations of Europe, Japan, and the US formally met to plan the inception of an International Conference. In the meeting delegates also discussed the broader implications and terms of reference of ICH. Canada was involved as an observer from the beginning. At the very first ICH Steering Committee (SC) meeting the Terms of Reference were agreed upon, and it was decided that the topics selected for harmonization would be divided into Safety, Quality and Efficacy to reflect the three criteria which are the basis for approving and authorizing new medicinal products.

Evolution of ICH

Since ICH's inception in 1990, the regulatory process has gradually evolved. In the first decade, ICH's showed significant progress in the development of Tripartite ICH Guidelines on Safety, Quality and Efficacy topics. Development of some critical multidisciplinary topics, like MedDRA (Medical Dictionary for Regulatory Activities) and the CTD (Common Technical Document) was also undertaken. Throughout the second decade, ICH Guidelines continued to be developed with more attention given to the need to maintain already existing Guidelines relevant as science and technology continued to evolve. The need to leverage with other organizations was also acknowledged, particularly for the development of electronic standards. The SC recognized the benefits afforded by collaboration with Standards Development Organisations, not only from the perspective of having a larger available pool of technical expertise but also the opportunity to progress ICH standards as global standards. As ICH started into the new millennium, the need to expand communication and dissemination of information on ICH guidelines with non-ICH regions became a key focus. Attention was directed toward facilitating the implementation of ICH guidelines in ICH's regions. Active participation of non-ICH regions in guideline development is also seen as a crucial factor in this effort.

MISSION OF ICH

- Contribute towards protection of public health from an international perspective;
- To improve the efficiency of new drug development and registration process;
- To facilitate the adoption of new or improved technical research and development approaches updating and replacing current practices, permitting a more economical use of human, animal and material resources without compromising safety;

- To prevent duplication of clinical trials in humans and minimize the use of animal testing without compromising safety and efficacy;
- To maintain a forum for constructive dialogue between regulatory authorities and the pharmaceutical industry on the real and perceived differences in the technical requirements for product registration.
- To ensure secure and speedy introduction of new medicinal products and their availability to patients;
- To monitor and update harmonized technical requirements intended to guide towards substantial mutual acceptance of research and development data between the regulatory agencies of different countries;
- To harmonize divergent regulatory requirements of selected topics generated as a result of therapeutic advances and development of new technologies for the production of medicinal products;
- To facilitate dissemination of information and effective communication on harmonized guidelines and their use encouraging implementation and integration of common standards.

ORGANIZATION OF ICH

Before reform in 2015 the governance structure of ICH was (Fig. 3.1):
- Steering Committee
- Global Cooperation Group
- MedDRA Management Board
- Secretariat and the Coordinators
- ICH Working Groups
  - Quality (Q)
  - Safety (S)
  - Efficacy (E)
  - Multi-disciplinary (M)

The Steering Committee (SC)

The SC is the governing body that oversees the harmonization activities. Established in

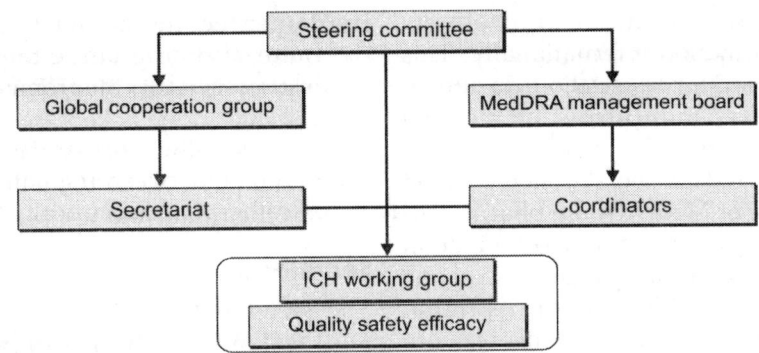

Fig. 3.1: The organizational structure of the International Conference on Harmonisation (ICH)

1990, each of its six cosponsors of SC has had two seats. The six cosponsors are European Union (EU), EFPIA, Ministry of Health, Labour and Welfare (MHLW), Japan Pharmaceutical Manufacturers Association (JPMA), US Food and Drug Administration (USFDA) and Pharmaceutical Research and Manufacturers of America (PhRMA). Other parties are having a significant interest in ICH and have been invited to nominate Observers to the SC. The three observers are the WHO, Health Canada and the European Free Trade Association (EFTA). The IFPMA participates as a nonvoting member of the SC.

Global Cooperation Group (GCG)

In response to a growing interest in the use of ICH guidelines by the countries beyond the ICH regions, the ICH Steering Committee took the first step in 1999 by establishing the ICH-GCG as a subcommittee of the ICH SC. In 2003, new terms of reference and rules were endorsed for the GCG with the aim of establishing partnerships beyond ICH regions to promote a better understanding of ICH guidelines. The scope of activities undertaken by the GCG is embodied in the mission statement adopted by all parties in 2005: *"To promote a mutual understanding of regional harmonisation initiatives in order to facilitate the harmonization process related to ICH Guidelines regionally and globally, and to facilitate the capacity of drug regulatory authorities and industry to utilise them."*

In 2005, five Regional Harmonisation Initiatives (RHIs) from across the globe were invited to participate in the GCG discussions, namely APEC, ASEAN, EAC, GCC, PANDRH, and SADC. The GCG was further expanded with the decision of the SC in 2007 and invited the participation of representatives from Drug Regulatory Authorities (DRAs)/Department of Health (DoH) from countries with a history of ICH guideline implementation. The countries like Australia, Brazil, China, Chinese Taipei, India, Republic of Korea, Russia and Singapore having major pharma production and clinical research setups were also invited. Besides, as per a decision of the SC in 2010, invited RHIs and DRAs/DoH may also nominate technical experts as active members of ICH Expert Working groups. RHI and DRAs/DoH representatives are invited to participate in the GCG meeting and listen to technical topics at the level of the Steering Committee at the biannual ICH meetings.

MedDRA

The MedDRA Management Board, appointed by the ICH SC, has overall responsibility for the direction of MedDRA, an ICH standardized dictionary of medical terminology. MedDRA is a highly specific standardized medical terminology developed by ICH to facilitate sharing of medical products regulatory information internationally. This information is used for registration, documentation and safety monitoring of medical products both before and after a drug product has been authorized for sale. Products covered under the scope of MedDRA are pharmaceuticals, vaccines, and drug-device combination products. MedDRA is now open to everyone intended to use it, although, on its initial implementation in 1999, most users were based in Europe, Japan, and the USA. Today, worldwide regulatory authorities, global pharmaceutical companies, clinical research organizations, and health care professionals are using these guidelines. The MSSO (Maintenance and Support Services Organization), contracted by ICH with technical and financial oversight by the MedDRA Management Board, is tasked to maintain, develop and distribute MedDRA terminologies. The terminology documents are free for all regulators worldwide, academics, and health care providers while paid subscriptions are on a sliding scale linked to an annual turnover of companies.

MedDRA is continuously evolving to meet the evolving needs of regulators and industries around the world under the governance of the ICH MedDRA Management Board. The current ICH M1 (Multidisciplinary Guidelines: MedDRA Terminology M1), Working Groups, develop and maintain documents on the use of MedDRA for data entry (coding) and data retrieval/analysis. Data retrieval provide guidance on the use of Standardised MedDRA Queries, as powerful tools for assisting the safety signal detection. With every MedDRA release, both the documents are updated twice a year. To further facilitate its implementation and correct use, free training is offered, and MedDRA is available today in many translations of the original English version—Chinese, Czech, Dutch, French, German, Hungarian, Italian, Japanese, Portuguese and Spanish. MedDRA is fully implemented in the WHO global safety database allowing entry and retrieval of information in either MedDRA or WHO-ART. A mapping bridge is kept updated by WHO and ICH, to allow conversion of WHO-ART coded data into MedDRA, allowing users to convert their data and use MedDRA readily.

Secretariat

The Secretariat of ICH is located in Geneva, Switzerland. Staff members appointed perform regular works like preparations of documentation, SC and Working Groups (WG) meeting conduction and provides administrative support to the ICH GCG and MedDRA.

Coordinators

Each of the six cosponsors appoints a Coordinator to act as the primary contact point with the ICH Secretariat. Coordinators ensure proper distribution of documents to the appropriate persons from their counterpart (SC members, Topic Leaders, Experts) and are responsible for proper follow up on actions within assigned deadlines.

Working Groups (WG)

WG members do not have a fixed membership. In the first phase of harmonization process, each technical topics selected for implementation is assigned to a WG appointed SC to review the differences in requirements between the three regions and develop scientific consensus required to reconcile those differences. Each of the six parties nominates WG members as Topic Leader (or a Deputy Topic Leader) depending on the topic content. WG members are invited from ICH Observers, Pharmacopoeia authorities, representatives from industry to participate. Different types of WGs are:

- Expert Working Group (EWG) is charged with developing a harmonized guideline that meets the objectives in the Concept Paper and Business Plan.

- Implementation Working Group (IWG) is tasked to develop Questions and Answer to facilitate implementation of existing guidelines.
- Informal Working Group is formed before any official ICH harmonization activity with the objectives of developing/finalizing a concept paper and for developing business plan.
- Discussion Group is formed to discuss specific scientific considerations or views like Gene Therapy Discussion Group, Women Discussion Group, etc.

ICH REFORM AND ORGANIZATIONAL CHANGE

International Conference on Harmonisation was reformed as International Council for Harmonisation (ICH), in the inaugural Assembly meetings held on 23 October 2015 establishing ICH as an international association with a legal entity under Swiss law. The reformation with organizational changes was aimed at reinforcement of the foundations of ICH to make it better-equipped to face the challenges of global pharmaceutical development and regulation. The primary focus of reformed ICH is to improve transparency and openness in its processes, extensive international outreach with increased participation of regulators and global industry sectors, secure alternative funding model with less dependence on industry and most importantly to become a legal association under Swiss law. The organizational structure was reformed to have a more stable operating system. As a legal association ICH has established a new Assembly, as the over-arching governing body that will be instrumental in facilitating future growth through the participation of new members. More involvement from regulators around the world was ensured, especially from counterparts from Europe, Japan, USA, Canada, and Switzerland were invited to join as ICH regulatory members (Fig. 3.2).

Membership under new legal entity is as:
- Permanent members
  - Founding members: United States Food and Drug Administration (US FDA), European Union (EU), Pharmaceuticals and Medical Devices Agency, Japan (PMDA)/Ministry of Health, Labour and Welfare (Japan) (MHLW), PhRMA, European Federation of Pharmaceutical Industries and Associations (EFPIA), Japan Pharmaceutical Manufacturers Association (JPMA)
- Standing members: Health Canada, Swissmedic
- Other
  - Standing observers: World Health Organisation (WHO), IFPMA
  - Future members and observers

The governance structure of ICH under new legal entity after reform in 2015 is:
- ICH Assembly
- Management Committee
- MedDRA Management Committee
- Secretariat and the Coordinators
- ICH Working Groups
  - Quality (Q)
  - Safety (S)
  - Efficacy (E)
  - Multi-disciplinary (M)
- Auditors

ICH Members and Observers are committed to attending the meeting in a self-financed mode with an expectation of continuity and stable participation. The Permanent Members previously ensured the funding of ICH operations (secretariat, meetings, etc.) but now it is expected to be self-funded through membership fees approved by the Assembly.

Assembly

Assembly is the overarching body that brings together all Members and Observers of the

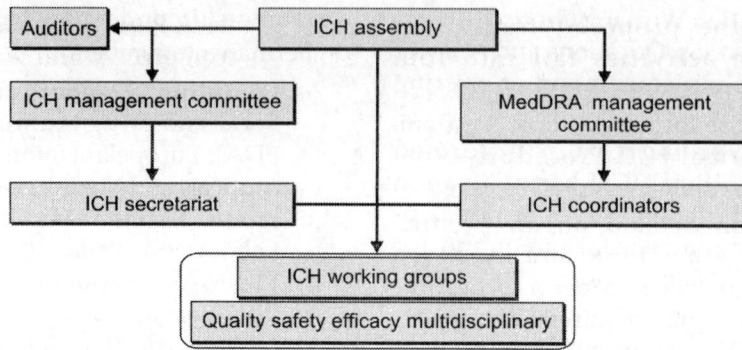

Fig. 3.2: The organizational structure of the International Council for Harmonisation (ICH)

ICH Association. Assembly includes the drug regulatory authorities and international pharmaceutical industry associations those who apply to become an ICH member and following fulfilment of the eligibility criteria they can become a member of the Assembly. Assembly has decision-making power on matters in particular to the Articles of Association, admission of new members and observers and adoption of guidelines on a consensus basis. The ICH Assembly meets biannually, and the meeting agendas and reports are made available on the ICH website summarising the main decisions.

The Management Committee (MC)

Management Committee includes all the current members of the SC initially as permanent members and subsequently also elected members. The ICH MC has representatives from the six founding members (Europe EC, EFPIA, US FDA, MHLW, Japan PMDA, and PhRMA), standing regulatory members (Health Canada and Swissmedic, Switzerland) as well as Standing Observers (IFPMA, WHO). MC is incharge of administrative matters on behalf of all Members, including administrative and financial matters and oversight of the WGs. MC determines ICH policies and procedures, decides on adoption of ICH projects, select topics for harmonization, endorse the creation of expert WGs, monitors and facilitates the progress of

expert WGs. The MC submit recommendations and proposals to the Assembly in preparation of Assembly discussions. The minutes of ICH MC meetings and summary reports are published on the ICH website summarising the main decisions taken.

Subcommittees

- Rules of procedure
- Financial
- Membership
- Communication
- Secretariat liaison

Auditors

The ICH Assembly has appointed an auditing firm as Auditors in line with Articles 55 and 56 of the ICH Articles of Association. Auditors are appointed for two years and further be reappointed. The responsibility of the Auditors is to audit the financial statements of the Association upon conclusion of each fiscal year. They should ensure that the accounting of the association complies with Swiss law and generally accepted Swiss accounting principles.

HARMONISATION PROCESS

Harmonisation activity is initiated by a concept paper which is a summary of the proposal and in some cases a business plan outlining the costs and benefits of harmonizing the proposed topic. ICH harmonization activities fall into four categories:

- Requisite arise for a New topic harmonization—**Formal ICH Procedure**—concept paper and business plan required
- Clarification needed on an existing guideline—**Questions and Answers Procedure**—concept paper and in some cases business plan required
- The content of an existing guideline outdated or invalid or new information needed to be incorporated in an existing guideline—**Revision Procedure**—concept paper required
- Changes are required in Q3 guideline or M2 recommendation—**Maintenance Procedure**—concept paper required for Q3 but not for M2

Formal ICH Procedure

The ICH Assembly endorses the Concept Paper and Business Plan to initiate this procedure with subsequent establishment of an Expert WG (EWG). The EWG develops draft guideline and pass it through the various steps of the procedure to Step 5, that is the implementation of Harmonised Guideline in the ICH regions.

Step 1: Consensus building—technical document

Step 2a: ICH parties consensus on Technical Document

Step 2b: Draft guideline adoption by ICH regulatory parties

Step 3: Regulatory consultation and discussion

Step 4: Adoption of ICH harmonised guideline

Step 5: Implementation

Step 1: Consensus building

The EWG works to prepare a draft of the Technical Document by the objectives set out in the Concept Paper in communication via e-mail, teleconferences and web conferences.

EWG can also meet at the time of the biannual assembly meetings following endorsement of the ICH MC. Interim reports on the progress of the draft are communicated regularly to the assembly. The technical experts of the EWG sign the Step 1 Experts sign-off sheets when consensus on the draft is reached. The Experts Technical Document of Step 1 with EWG members signatures is then submitted to the Assembly with request to progress under Step 2.

Step 2a: Confirmation of consensus on the Technical Documents

Ensuring sufficient scientific consensus on the technical issues the assembly agrees to proceed with the Technical Document to the next stage of Step 2a regulatory consultation based on the report of the EWG.

Step 2b: Adoption of draft Guideline by Regulatory Members

ICH Regulatory Members develop the draft guideline by the technical document, and Step 2b is reached with the endorsement of draft guideline by the regulatory members.

Step 3: Regulatory Consultation and Discussion

Step 3 has three distinct stages as regulatory consultation followed by discussion, and finalization of the Expert Draft Guideline.

Stage I: Regional regulatory consultation: The guideline embodying the scientific consensus come out of internal ICH process and becomes subject of wide-range regulatory consultation in the ICH region. Regulatory authorities and industry associations in non-ICH regions can also comment on the draft consultation documents by providing comments to the ICH Secretariat.

Stage II: Discussion on regional consultation comments: The EWG works to address all the comments obtained from the consultation process, and reaches consensus on the Step 3 Experts Draft Guideline.

Stage III: Finalisation of Step 3 Experts Draft Guideline: The Step 3 Expert Draft Guideline is signed by the experts of the ICH Regulatory Members when consensus is reached on the revised version of the Step 2b draft guideline after due consideration of the consultation results by the EWG. Following signature of EWG, the Step 3 Expert Draft Guideline is submitted to the Regulatory Members of the Assembly to request adoption as Step 4 of the ICH process.

Step 4: Adoption of an ICH Harmonised Guideline

The Step 4 Final Document is adopted by the Regulatory Members of the Assembly as an ICH Harmonised Guideline when the assembly agrees that there is sufficient consensus on the draft guideline.

Step 5: Implementation

The harmonized guideline moves immediately to the final step of the regulatory implementation process. Step 5 is executed according to the same national/regional procedures applicable to the regional regulatory guidelines and requirements, in the ICH regions.

Question and Answer Procedure

This procedure is followed when additional guidance is considered necessary to help the interpretation of certain ICH harmonized Guidelines to ensure smooth and consistent implementation. This additional guidance is usually developed in the form of "Questions and Answers". The procedure is initiated with the endorsement of concept paper by the assembly. The assembly may also consider the need for business plan, in case of significant implementation activities with subsequent establishment of Implementation Working Group (IWG).

The procedure is driven by questions/issues raised by stakeholders, which serves as the basis for the development of model questions for which standard answers are developed. Stakeholders are invited to submit their questions on a specific guideline assisting the process via the ICH website. The IWG functions to reach consensus on a draft questions and answers document and forward recommendation to the Assembly on whether the document should be in Step 2b draft document published for consultation or in Step 4 final document published without consultation based on the level of information provided by the answers. The document then follows the usual path of a Step 2/Step 4 document as per the formal ICH procedure.

Revision Procedure

The revision procedure is followed for an existing document with scientific/technical content that is no longer up-to-date or valid, or in cases, new information is required to be added with no amendments to the existing ICH Guideline. All new information is added in the form of Addendum or Annex to the Guideline in question. The procedure is initiated with the endorsement of concept paper by the ICH Assembly and subsequent establishment of Expert Working Group (EWG). The revision procedure is almost identical to 5-step Formal ICH Procedure with the only difference that the outcome is a revised version of an existing guideline, instead of a new guideline. After the common denomination of the guideline, the revised version is designated by letter R1, and following subsequent revision of the document is named R2, R3, R4. Addendum or Annex is normally added to the existing guideline proceeding as a revised guideline upon reaching Step 4.

Maintenance Procedure

Currently, maintenance procedure applies only to changes in the Q3C and Q3D Guidelines and M2 Recommendations when new information is required to be added, or the scientific/technical content is out-of-date or no longer valid.

Maintenance procedure for Q3C and Q3D guideline: The maintenance procedure for Q3C/Q3D is followed when there is a proposal for inclusion of permitted Daily Exposure (PDE) for a new solvent/elemental impurity or revision in PDE for an already classified solvent/elemental impurity. Like the formal ICH Procedure, this procedure similarly follows the 5 steps.

Maintenance procedure for M2 recommendations: The M2 EWG works on Electronic Standards for the Transfer of Regulatory Information (ESTRI) and can suggest for inclusion of some recommendations. Recommendations need not to undergo the formal ICH process steps. The EWG agrees on and subsequently got approved by the ICH assembly following signature by all EWG members. A different version number designates each new version of the M2 recommendations.

ICH TOPICS AND HARMONIZED TRIPARTITE GUIDELINES

ICH develop and implement harmonized tripartite guidelines to be adopted by the regulatory agencies in the three ICH regions. ICH addressed topics are broadly grouped under the general headings of "Quality" (pharmaceutical development and specifications),"Safety"(pre-clinical toxicity and related tests), "Efficacy" (clinical testing programs and safety monitoring) and "Multidisciplinary"(topics impacting more than one area, such as regulatory communications, including electronic communication, timing of toxicity studies in relation to clinical studies and the common technical document.

Quality Guidelines

Harmonization initiatives in the quality segment are of pivotal importance for the conduct of stability studies, defining relevant thresholds for impurity testing with a more flexible approach to pharmaceutical quality based on good manufacturing practice (GMP) and risk management. Quality guidelines provided recommendations in crucial areas like stability and impurities. Previously stability studies were typically conducted at "room temperature" or as defined by the company concerned with or without humidity control. This required generation of new stability data for registrations in different climatic regions where the original study had been conducted. ICH harmonization guidelines provide standard sets of stability conditions taking account of the climatic zones in each of the three regions so that data generated on stability in any one of the three regions are mutually acceptable omitting expense of duplicate testing. The impurities guidelines provide scientific agreement on the recording and reporting of impurity levels like the threshold limits for impurity qualification and impurity identification. Changes in impurity profile throughout a development program can be managed following a single specification for any drug substance or product that is acceptable across the three ICH regions. The guidelines have made the supply chain far simpler and minimized error. The guidelines cover the specific issues associated with biotechnological products having a significant favorable impact on both development and resource utilization in biotechnology industry. The latest quality guideline Q12 provides a framework for management of post-approval chemistry, manufacturing and controls (CMC) changes over the product lifecycle.

Quality: 14 topics/50 guidelines

1. Stability: Q1A–Q1F

1.1 Q1A(R2): Stability Testing of New Drug Substances and Products: This guideline reached Step 4 of the ICH process after second revision in 2003. This guideline provides recommendations on temperature, humidity, and trial duration parameters of stability testing protocols for climatic Zone I and II. The revised document described requirements for stability testing in climatic zones III and IV to minimize the different storage conditions for submission of a global dossier.

1.2 Q1B Stability Testing: Photostability Testing of New Drug Substances and Products: Guideline finalized under Step 4 in 1996 forms an annex to the main stability guideline and gave guidance on the basic testing protocol required to evaluate the light sensitivity and stability of new drugs and products.

1.3 Q1C Stability Testing for New Dosage Forms: It defines the stability guideline for new formulations of previously approved medicines and defines the circumstances under which compressed stability data can be accepted.

1.4 Q1D Bracketing and Matrixing Designs for Stability Testing of New Drug Substances and Products: The general principle of bracketing and matrixing designs for stability testing are described in this guideline for reduced stability testing time of new drugs.

1.5 Q1E Evaluation of Stability Data: Finalized under Step 4 in 2003, this document is an extension of the main guideline, explaining possible situations where extrapolation of retest periods/shelf-lives beyond the real-time data may be appropriate. It also provides examples of statistical approaches to stability data analysis.

1.6 Q1F Stability Data Package for Registration Applications in Climatic Zones III and IV: The ICH Steering Committee endorsed withdrawal of this guideline in Yokohama, 2006 meeting and decided to leave the definition of storage conditions in climatic zones III and IV to the respective regions and WHO.

2. Analytical Validation Q2

Q2(R1) Validation of Analytical Procedures: Text and Methodology: The tripartite harmonized ICH guideline (previously coded Q2A) was finalized under Step 4 in 1994. This guideline identifies validation parameters for variety of analytical methods included as part of registration applications. The guideline on methodology (previously coded Q2B) was finalized under Step 4 in 1996, extending Q2A guideline to include required actual experimental data along with statistical interpretation for analytical procedures validation. Methodology guideline was incorporated Q2 in 2005 and renamed Q2(R1), without any changes in the contents.

3. Impurities Q3A–Q3D

3.1 Q3A(R2) Impurities in New Drug Substances: This guideline was revised under Step 2 of the ICH process in 1999 and finalized under Step 4 on 2002 (Q3A-R1). This guideline addresses the chemistry and safety aspects of impurities with identification and qualification. It includes listing of impurities specifications and defines the thresholds for reporting. The revision of the guideline has clarified inconsistencies in the decision tree revision, harmonization with Q3B and other editorial issues.

3.2 Q3B(R2) Impurities in New Drug Products: This guideline has been first revised and finalized under Step 4 in 2003, providing advice regarding impurities in products containing new, chemically synthesized drug substances. The guideline deals explicitly with the impurities came out as degradation products of the drug substance or interactions between drug substance and excipients or components of primary packaging materials. Based on the scientific appraisal of likely and actual impurities observed, and of the safety implications, this guideline sets out the rationale for the reporting, identification, and qualification of such impurities. Threshold values for reporting and control of impurities are proposed based on the maximum daily dose of the drug product.

3.3 Q3C(R6) Impurities: Guideline for Residual Solvents: This core tripartite harmonized guideline was finalized under Step 4 in 1997, that recommends the use of less toxic solvents in the manufacturing of drug substances and dosage forms, and sets pharmaceutical limits for residual solvents (organic volatile impurities) in drug products.

Maintenance Process: The maintenance process revised Permitted Daily Exposure (PDE), as new toxicological data for solvents are released. Limit values for three residual solvents were revised on the basis of the newly recognized toxicity data; lower PDE for N-methylpyrrolidone (NMP) being kept in Class 2 (limited by health-basis) and placed Tetrahydrofuran (THF) and Cumene from Class 3 to Class 2 (no health-based). A corrigendum to calculate the formula for NMP was subsequently approved in 2002, and incorporated into the core guideline in 2005, as per the new coding rule. In 2009, Table 2, Table 3 and Appendix 1 of the core guideline were updated to reflect the revision of the PDEs for NMP and THF (Q3C-R4). The revision of the PDE for Cumene reached Step 4 of the process in 2011 and was integrated as part IV in the core guideline (Q3C-R5).

Q3C(R4) Revised PDE for N-methyl-pyrrolidone (2002)

Revised PDE for Tetrahydrofuran (2002)

Q3C(R5) Revised PDE for Cumene (2011)

Q3C (R6) Revised PDE for methyl isobutyl ketone (2016)

The current version of Q3C (R6) maintenance guideline, revise the PDE for methyl isobutyl ketone (MIBK) and add Triethylamine (TEA) was included in Class 3 (solvents with low toxic potential) as a new solvent. MIBK was moved from Class 3 (solvents with low toxic potential) to Class 2 (solvents to be limited) based on new data.

3.4 Q3D Impurities: Guideline for Elemental Impurities: ICH Q3D guideline aims for the control of elemental impurities in new drug products and establishes PDEs for 24 Elemental Impurities (EIs) for drug products administered by the oral, parenteral and inhalation routes. The ICH Steering Committee in 2009 endorsed this topic. This guidance provides global policy for limiting metal impurities qualitatively and quantitatively in drug products and ingredients. The existing Q3A guideline classifies impurities as organic, inorganic, and residual solvents. The Q3C guideline was developed to provide clarification on the requirements for residual solvents, whereas the Q3D provides similar clarification on requirements for metals included as inorganic impurities. Classification has reached Step 4 of the ICH process in 2014.

3.5 Q3D Training: Implementation of Guideline for Elemental Impurities: The ICH Steering Committee in 2014 endorsed this Implementation Working Group (IWG) guideline. Throughout the development of the Q3D guideline, complexity of the implementation approaches were regularly communicated between external audiences, constituents countries, and interested parties. This guideline does not provide detailed example covering potential case studies for drug products. Consequently, ICH SC considered development of a comprehensive training programme and supporting documentation necessary to ensure proper interpretation and effective utilization by industry and regulators to enable harmonized and smooth implementation of Q3D on global basis.

4. Pharmacopoeias Q4A-Q4B

4.1 Q4 Pharmacopoeias: Q6A activity provided the framework to set specifications for drug substances to address how regulators and manufacturers might avoid setting or agreeing to conflicting standards for the same product, as part of the registration in different regions. The resulting ICH Q6A guideline provides harmonized guidance on chemical substances. Harmonization of several compendial test chapters has been considered as critical by the ICH Steering Committee. These chapters are at various stages of harmonization among the three pharmacopoeial organizations (USP, JP, and EP). The three organizations conduct their harmonization efforts through a tripartite pharmacopoeial harmonization program known as the Pharmacopoeial Discussion Group (PDG).

4.2 Q4A Pharmacopoeial Harmonisation: The pharmacopoeial authorities, working together through the PDG, is closely involved with the work of ICH since the outset harmonization initiatives between the major pharmacopoeias. The ICH Steering Committee reviews regular reports on the status of pharmacopoeial harmonization at its meetings.

4.3 Q4B Evaluation and Recommendation of Pharmacopoeial Texts for Use in the ICH Regions: The tripartite harmonized ICH Guideline was finalized under Step 4 in 2007. This document describes the process for the evaluation and recommendation on selected Pharmacopoeial texts for use as interchangeable in the ICH regions and since 2010 in Canada by the Q4B EWG to facilitate recognition by regulatory authorities. Following favorable evaluations, ICH issues topic specific annexes with information on Pharmacopoeial texts and other relevant details on implementation intended to avoid redundant testing by industry.

4.4 Q4B Annex 1R1 Residue on Ignition/Sulphated Ash

4.5 Q4B Annex 2R1 Test for Extractable Volume of Parenteral Preparations

4.6 Q4B Annex 3R1 Test for Particulate Contamination: Sub-visible Particles

4.7 Q4B Annex 4AR1 Microbiological Examination of Non-Sterile Products: Microbial Enumeration Tests

4.8 Q4B Annex 4BR1 Microbiological Examination of Non-Sterile Products: Tests for Specified Micro-organisms

4.9 Q4B Annex 4CR1 Microbiological Examination of Non-sterile Products: Acceptance Criteria for Pharmaceutical Preparations and Substances for Pharmaceutical Use: This annex of pharmacopoeial text for microbiological examination of non-sterile products is non-mandatory and provided for informational purposes only for the regulatory region.

4.10 Q4B Annex 5R1 Disintegration Test

4.11 Q4B Annex 6R1 Uniformity of Dosage Units

4.12 Q4B Annex 7R2 Dissolution Test

4.13 Q4B Annex 8R1 Sterility Test

4.14 Q4B Annex 9R1 Tablet Friability

4.15 Q4B Annex 10R1 Polyacrylamide Gel Electrophoresis

4.16 Q4B Annex 11 Capillary Electrophoresis

4.17 Q4B Annex 12 Analytical Sieving

4.18 Q4B Annex 13 Bulk Density and Tapped Density of Powders

4.19 Q4B Annex 14 Bacterial Endotoxins Test

Q4B FAQs Frequently Asked Questions

5. Quality of Biotechnological Products Q5A-Q5E

5.1 Q5A(R1) Viral Safety Evaluation of Biotechnology Products Derived from Cell Lines of Human or Animal Origin: Guideline finalized under Step 4 in 1997 is concerned with testing and evaluation of viral safety of biotechnology products derived from characterized human or animal cell lines. This guideline provides a general framework and design of virus testing experiments for evaluation of virus clearance studies.

5.2 Q5B Analysis of the Expression Construct in Cells Used for Production of r-DNA Derived Protein Products: The guideline was finalized under Step 4 in 1995, to advice on the types of information that are considered valuable in assessing the structure of the expression construct used to produce recombinant DNA derived proteins.

5.3 Q5C Stability Testing of Biotechnological/Biological Products: This document augments the Q1A stability guideline with a particular focus on stability test procedures required for products having active components typically proteins and/or polypeptides of particular characteristics.

5.4 Q5D Derivation and Characterisation of Cell Substrates Used for Production of Biotechnological/Biological Products: This document provides broad guidance on appropriate standards for human and animal cell lines and microbes used for the preparation of biotechnological/biological products and characterization of cell banks.

5.5 Q5E Comparability of Biotechnological/Biological Products Subject to Changes in their Manufacturing Process: The principles for assessing comparability of biotechnological/biological products before and after making changes in the manufacturing process of a drug substance or drug product is addressed in this document. This document does not prescribe any particular analytical, nonclinical or clinical strategy but primarily emphasis on quality aspects. This guideline assists in relevant technical information collection that serves as evidence to justify that changes in the manufacturing process do not have an adverse impact on the quality, safety, and efficacy of the drug product

Specifications Q6A-Q6B

6.1 Q6A Specifications: Test Procedures and Acceptance Criteria for New Drug Substances and New Drug Products Chemical Substances: Guideline finalized under Step 4 in 1999, addresses the process of selecting tests and methods and setting specifications for the testing of drug substances and dosage forms. The account has been taken for considerable

guidance and background information which are present in existing regional documents.

6.2 Q6B Specifications: Test Procedures and Acceptance Criteria for Biotechnological/Biological Products: This document guides on setting justification and specifications for proteins and polypeptides derived from recombinant or non-recombinant cell cultures. Although the scope is limited to well-characterized biotechnological products, the concepts may apply to other biologicals as appropriate. Given the nature of the products, this topic of specifications include in-process controls, bulk drug, the final product, and stability specifications. This document give guidance for a harmonized approach for determining appropriate specifications based on safety, process consistency, purity, analytical methodology, product administration, and clinical data considerations.

7. Good Manufacturing Practice Q7

7.1 Q7 Good Manufacturing Practice Guide for Active Pharmaceutical Ingredients: Earlier, the ICH process has agreed on adequate international harmonization of Good Manufacturing Practices (GMP) technical aspects for Pharmaceutical Products, but need to formalize GMP requirements for the components of pharmaceutical products—both active and inactive arises. In 1998, the ICH SC agreed on adoption of ICH Topic on GMP for Active Pharmaceutical Ingredients (APIs). While adopting this topic, the Steering Committee ensured due accounting of works already in progress with PIC/S, FDA, and other parties. Given the unusually wide implications of this topic, a much extended EWG has been established which includes, in addition to the six ICH parties and the Observers, experts representing IGPA (generics industry), WSMI (self-medication industry) and PIC/S. Concerning the latter representatives from China, India, and Australia have been invited to participate.

7.2 Q7 Questions and Answers: Good Manufacturing Practice Guide for Active Pharmaceutical Ingredients: The guideline reached Step 4 of the ICH process on 2015. Since the finalization of ICH Q7 guideline in 2000, experience gained on implementation shows existence of uncertainties related to the interpretation of some sections. Technical issues about GMP of APIs, also in context with new ICH guidelines, are addressed in this Question and Answer document in order to harmonize expectations during inspections, to remove ambiguities and uncertainties and also to harmonize the inspections of both small molecules and biotech APIs.

8. Pharmaceutical Development Q8

8.1 Q8(R2) Pharmaceutical Development: The core tripartite harmonized ICH guideline was finalized under Step 4 in 2005. This guideline guides on the contents of drug products. Pharmaceutical Development as defined in the scope of Module 3 of the CTD (ICH topic M4) but does not apply to the clinical research stages of drug development. The applicability of this guideline concerned to a particular type of product is decided based on consultation with the appropriate regulatory authorities.

The annex to the tripartite harmonized ICH text was finalized under Step 4 in 2008 and incorporated into the core guideline, which was then renamed Q8(R1). The annex provides further clarification of fundamental concepts outlined in the core Guideline along with principles of quality by design (QbD). Though this annex is not intended to establish new standards, it guides on practice of concepts and tools to enhance science and risk-based regulatory approaches (e.g. design space) outlined in the parent Q8 document when quality by design and quality risk management (Q9: Quality Risk Management) systems are applied linked to appropriate pharmaceutical quality system.

8.2 Q8/9/10 Questions and Answers R4 Q8/ Q9/Q10—Implementation: All parties within the ICH regions have experienced the need for some clarification with the implementation of the ICH Q8 (R2), Q9 and Q10 Guidelines. These Questions and Answers developed by the Quality Implementation Working Group (IWG) are intended to facilitate the implementation of the Q8(R2), Q9 and Q10 guidelines, by clarifying key issues. Covering the topics of Q8(R2), Q9 and Q10, the ICH Quality IWG also prepared some 'Points to Consider' which supplement the existing Questions & Answers and workshop training materials relevant to the implementation.

9. Quality Risk Management Q9

9.1 Q9 Quality Risk Management: The tripartite harmonized ICH Guideline was finalized under Step 4 in 2005. This guideline provides principles with relevant examples of quality risk management tools targeted to be applied to all pharmaceutical quality aspects including development, manufacturing, distribution, and inspection. The submission/ review processes throughout the lifecycle of drug substances and drug (medicinal) products, including the use of raw materials, solvents, excipients, packaging and labeling materials, biological and biotechnological products are also covered.

9.2 Q8/9/10 Questions and Answers R4 Q8/ Q9/Q10—Implementation: Reaching Step 4 of publication within the ICH regions, the Questions and Answers developed by the Quality IWG are intended to facilitate the implementation of the Q8(R2), Q9 and Q10 guidelines, by clarifying key issues.

10. Pharmaceutical Quality System Q10

10.1 Q10 Pharmaceutical Quality System: This is applicable throughout the product lifecycle to the pharmaceutical drug substances and drug products, biotechnology and biological products, The elements of Q10 are applied in an appropriate and proportionate manner to the product lifecycle stages, recognizing the differences among, and the different goals of each stage.

10.2 Q8/9/10 Questions and Answers R4

Q8/Q9/Q10—Implementation: Implements the Questions and Answers developed by the Quality IWG to facilitate the clarification on issues related to the Q8(R2), Q9 and Q10 guidelines.

11. Development and Manufacture of Drug Substances Q11

Q11 Development and Manufacture of Drug Substances (Chemical Entities and Biotechnological/Biological Entities): The Q11 draft guideline has been released for consultation under Step 2 of the ICH process in May 2011. This guideline is proposed for harmonization of scientific and technical principles relating to the description and justification of the development and manufacturing process of Active Pharmaceutical Ingredients (APIs) from both chemical and biotechnological/biological entities.

12. Life Cycle management Q12

Q12 Technical and Regulatory Considerations for Pharmaceutical Product Lifecycle Management: This topic was endorsed by the ICH SC in 2014, intended to complement the Q8 to Q11 guidelines. This guideline provides guidance framework on facilitation of the changes in the management of post-approval Chemistry, Manufacturing, and Controls (CMC) more predictably and efficiently across the product lifecycle. Adoption of this new ICH guideline is intended to promote innovation and continual improvement and strengthen quality assurance and reliable supply of product, including proactive planning of supply chain adjustments. It is to allow regulators (assessors and inspectors) to better understand the firms Pharmaceutical Quality Systems (PQSs) for management of post-approval CMC changes.

13. Continuous Manufacturing of Drug Substances and Drug Products

Endorsed in June 2018, this topic is proposed to harmonise cGMP elements specific to continuous manufacturing (CM). This enables drug manufacturers to employ flexible approaches to develop, implement or integrate CM for the manufacturing of small molecules and therapeutic proteins for new and existing drug products. This also provides guidance to industry and regulatory agencies regarding regulatory expectations on the development, implementation and assessment of CM technologies.

14. Analytical Procedure Development

Development of concept paper and business plan is under development.

Safety Guidelines

To uncover any potential risks of toxicity, i.e. carcinogenicity, genotoxicity, reprotoxicity of drug products, iCH has produced a comprehensive set of safety guidelines. In concern to safety, registration of New Chemical Exclusivity (NCE) requires extensive preclinical toxicity testing. Before the ICH initiative industries would do the types of preclinical studies as agreed by the regulators as part of a registration package. There was little agreement between the regulators of different countries regarding study length, content, species requirements, dose selection and exposure levels for assessment of risk/benefit ratio of NCE. Regional differences have laid to a considerable amount of repeat testing not only wasting time and resources but also evoking ethical and politically sensitive issues. Harmonization has minimized requirements for repeat studies significantly savings both experimental animals, the time delay in drug registration and funding in development programs. Safety guideline was also implemented for non-clinical testing and assessing the QT interval prolongation liability of a drug which is the single most important cause of drug withdrawal. A recent breakthrough is the adoption of a guideline to support pediatric drug development recommending conditions under which nonclinical juvenile animal testing is considered necessary to support pediatric clinical trials.

Safety: 11 topics/19 guidelines

1. Carcinogenicity Studies S1A - S1C

1.1 S1 Rodent Carcinogenicity Studies for Human Pharmaceuticals: This topic on rodent carcinogenicity testing was endorsed by the ICH SC in 2012 to introduce a more comprehensive and integrated approach for addressing the risk of pharmaceuticals concerned to human carcinogenicity and to set criteria for the conduct of a two-year rodent carcinogenicity study of a given pharmaceutical for value addition to risk assessment. The SC has endorsed revision of both the S1 concept paper and business plan to provide clarification concerning integration of prospective data gathering period into the normal ICH process steps. The revised S1 concept paper and business plan describes the S1 strategy for preparing a draft "Regulatory Notice for Public Input" document first time. This was issued by each ICH regulatory health authority to solicit comments from the public on the proposal, the procedure, and the specific weight-of-evidence criteria. In 2016, an update to the Regulatory Notice Document (RND) had been posted following discussions by the S1 Expert Working Group at the ICH Meeting held in 2015. The S1 EWG has completed Prospective Evaluation Period Status Report with a brief overview of the study progress and actions taken by the EWG ensuring successful completion of the study.

1.2 S1A Need for Carcinogenicity Studies of Pharmaceuticals: Guideline finalized Step 4 in 1995 defines the circumstances under which it is necessary to undertake carcinogenicity studies of new drugs. This guideline provides recommendations about the known risk factors as well as the intended indications and duration of exposure.

1.3 S1B Testing for Carcinogenicity of Pharmaceuticals: Finalized Step 4 in 1997, this document provides guidance on the need to carry out carcinogenicity studies in both mice and rats, and guidance is also given on alternative testing procedures which may be applied without jeopardizing safety.

1.4 S1C(R2) Dose Selection for Carcinogenicity Studies of Pharmaceuticals: The addendum on "Addition of a Limit Dose and Related Notes,"was finalized in 1997, and incorporated into the core guideline in 2005, renamed S1C(R1). The second revision was approved by the ICH SC directly under Step 4 in 2008. This document addresses the criteria for the selection of the high doses to be used in carcinogenicity studies of new therapeutic agents to harmonize current practices and improve the study design. The pharmacokinetic endpoint is applicable also for pharmaceuticals with positive genotoxicity signals. This change has a positive implication on "Refinement" (one of the 3Rs principles of animal research) enhancing the animal welfare by reducing the pain or discomfort at the maximally tolerated dose (MTD).

2. Genotoxicity Studies S2

S2(R1) Guidance on Genotoxicity Testing and Data Interpretation for Pharmaceuticals Intended for Human Use: The tripartite harmonized ICH guideline was finalized under Step 4 in 2011. This provides specific guidance for *in vitro* and *in vivo* tests and recommendations on the evaluation of test results. S2(R1) has a glossary of terms for genotoxicity testing to improve consistency in applications.This guidance replaces and also combines the ICH S2A and S2B guidelines.

S2A: Guidance on Specific Aspects of Regulatory Genotoxicity Tests for Pharmaceuticals: The tripartite harmonized ICH guideline was finalized under Step 4 in 1995, having a glossary of terms related to genotoxicity tests.

S2B Genotoxicity:A Standard Battery for Genotoxicity Testing for Pharmaceuticals: Guideline was finalized under Step 4 in 1997. This document addresses the fundamental areas of genotoxicity testing; identification of a standard set of assays to be conducted for registration, and the extent of confirmatory experimentation in any particular genotoxicity assay in the standard battery. Revision of this combined Guideline optimizes the standard genetic toxicology battery for prediction of potential human risks and interpretation of results. The ultimate goal is to improve risk characterization related to carcinogenic effects based on changes in the genetic material. The revised guidance describes internationally agreed standards for follow-up testing and interpretation of *in vitro* and *in vivo* positive results of the standard genetic toxicology battery, including assessment of non-relevant findings.

3. Toxicokinetics and Pharmacokinetics S3A-S3B

3.1 S3A Note for Guidance on Toxicokinetics: The Assessment of Systemic Exposure in Toxicity Studies: This guideline was finalized Step 4 in 1994, that gives guidance on developing test strategies in toxicokinetics and the need to integrate pharmacokinetics into toxicity testing, in order to aid in the interpretation of the toxicology findings and promote rational study design development.

3.2 S3A Questions and Answers: Note for Guidance on Toxicokinetics: The Assessment of Systemic Exposure—Focus on Microsampling: This IWG was endorsed by the ICH SC in 2014 since reaching Step 4 and publication within the ICH regions, experiences by all parties with the implementation of the S3A guideline on toxicokinetics have

resulted in the need for some clarification. The Questions and Answers developed by the S3A Implementation Working Group (IWG) are intended to facilitate the implementation of the S3A Guideline and especially to address the benefit and use of microsampling techniques in main study animals.

3.3 S3B Pharmacokinetics: Guidance for Repeated Dose Tissue Distribution Studies: The tripartite harmonized ICH Guideline was finalized Step 4 in 1994. This document gives guidance on circumstances for consideration of repeat dose tissue distribution studies (i.e. when appropriate data cannot be derived from other sources) and also provides recommendations on the conduct of such studies.

4. Toxicity Testing S4

4.1 S4 Duration of Chronic Toxicity Testing in Animals (Rodent and Non-Rodent Toxicity Testing): The recommendations given in this harmonized guideline finalized under Step 4 in 1998 are similar to those of the consultation draft issued in 1997. The text additionally incorporates the guidance for repeat-dose toxicity tests that was agreed at the time of ICH 1, in 1991 (reduction of the duration of repeat dose toxicity studies in the rat from 12 to 6 months).

5. Reproductive Toxicology S5

5.1 S5(R2) Detection of Toxicity to Reproduction for Medicinal Products and Toxicity to Male Fertility: This document finalized Step 4 in 1993 provides guidance on reproductive toxicity studies. It defines the periods of treatment required in animals to better reflect human exposure to medicinal products and more specific identification of risk stages. The addendum to the core ICH guideline S5 concerning male fertility studies was finalized in Step 4 in 1995, and amended in 2000, under the Maintenance Process. The amendments specially provide a better description of the testing concept addressing flexibility, pre-mating treatment duration, and recommendations on observations.

5.2 S5 (R3) Revision of S5 Guideline on Detection of Toxicity to Reproduction for Human Pharmaceuticals: The ICH SC endorsed this topic in 2015 based on experience gained with S5(R2) guideline adoption for reproduction toxicity testing of pharmaceuticals using the current and novel testing paradigms. Scientific, technological and regulatory knowledge has evolved significantly, with consequent new opportunities for modernizing testing paradigms to enhance human risk assessment, while potentially reducing animal use. The guideline has scopes to be revised or amended for greater clarity and full alignment with other recent ICH Guidelines, such as M3(R2), S6(R1) and S9.

6. Biotechnological Products S6

S6(R1) Preclinical Safety Evaluation of Biotechnology-Derived Pharmaceuticals: This document finalized under Step 4 in 1997, covers the pre-clinical safety testing requirements for biotechnological products. It addresses the issues related to the use of animal models of disease, determination of genotoxicity assays and carcinogenicity studies performance need and impact of antibody formation on the duration of toxicology studies. Scientific advances and experience gained from the original ICH S6 guideline call for this addendum. This addendum provides clarification on S6 and update of the following topics discussed in the original ICH S6 guideline, i.e. species selection, study design, immunogenicity, reproductive toxicity, developmental toxicity and assessment of carcinogenic potential. The harmonized addendum provides further complementary guidance to the S6 Guideline and helps to define the current recommendations and reduce the likelihood that substantial differences that exist among regions. The addendum reached Step 4 of the harmonization process in 2011 and was integrated as part II in the core Guideline that was then renamed S6(R1).

7. Pharmacology Studies S7A-S7B

7.1 S7A Safety Pharmacology Studies for Human Pharmaceuticals: This guideline reached Step 4 of the ICH process in 2000. This document gives definition, objectives, and scope of safety pharmacology studies. It also addresses the studies needed before the initiation of Phase 1 clinical studies as well as information needed for marketing.

7.2 S7B The Non-Clinical Evaluation of the Potential for Delayed Ventricular Repolarization (QT Interval Prolongation) by Human Pharmaceuticals: The guideline reached Step 4 of the ICH process on 2005, describes the non-clinical testing strategy for assessing the potential of a test substance to delay ventricular repolarization. This guideline includes information concerning non-clinical assays and integrated risk assessments.

8. Immunotoxicology Studies S8

S8 Immunotoxicity Studies for Human Pharmaceuticals: This guideline reached Step 4 of the ICH process on 2005. It provides recommendations on nonclinical immunosuppression potential testing for low molecular weight non-biologicals drugs intended for human use. This guidance is applicable to new pharmaceuticals as well as changes in marketed drug products for new indications or other variations on the current product label resulting in unaddressed and relevant toxicologic issues. Besides, the guideline might also apply to drugs in which clinical signs of immunosuppression are observed during clinical trials and the following approval to market. The term immunotoxicity in this guideline primarily refers to immunosuppression, i.e. increased susceptibility to infections or the development of tumours. This guideline does not provide specific guidance on how each immunotoxicity study should be performed.

9. Nonclinical Evaluation for Anticancer Pharmaceuticals S9

9.1 S9 Nonclinical Evaluation for Anticancer Pharmaceuticals: This guideline reached Step 4 on 2009, provides information for both small molecule and biotechnology-derived pharmaceuticals only intended to treat cancer in patients with late-stage or advanced disease regardless of the route of administration. It describes the type of studies and proposed duration of nonclinical studies needed for the development of anti-cancer pharmaceuticals and reference to other guidance as appropriate.

9.2 S9 Questions and Answers: Nonclinical Evaluation for Anticancer Pharmaceuticals: The ICH Steering Committee in 2014 endorsed this IWG guideline. Since reaching Step 4 and publication within the ICH regions implementation of the S9 guideline generates need for some clarification. The Questions and Answers developed by the S9 IWG are intended to facilitate the implementation of the S9 guideline clarifying its scope as well as its interpretation and implementation.

10. Photosafety Evaluation S10

S10 Photosafety Evaluation of Pharmaceuticals: The tripartite harmonized ICH Guideline reached Step 4 of the ICH process on 2013. This guideline provides international standards for photosafety assessment, harmonizes assessments parameters of photosafety in clinical trials and marketing authorizations for pharmaceuticals. It includes factors for initiation of and triggers for additional photosafety assessment and should be read in conjunction with ICH M3(R2), Section 14 on Photosafety Testing.

11. Nonclinical Paediatric Safety S11

S11 Nonclinical Safety Testing in Support of Development of Pediatric Medicines: This S11 topic was endorsed by the ICH SC in 2014 providing direction on the essential nonclinical safety studies supporting pediatric development program. It recommends standards for the conditions under which nonclinical juvenile animal testing is considered informative and necessary to support pediatric clinical trials and also provide guidance on the design of the studies. It is intended to streamline drug development and higher scientific rigor while minimizing the unnecessary use of animals.

Efficacy Guidelines

The guidelines developed under the efficacy heading is concerned with the designing, conduction, and reporting of clinical trials. It also covers novel types of medicines derived from biotechnological processes and the use of pharmacogenetics/pharmacogenomics techniques to produce better targeted medicines. All the 19 efficacy guideline topics address significant issues in the area of clinical trials, and is of particular importance to the industry. Until the introduction of the guideline 'Ethnic Factors' (E5) in 1998, there was a repetition of intensive phase III clinical trials when a drug is marketed in more than one region making the marketing approval costly and time consuming. Data collected from a foreign clinical trials conducted following guidance on the influence of ethnic factors (E5 and E10), and the principles of 'GCP' (E6) may be submitted for approval in any ICH region. Utilizing this guideline Pfizer successfully got the approval of Viagra® in Japan by conducting a bridging study (a vital part of the E5 guideline), rather than a repeated clinical trial(s).

E3 led to harmonization of reporting in the three regions by establishing a common format for clinical study reports providing the basic framework for the current CTD. As an international standard, wide acceptance of 'GCP' (E6) is a major achievement of ICH that formed the base for other national and international GCP guidelines. 'General Considerations for Clinical Trials' (E8) provides principles of trial design and further E9 'Statistical Principles for Clinical Trials' describe a framework for planning, conducting and interpreting sensitivity analyses of clinical trial data. 'Clinical Trials in Pediatric Populations'(E11) addressed issues like the timing of pediatric study initiation during medicinal product development, types of studies that can be conducted, age categories and most importantly ethical relevancy. 'Definitions in Pharmacogenetics/Pharmacogenomics' (E15), 'Qualification of Genomic Biomarkers' (E16) and the currently implemented 'Genomic Sampling' (E18) enumerates process to be adopted during the clinical trial for validation and qualification of genomic biomarkers along with evidence for their intended use and acceptance criteria. With the globalization of drug development, it has become evident that data from multi-regional clinical trials (MRCTs) is needed to be accepted by regulatory authorities for marketing approval of drugs. 'Multi-Regional Clinical Trials'(E17) provides general principles for the planning and design of MRCTs for acceptability in global regulatory submissions. The latest efficacy guideline Safety Data Collection E19 provides a concept for targeted approach while data collection in late-stage pre-marketing or post-marketing studies to reduce the burden of unnecessary data collection in favor of patient welfare.

Efficacy: 19 topics / 32 guidelines

1. Clinical Safety for Drugs used in Long-term Treatment E1

E1 The Extent of Population Exposure to Assess Clinical Safety for Drugs Intended for Long-Term Treatment of Non-Life Threatening Conditions: Finalized under Step 4 in 1994, this document gives recommendations on the numbers of patients and duration of exposure for the safety evaluation of drugs intended for the long-term treatment of non-life-threatening conditions.

2. Pharmacovigilance E2

2.1 E2A Clinical Safety Data Management: Definitions and Standards for Expedited Reporting: This document gives standard definitions and terminology for critical aspects of clinical safety reporting. It also gives guidance on the handling of expedited (rapid) reporting of adverse drug reactions in the investigational phase of drug development.

2.2 E2B(R3) Maintenance of the Clinical Safety Data Management including Data Elements for Transmission of Individual Case Safety Reports: The harmonized guideline was finalized as E2B under Step 4 in 1997 and amended for Maintenance as E2B(R1) on 2000. Post Step 4 editorial corrections were given in 2001 second revision and renamed E2B(R2).

E2B Questions and Answers (R5) Clinical Safety Data Management Questions and Answers: Experiences on the implementation of the First Revision of E2B guideline have resulted in the need for some clarification, supplementing the Questions and Answers document intends to clarify key issues.

E2B(R3) Clinical Safety Data Management: Data Elements for Transmission of Individual Case Safety Reports: In 2005, the ICH E2B(R3) guideline was released for consultation at Step 2 of the ICH process. Changes proposed to the E2B(R2) guideline included the provision of additional fields, greater granularity of some fields, and the greater use of controlled vocabularies. In 2006, the ICH Steering Committee took a critical decision that technical specifications should no longer be developed solely within ICH, but should be created in collaboration with Standards Development Organisations (SDOs) to enable extensive interoperability across regulatory and healthcare communities. This guideline was subsequently submitted to ISO for development under this process. The E2B(R3) Step 2 guideline was updated based upon feedback received during consultation in 2005, as well as additional considerations following its submission to ISO for development as an International Standard. Key parts of this updated guideline were incorporated into the ICH Implementation Guide for Electronic Transmission of Individual Case Safety Reports Message Specification which is currently undergoing development as an ISO standard.

E2B (R3) IWG Implementation: Electronic Transmission of Individual Case Safety Reports: In 2013, the ICH Steering Committee endorsed the establishment of the IWG on E2B(R3) to assist with the implementation of the E2B(R3). Implementation Guide (published in 2013) helped to facilitate the transition from E2B (R2) to E2B (R3) supporting its tasks for the use of constrained ISO IDMP terminologies in ICSRs, as well as maintenance of technical documents related to E2B (R3). In 2014, the IWG finalized the first version of Questions and Answers to clarify questions and comments for E2B (R3) implementation.

2.3 E2C(R2) Clinical Safety Data Management: Periodic Safety Update Reports for Marketed Drugs: This is a crucial document providing guidance on the format and content of safety updates, need to be provided at intervals to regulatory authorities after marketing approval of drug products. The guideline is intended to ensure that worldwide safety related information is provided to authorities with maximum efficiency at a defined time interval after marketing of drug product to avoid duplication of testing effort. Based on the comments made by the members of the Expert Working Group on CIOMS V recommendations and the PhRMA-EFPIA working document, an addendum has been finalized and reached Step 4 in 2003. The addendum further clarifies guidance for the preparation of PSURs as specified in E2C. Additionally, the document addresses some new concepts, not in E2C reflecting current pharmaco-

vigilance practice needs, including Proprietary Information (Confidentiality), Executive Summary, Summary Bridging Report, Addendum Reports and Risk Management Program.

Addendum: Periodic Safety Update Reports for Marketed Drugs

E2C(R2) Periodic Safety Update Reports for Marketed Drugs: This revision was endorsed by the ICH SC in 2010. The newly created E2C(R2) Expert Working Group (EWG) is to evaluate the ICH pharmacovigilance documentation, conduct a gap and possible improvement analysis of ICH E2C, E2E and E2F and draft a new ICH guideline E2C(R2) covering periodic benefit risk evaluation reporting.

E2C (R2) Questions and Answers: Periodic Benefit-Risk Evaluation Report: The ICH SC endorsed the establishment of the IWG on E2C(R2) to assist with the implementation of the new revision (R2) of the E2C guideline, that was finalized under Step 4 of the ICH process in 2012. The revision has introduced new concepts and principles linked to the evolution of the traditional PSUR from an interval safety report to cumulative benefit-risk report and with a change in focus from individual case reports to more aggregate data evaluation. This supplementary Questions and Answers document was finalized under Step 4 in 2014 intending to clarify key issues.

2.4 E2D Post-Approval Safety Data Management: Definitions and Standards for Expedited Reporting: This document finalized under Step 4 in 2003, provides a standardized procedure for post-approval safety data management including expedited reporting to the relevant authority. The definition of the terms and concepts specific to the post-approval phase are also provided. Clinical safety data management definitions of E2A were maintained in this document as post-approval safety data management as off seriousness definition. The data management practices were standardized in the processing of cases obtained from consumers, literature and internets specific to post-approval safety data. Good Case Management practice was focused and recommended for expedited reporting with clear definitions.

2.5 E2E Pharmacovigilance Planning: This guideline aids in planning pharmacovigilance activities, especially preparation for the early postmarketing period of a new drug (in this Guideline, the term "drug" denotes chemical entities, biotechnology-derived products, and vaccines). Main focus of this guideline is on Safety Specification, and Pharmacovigilance Plan submitted at the time of license application.

2.6 E2F Development Safety Update Report (DSUR): The main focus of the DSUR is to acquire data from interventional clinical trials (referred to in this document as "clinical trials") conducted by commercial or non-commercial sponsors on investigational drugs including biologicals, with or without marketing approval. Following the completion of the E2F as a Step 4 guideline, EWG developed DSUR examples to help commercial and non-commercial sponsors on proper use of the guideline.

3. Clinical Study Reports E3

3.1 E3 Structure and Content of Clinical Study Reports: This document finalized under Step 4 in 1995, provides the format and content of study report acceptable in all three ICH region. It guides on the format of core report suitable for all submissions and appendices that are needed to be available but not to be submitted for all cases.

3.2 E3 Questions and Answers: Structure and Content of Clinical Study Reports: In 2011, the ICH Steering Committee endorsed the establishment of an E3 Implementation Working Group to clarify issues identified since the implementation of the ICH E3 Guideline in 1996 that hinder consistent implementation of that guideline.

4. Dose-Response Studies E4

E4 Dose-Response Information to Support Drug Registration: This document recommendations on the design and conduct of dose relationship studies assessing blood level and clinical responses throughout the clinical development of a new drug.

5. Ethnic Factors E5

5.1 E5(R1) Ethnic Factors in the Acceptability of Foreign Clinical Data: This document finalized under Step 4 in 1998, addresses the intrinsic characteristics of the drug recipient and extrinsic characteristics associated with environment and culture that could affect the results of clinical studies carried out in particular geographic regions. It describes the concept of the "bridging study" as a new region may request to determine whether data from one region are applicable to the population of another region.

5.2 E5 Questions and Answers (R1): Ethnic Factors in the Acceptability of Foreign Clinical Data: Since reaching Step 4 and publication within the ICH regions, this supplementary Questions and Answers document intends to clarify key issues.

6. Good Clinical Practice E6

E6(R2) Good Clinical Practice (GCP): This GCP document describes the responsibilities and expectations of all participants involved in clinical trials conduction, i.e. investigators, monitors, sponsors, and IRBs. The guideline covers all aspects of clinical trial monitoring, reporting and archiving and incorporating addenda on the Essential Documents and on the Investigator's Brochure which had been agreed earlier through the ICH process. This harmonized guideline was amended in 2016 with an integrated Addendum to encourage implementation of improved and more efficient approaches to clinical trial design, conduct, oversight, recording and reporting while continuing to ensure human subject protection and reliability of trial results.

Electronic records and standard essential documents intended to increase clinical trial quality and efficiency was also updated.

7. Clinical Trials in Geriatrics Population E7

7.1 E7 Studies in Support of Special Populations: Geriatrics: The E7 recommendations on the special considerations applicable for design and conduct of clinical trials of medicines having significant use in the elderly.

7.2 E7 Questions & Answers: Studies in Support of Special Populations: Geriatrics: This supplementary Questions and Answers document clarify important issues regarding implementation of the E7 guideline.

8. General Considerations for Clinical Trials E8

This document sets out the general scientific principles for the conduct, performance, and control of clinical trials. The guideline addresses all aspects of the clinical trial design and execution widely.

9. E9 Statistical Principles for Clinical Trials

9.1 E9 (R1) Addendum: Statistical Principles for Clinical Trials: This topic was endorsed by the ICH SC in 2014. This addendum provides clarification on E9 and gives an update on clinical trials agreed framework for planning, conducting and interpreting sensitivity analyses of clinical trial data. This addendum focuses on statistical principles related to estimands and sensitivity analysis but not the use or acceptability of specific statistical procedures or methods. The primary focus of the addendum is confirmatory clinical trials through a variety of mid- and late-stage clinical trials may also be in scope. It promotes harmonized standards on a framework for planning, conducting and interpreting sensitivity analyses of clinical trial data.

9.2 E9 Statistical Principles for Clinical Trials: This biostatistical guideline describes the essential design and analysis considerations of clinical trials, primarily the 'confirmatory' (hypothesis testing) trials that are the basis for demonstrating effectiveness.

10. Choice of Control Group in Clinical Trials E10

E10 Choice of Control Group and Related Issues in Clinical Trials: Step 4 in 2000, this document addresses the issues related to control group choices in clinical trials considering the ethical and inferential properties. Limitations concerned to the choice of different kinds of control groups are also discussed. It points out the assay sensitivity problem in active control equivalence/non-inferiority trials that may limit the usefulness of trial design in many circumstances.

11. Clinical Trial in the Pediatric Population E11

11.1 E11 Clinical Investigation of Medicinal Products in the Pediatric Population: This document guides on the conduct of clinical trials in pediatric populations. This document facilitates in the development of safe and effective use of the medicinal product in pediatrics.

11.2 E11 (R1) Addendum: Clinical Investigation of Medicinal Products in the Pediatric Population: This topic was endorsed by the ICH Steering Committee in 2014, since the adoption of the E11 guideline in 2000, pediatric drug development has been enhanced by advancements in several areas of general adult drug development. Targeted scientific and technical issues relevant to pediatric populations, regulatory requirements for pediatric study plans, and infrastructures for undertaking complex trials in pediatric patient populations have been considerably advanced in the last decade, without a parallel development of harmonized guidance in these areas. This addendum is proposed to address new scientific and technical knowledge advances in pediatric drug development.

12. Clinical Evaluation by Therapeutic Category E12

E12 Principles for Clinical Evaluation of New Antihypertensive Drugs: This document provides guidance on clinical evaluation of new antihypertensive drugs. A set of general 'principles' was agreed upon by all three ICH regions covering the study endpoints and trial designs. Since there are a few differences in the requirements of the three regions that have not been harmonized, this document is considered an "ICH Principle Document" rather than an "ICH Guideline."

13. Clinical Evaluation E14

13.1 E14 The Clinical Evaluation of QT/QTc Interval Prolongation and Proarrhythmic Potential for Non-Antiarrhythmic Drugs: This document provides recommendations concerning the design, conduct, analysis, and interpretation of clinical studies intended to assess the potential of a drug to delay cardiac repolarization. Assessment drugs effects on cardiac repolarization are the subject of active investigation. This assessment includes testing the effects of new agents on the QT/QTc interval as well as data collection on any other cardiovascular adverse events. Investigational approach for a particular drug should be individualized depending on the pharmacodynamic, pharmacokinetic and proposed clinical use and safety characteristics of the product. This document may be reevaluated and revised in future following accumulation of additional non-clinical and clinical data.

13.2 E14 Questions and Answers (R3): The Clinical Evaluation of QT/QTc Interval Prolongation and Proarrhythmic Potential for Non-Antiarrhythmic Drugs: The revision of the E14 Questions and Answers document was endorsed by the ICH SC in 2010. This new document is intended to clarify some issues which are not explicated clearly in the ICH E14 guideline or the following Questions and Answers document that was generated in 2008.

E14 Questions and Answers (R1): In 2012, the second set of Questions and Answers was developed and approved by the Steering Committee for integration.

E14 Questions and Answers (R2): In 2014, the third set of Questions and Answers was developed.

E14 Questions and Answers (R3): In 2015, the E14 Questions and Answers(R2) was revised to generate harmonized guidance on how concentration response modeling could be used for regulatory decision making.

14. Definitions in Pharmacogenetics/ Pharmacogenomics E15

E15 Definitions for Genomic Biomarkers, Pharmacogenomics, Pharmacogenetics, Genomic Data, and Sample Coding Categories: This Guideline defines key terms of pharmacogenomics and pharmacogenetics discipline, namely genomic biomarkers, pharmacogenomics, pharmacogenetics, genomic data, and sample coding categories. Validation and qualification of genomic biomarkers, evidence for their intended use and acceptance criteria across ICH regions are outside of the scope of this guideline. As per new scientific knowledge in the discipline of pharmacogenomics and pharmacogenetics emerges, the current guidance has been reviewed and expanded as appropriate.

15. Qualification of Genomic Biomarkers E16

E16 Biomarkers Related to Drug or Biotechnology Product Development: Context, Structure, and Format of Qualification Submissions: The harmonized guideline was finalized under Step 4 in 2010. As defined in ICH E15, this document describes recommendations on context, structure, and format of regulatory submissions for qualification of genomic biomarkers.

16. Multi-Regional Clinical Trials E17

E17 General principle on planning/designing Multi-Regional Clinical Trials: This topic was endorsed by the ICH Steering Committee in 2014 to provide guidance on general principles on planning/designing Multi-Regional Clinical Trial (MRCT). Regulatory agencies are currently facing challenges in evaluating data from MRCTs for drug approval, and it is necessary to develop a harmonized international guideline to promote conducting MRCT appropriately, mainly focusing on scientific issues in planning/designing MRCTs. This new Guideline complement the guidance on MRCTs provided in E5(R1) guideline and facilitate MRCT data acceptance by multiple regulatory agencies.

17. E18 Genomic Sampling E18

E18 Genomic Sampling and Management of Genomic Data: Endorsed by the ICH Steering Committee in 2014, this new guidance is proposed to provide guidance on genomic sample collection to evaluate the efficacy and safety of a drug for regulatory approval. In recent years, genomic information is increasingly included in drug label relevant for the benefit/risk evaluation. To accumulate such data during drug development and throughout the product lifecycle, genomic samples should be collected in clinical trials and other studies following a particular methodology and be stored for certain periods. It has been noted that the collection rate of such samples is still low in many ICH regions and was deemed necessary to harmonize the guidance that was already published independently by the different ICH regulatory authorities. Harmonization across regions on this topic is intended to maximize

the information gathered from the studies, e.g. sample collection and analysis (including ethical considerations) and facilitate implementation of pharmacogenomics for the benefit of all stakeholders.

18. E19 Safety Data Collection

E19 Optimisation of Safety Data Collection: Endorsed in 2016, this new guideline is proposed to provide harmonized guidance on when it would be appropriate to use a targeted approach to safety data collection in some late-stage pre-marketing or post-marketing studies, and how such an approach would be implemented. Patient welfare protection during drug development is critically important. Unnecessary data collection is always burdensome to patients and also serve as a disincentive to clinical research participation. Patients burden can be reduced by tailoring safety data collection. The proposed guideline is consistent with risk-based approaches and quality-by-design principles.

19. E20 Adaptive Clinical Trials

ICH assembly endorsed this topic in June 2018. An informal WG was established in June 2019 to develop a concept paper and business plan.

Multidisciplinary Guidelines

These are the unique cross-cutting topics that do not conventionally fit into one of the Quality, Safety and Efficacy categories. The ICH medical terminology (MedDRA), the Common Technical Document (CTD) and the development of Electronic Standards for the Transfer of Regulatory Information (ESTRI) are some of them. Multidisciplinary topics impact the area such as regulatory communications, electronic communication, and timing of toxicity studies about clinical studies.

Multidisciplinary: 12 topics / 11 guidelines

1. MedDRA Terminology M1

1.1 MedDRA Medical Dictionary for Regulatory Activities: The ICH Steering Committee approved the development of a Medical Dictionary for Regulatory Activities in 1997 and the terminology launched in 1999. All information about MedDRA and the 'Points to Consider' documents developed for every MedDRA version developed over the years are available on the MedDRA page under the Work Products.

2. Electronic Standards M2

2.1 Electronic Standards for the Transfer of Regulatory Information: The ICH Steering Committee established the M2 EWG in 1994 with the objective of facilitating international electronic communication by evaluating and recommending, Electronic Standards for the Transfer of Regulatory Information (ESTRI) that is intended to meet the requirements of the pharmaceutical companies and regulatory authorities. The M2 EWG is involved in a number of activities:

- Recommendation for use by open international standards (M2 Recommendations),
- Development of specifications for electronic messages of the E2B(R2),
- Guideline on Clinical Safety Data Management,
- Data Elements for Transmission of Individual Case Safety Reports,
- Development of M4 Common Technical Document (CTD),
- Input on the technical provision of ICH E2B(R3), and
- Through M5 EWG progress for respective standards of the Standards Development Organisation (SDO) process.

In 2010, the ICH SC modified the mandate of the M2 EWG. Notable changes included a newly established M8 EWG undertakes agreement on Electronic Common Technical Document (eCTD). The M2 EWG is no longer directly involved in the development of technical solutions in relation to E2B(R3) and M5 topics, but instead, provide a framework for the efficient and effective development of the solutions to these topics. As per the new mandate, the M2 EWG is responsible for evaluation and recommendation on standards and is also responsible for SDO relationship management.

3. Nonclinical Safety Studies M3

3.1 M3(R2) Guidance on Nonclinical Safety Studies for the Conduct of Human Clinical Trials and Marketing Authorization for Pharmaceuticals: The recommendations of this revised guidance further harmonize the nonclinical safety studies to support the various stages of clinical development among the regions of the European Union (EU), Japan, and the United States. The existing guidance represents the consensus that exists regarding the type and duration of nonclinical safety studies and their timing to support the conduct of human clinical trials and marketing authorization for pharmaceuticals.

3.2 M3(R2) Questions and Answers: Guidance on Non-Clinical Safety Studies for the Conduct of Human Clinical Trials and Marketing Authorization for Pharmaceuticals: The complexity of the M3(R2) guidance with its broader scope and numerous changes in recommendations from the M3(R1) guidance have generated questions. To clarify the crucial issues of this document, the SC has endorsed the establishment of an M3(R2) IWG for development of Questions and Answers. The document with the first set of Questions and Answers addressing Limit Dose for Toxicity Studies, Metabolites and Reversibility of Toxicity was finalized under Step 4 in 2011.

4. Common Technical Document M4

The M4 CTD was agreed upon by the SC in 2000, and all information about this is available on the CTD page under the Work Products.

5. Data Elements and Standards for Drug Dictionaries M5

The lack of internationally harmonized standards related to core sets of medicinal product information and medicinal product terminology is hindering the scientific evaluation and comparison of product data. This applies in particular to the area of pharmacovigilance, where the exchange and management of medicinal product information in expedited and periodic adverse reaction reports at the international level are vital aspects of ensuring drug safety. In 2004, the ICH Steering Committee approved the development of the ICH M5 guideline with the aim of providing guidance on the harmonized standards being proposed by the ICH M5 EWG to facilitate the exchange and practical use of medicinal product data by regulators and pharmaceutical industry. In 2005, the ICH M5 guideline was released for consultation at Step 2 of the ICH process, along with controlled vocabularies, lists for Routes of Administration and Units of Measurement.

In 2006, the ICH SC took a critical decision that technical specifications should no longer be developed solely within ICH, but should be created in collaboration with Standards Development Organisations (SDOs) to enable broader interoperability across regulatory and healthcare communities. This guideline was subsequently submitted to ISO, for development under this process. The M5 Step 2 guideline was updated based upon feedback received during consultation in 2005, as well as additional considerations following its submission to ISO for development as an International Standard. Key parts of this updated guideline were incorporated into the ICH Implementation Guide for Identification of Medicinal Products (IDMP) which has been developed as five different ISO IDMP standards. The fourth one ISO 11616:2017 'Regulated pharmaceutical product information' standards document was published in October 2017.

6. Gene Therapy M6

M6 Virus and Gene Therapy Vector Shedding and Transmission: This topic was endorsed by the ICH SC in 2009 to provide recommendations to industry and regulators on non-clinical, and clinical studies and guidance on the use of analytical assays for the detection and characterization of shed virus. This guideline also provides recommendations on how to use and interpret non-clinical data in order to determine whether or not a virus and gene therapy vector shedding studies are necessary. The assessment of shedding can be utilized to estimate the likelihood of transmission of virus and gene therapy vectors to third parties, such as healthcare workers and family members.

7. Genotoxic Impurities M7

M7 (R1) Assessment and Control of DNA Reactive (Mutagenic) Impurities in Pharmaceuticals to Limit Potential Carcinogenic Risk: The ICH M7 guideline was finalized in 2014 offering guidance on the analysis of Structure Activity Relationships (SAR) for genotoxicity. This is proposed to offer guidance on the analysis of structure-activity relationships (SAR) for genotoxicity. This guideline is intended to resolve questions such as whether impurities with similar alerts potential and having a similar mechanism of action can be combined in calculating a Threshold of Toxicological Concern (TCC) and whether the TTC may differ based on differences in the approved duration of use.

8. Electronic Common Technical Document (eCTD) M8

In 2010, the ICH SC endorsed the establishment of an EWG/IWG for the eCTD and assigned the topic code "M8". Previously eCTD work was undertaken by the M2 EWG. The M8 supports the progression of the eCTD through the Standards Development Organisation (SDO) process contributing to developing the eCTD as an International Standard. As the 2008 Steering Committee decision the next major version of the eCTD was developed in collaboration with SDOs, first as a Health Level Seven (HL7) standard, and then as an ISO standard. The M8 works to maintain the current ICH specifications for the eCTD and Study Tagging File.

CTD Quality Implementation Working Group: In 2007, the ICH SC endorsed the establishment of a CTD Quality Implementation Working Group to assist the then M2 eCTD IWG subgroup with addressing Questions/Change Requests received about the organization of the Quality section of the eCTD (Modules 2 and 3). This group continues to work to address the quality issues which have been identified for integration as Questions and Answers into the Change Request/Questions and Answers document available on the ESTRI page.

9. Biopharmaceutics Classification System-based Biowaivers M9

The ICH Management Committee in 2016 endorsed this topic. This new multidisciplinary guideline is proposed to address the Biopharmaceutics Classification System (BCS)-based biowaivers. BCS-based biowaivers are applicable to BCS Class I and III drugs but are not recognized worldwide. The pharmaceutical companies have to follow different approaches in different regions. This guideline provides recommendations to support the biopharmaceutics classification of medicinal products and provide recommendations to support the waiver of bioequivalence studies for better harmonization of current regional guidelines/guidance and support streamlined global drug development.

10. Bioanalytical Method Validation M10

This topic was endorsed by the ICH Management Committee in 2016. This new multi-disciplinary guideline is applicable to bioanalytical method validation for analyses of non-clinical and clinical study samples. Reliable data derived through validated bioanalytical methods are essential for the review of the marketing authorization application. This guideline provides recommendations on the scientific, regulatory requirements for bioanalysis conducted during the development of drugs of both chemical and biological origins. It also addresses issues on method validation by considering the characteristics of the analytical methods used in bioanalysis, e.g. chromatographic assay and ligand binding assay. The harmonized bioanalytical method validation guideline promote the prompt, rational and effective non-clinical and clinical studies, thereby advancing the mission of the ICH.

11. M11 Clinical Electronic Structured Harmonised Protocol (CeSHarP)

This topic endorsed by the ICH Management Committee in November 2018 proposed to provide a template to include identification of Headers, common text and a set of data fields and terminologies for efficient data exchange. It also provides technical specification to be used as open non-proprietary standard to enable electronic exchange of clinical protocol information.

12. M12 Drug Interaction Studies

An informal WG was established in June 2019 to develop a concept paper and business plan on this topic.

The Guidelines Currently Undergoing Public Consultations

E9 (R1) EWG: Estimands and Sensitivity Analysis in Clinical Trial and Manufacture of Drug Substances: This addendum provides clarification on E9 and updates on the estimand choice for sensitivity analyses of clinical trial data describing an agreed framework for planning, conducting and

Table 3.1: The International Conference of Harmonisation (ICH) comprehensive working group guidelines

Quality	Safety	Efficacy	Multidisciplinary
Q1 Stability Q1A–Q1F	S1 Carcinogenicity Studies S1A–S1C	E1 Clinical Safety for Drugs used in Long-Term Treatment E1	M1 MedDRA Terminology M1
Q2 Analytical Validation Q2	S2 Genotoxicity Studies S2	E2 Pharmacovigilance E2A–E2F	M2 Electronic Standards M2
Q3 Impurities Q3A–Q3D	S3 Toxicokinetics and Pharmacokinetics S3A–S3B	E3 Clinical Study Reports E3	M3 Nonclinical Safety Studies M3
Q4 Pharmacopoeias Q4A–Q4B	S4 Toxicity Testing S4	E4 Dose-Response Studies E4	M4 Common Technical Document M4
Q5 Quality of Biotechnological Products Q5A–Q5E	S5 Reproductive Toxicology S5	E5 Ethnic Factors E5	M5 Data Elements and Standards for Drug Dictionaries M5
Q6 Specifications Q6A–Q6B	S6 Biotechnological Products S6	E6 Good Clinical Practice E6	M6 Gene Therapy M6
Q7 Good Manufacturing Practice Q7	S7 Pharmacology Studies S7A–S7B	E7 Clinical Trials in Geriatric Population E7	M7 Genotoxic Impurities M7
Q8 Pharmaceutical Development Q8	S8 Immunotoxicology Studies S8	E8 General Considerations for Clinical Trials E8	M8 Electronic Common Technical Document (eCTD) M8
Q9 Quality Risk Management Q9	S9 Nonclinical Evaluation for Anticancer Pharmaceuticals S9	E9 Statistical Principles for Clinical Trials E9	M9 Biopharmaceutics Classification System-based Biowaivers M9
Q10 Pharmaceutical Quality System Q10	S10 Photosafety Evaluation S10	E10 Choice of Control Group in Clinical Trials E10	M10 Bioanalytical Method Validation M10
Q11 Development and Manufacture of Drug Substances Q11	S11 Nonclinical Paediatric Safety S11	E11 Clinical Trials in Pediatric Population E11	M11 Clinical Electronic Structured Harmonised Protocol M11
Q12 Lifecycle Management Q12	–	E12 Clinical Evaluation by Therapeutic Category E12	M12 Drug Interaction Studies M12
Q13 Continuous Manufacturing of Drug Substances and Drug Products	–	E13 –	–
Q14 Analytical Procedure Development	–	E14 Clinical Evaluation of QT E14	–
–	–	E15 Definitions in Pharmaco-genetics/Pharmacogenomics E15	–
–	–	E16 Qualification of Genomic Biomarkers E16	–
–	–	E17 Multi-Regional Clinical Trials E17	–
–	–	E18 Genomic Sampling E18	–
–	–	E19 Safety Data Collection E19	–
–	–	E20 Adaptive Clinical Trials E20	–

interpreting. E9(R1) focuses on statistical principles for estimands and sensitivity analysis of clinical trial data.

S5 (R3) EWG: Detection of Toxicity to Reproduction for Human Pharmaceuticals: The revised S5 guideline is proposed to provide human safety assurance equivalent to that provided by current testing paradigms.

E2B(R3) IWG: In June 2013, the ICH SC endorsed the establishment of an E2B (R3) IWG to develop Questions and Answers document to help the transition from E2B(R2) to (R3), Individual Case Safety Report (ICSR) Implementation Guide released in 2013.

ICH: ADVANCING HARMONISATION FOR BETTER GLOBAL HEALTH

The purpose of ICH is to implement harmonization in the interpretation and application of technical guidelines and requirements for pharmaceutical product registration in order to reduce duplication of testing in the research and development of new medicines. Although ICH's initial focus was the development of guidelines for use in the ICH regions, where previously the vast majority of new pharmaceutical products were developed. The face of drug development has become increasingly global since ICH's inception in 1990. ICH through its harmonization initiatives is adding significant progress to drug development activities. ICH is doing ground breaking work in harmonizing drug regulatory requirements among the global partners. For three decades the ICH has achieved well-deserved success in developing scientific consensus between industry and regulatory experts and also persuaded commitment in the regulatory authorities towards implementation of the Tripartite Harmonised Guidelines and recommendations. In this third decade, most of the ICH activity was being directed towards extending the benefits of harmonization beyond the ICH regions. Till 2018, 112 guidelines have been produced by ICH

covering 56 significant topics that are currently being adopted and implemented by the regulatory agencies. WHO is playing a crucial role as observer in ICH by coordinating liaising between ICH and non-ICH countries to ensure information exchange between developed and developing countries.

Availability of internationally acceptable guidelines by ICH has facilitated the establishment of uniform procedures across the global organization, particularly for clinical study protocols and reports. ICH has promoted not only international harmonization but also facilitated intra-company globalization by the breakthrough adoption of common CTD and eCTD. CTD has enabled the industry to workout regulatory submissions far faster as a single technical dossier is required to be submitted to all competent authorities in ICH regions. Adoption of eCTD further streamlined the dossier preparation and submission process, augmenting resource and time savings. The M3 guideline directs on type and duration of nonclinical safety studies and their timing to support the conduct of human clinical trials and marketing authorization for pharmaceuticals having a positive impact on the drug development cycle. Clinical trials conducted following the ICH Ethnic Factors guideline facilitates simultaneous worldwide launch of new drugs. ICH guidelines also facilitate more comfortable management of the Product Life Cycle. Harmonized guideline on stability requirements for post-approval changes has significantly reduced the workload associated with multiple stability studies.

ICH has contributed significantly towards making the pharma regulatory guideline available and accessible in other non-ICH countries with a more comprehensive international understanding and acceptance. Unified and coordinated operating practices following the latest efficacy guidelines has enhanced patient safety in the clinical trials process. One of the most important outcomes of the harmonization initiative is in the efficacy area which has effectively reduced time and resources dedicated to new drug development. Implementation of the efficacy guidelines has reached out for faster and easier access to new drugs for the emerging markets such as Asia and Latin America. These markets have become increasingly important in the global economy, with the Asian market alone predicted to have contributed 15–20% of global pharmaceutical sales. Many pharmaceuticals are now conducting drug development following the principles of ICH guidelines. Most of the essential guidelines of ICH has been finalized in the past ten years going through a lengthy implementation process. Initial adoption and implementation of ICH guidelines is costly though on a long run its worth value for money. As new drugs pass through the development cycle in short period the actual benefits and value of the ICH process become obvious minimizing need for duplicate studies. A combined approach of ICH towards Quality, Safety, and Efficacy of drugs has streamlined the drug development process, and enabled to bring new drugs to the global market swiftly using fewer resources.

ICH in the last three decades has gone through the crucial stages of conception, initiation, establishment, expansion, and diversification with continuous, regular contribution and upgradation of guidelines. Maintenance of these high standard activities is essential for the thieving future of ICH. ICH has gone through significant reformation and organization changes in 2015, with the aim to promote broad participation and greater interaction between the competent authorities and industry associations. ICH now maintains a full-time secretariat functional with six members. Currently, in place of Steering Committee, Assembly has taken over to bring together both Member Representatives and Observer Delegates. Assembly is the new governing body which meets biannually to oversee both the maintenance process and the new initiatives. The Management Committee has 21 representatives from the six Founding Members to supervise operational aspects along with administrative and financial matters. ICH now provides a more adaptive common forum for communication to both regulators and industries. ICH harmonization process has proved to be tremendously beneficial for identifying the best scientific practice that stout to be applied uniformly across their regions. The harmonization process has improved the capacity of regulators through more efficient and collaborative use of resources. The impact of having led the regulatory agencies to adopt changes in practice and regulations far faster than would have been possible otherwise. In the absence of the ICH process, the regulatory agencies in the three major regions would continued to diverge in their practices and organizations engaged in drug development would have worked on regional rather than global basis. The time and resource saving have most importantly resulted in burden reduction on regulators leading to faster approval and delivering of new therapies to patients at a lower cost.

BIBLIOGRAPHY

1. Drug Benefits and Risks: International Textbook of Clinical Pharmacology, revised 2nd edition Edited by C.J. van Boxtel, B. Santoso, and I.R. Edwards. IOS Press and Uppsala Monitoring Centre, 2008. © 2008 The authors. All rights reserved.
2. Drug Regulation: History, Present, and Future1 Lembit Rägo, Budiono Santoso. Chapter 6.
3. EFPIA. www.efpia.org
4. EU. www.eudra.org
5. FDA. www.fda.gov
6. Health Canada. Overview and Reform of International Council for Harmonisation of technical requirements for pharmaceuticals for human use.www.ich-fda-rcc-nov2015-ccr-overview-apercu-eng.pdf.
7. ICH. http://www.ich.org/home.html.

8. Irs A, De Hoog TJ, Rägo L. Development of marketing authorization procedures for pharmaceuticals. In:Freemantle N, Hill S, editors. Evaluating pharmaceuticals for health policy and reimbursement. London: Blackwell BMJ Books; 2004. p. 3-24.

9. JPMA. www.jpma.or.jp/12english/index.html

10. MHW. www.mhw.go.jp/english/

11. PhRMA. www.phrma.org

12. Ratanwijitrasin S, Wondemagegnehu E. Effective drug regulation. A multi-country study. Geneva: World Health Organization; 2002.

13. Rägo L. ICH and global cooperation in the new millennium: WHO perspective. In: Cone M, editor. Proceedings of the fifth international conference on harmonization. San Diego, 2000. London: PJB Publications Ltd; 2001. p. 299–304.

14. The Value and Benefits of ICH to Industry. 2000. Caroline Nutley. Pharmaceutical Research and Manufacturers of America.

Basic Concept of Quality Control and Quality Assurance

CHAPTER OVERVIEW

KEY POINTS

- Depending upon the usability quality refers to the characteristics of a product. Quality of pharmaceutical products depends on adherence to purity, safety and efficacy parameters. Comprehensive Quality Control (QC) is a process employed to ensure a certain level of quality in a product or service. The basic objective of the pharmaceutical QC is to implement and practice procedure that ensures predefined desired quality standards in the finished product with minimum defect.
- QC laboratories are designed, developed and furnished with facilities as required by guidelines for the operations of testing of all raw, intermediate and finished products. The basic responsibility of the QC department is to approve or reject the finished products after testing as per procedures based on the specifications of quality, identity, and purity of drug product.
- Quality assurance (QA) guarantee the integrity of the quality management process by practicing concepts that impact the management plan concerning all matters that collectively influence the quality of the product. QA practices in accordance with the cGMP guidelines for the development of a globally competent quality compliance system in the pharmaceutical manufacturing facility.
- The amount spent towards efforts and maintenance works related to minimization of product quality deficiencies is called cost of quality. Six Sigma philosophy emphasizes on building quality into process striving for zero defect performance which can smooth out increased cost of quality by implementing better process control. The quality manual is prepared by the higher authorities of the company to describe the quality policy and the entire administration and employees are meant to work accordingly.
- Quality Management Programme (QMP) guideline describes the comprehensive quality systems model consistent with the cGMP regulatory requirements intended for the proper implementation of the quality system and risk management approaches. Total Quality Management (TQM) guideline enumerates appropriate approach of management to control quality in cost-effective manner. ICH Q10 guideline 'Pharmaceutical Quality System' recommends the requirements of a harmonized model for the pharmaceutical quality system to be followed by the pharmaceutical companies throughout the lifecycle of a product.

QUALITY

Quality is reflected as the features and characteristics of a product that in turn signifies its ability of customer satisfaction based on implied needs. Quality demonstrated notable product characteristics and performance excellence. Quality is relative to the product use criteria and the circumstances under which it is used. Quality is also subjective to personal discretion as each person has his or her definition of quality. Quality products ensure the survival of the companies in this era of cut-throat competition as quality plays a crucial role in differentiating an organization from its competitors. Pharmaceutical companies have to follow strict quality control guidelines not only for customers' satisfaction but are bound by the regulatory obligations.

Manufacturers View on Quality

1. Fulfilling all requirements as per the rules and regulations (Drugs and Cosmetic Act).
2. Fulfilling all requirements as per company's predecided quality objectives.
3. Fulfilling all requirements of consumer and providing consumer satisfaction.

Regulators Views on Quality

1. Drug or medicine should fulfill all requirements laid down in specifications (Drugs and Cosmetic Act.)
2. The product should be stable, and content should be the same as per label until the expiry of the product.

Doctors View on Quality

1. Medicine should be effective
2. Medicine should be easily available
3. Medicine should be safe

Consumers Views on Quality

1. Medicine should be efficient
2. Medicine should be effective
3. Medicine should be economic
4. Medicine should be safe
5. Medicine dosage form should be convenient to administer.

IMPORTANCE OF QUALITY

Definition and meaning of quality vary from person to person as every person looks at quality from a different point of view. Definition of quality especially for the medicinal products is a complex process since many people are involved. Quality of a product is measured based on performance, reliability, and durability, whereas the quality of pharmaceutical products depends on adherence to the parameters of purity, safety, and efficacy. Quality management methods such as Total Quality Management system or Six Sigma model have the common goal of delivering a high quality product. Quality management ensures the production of high quality products and services by eliminating defects and incorporating continuous changes and improvements in the system. High quality pharmaceutical products, in turn, lead to satisfied customers and high sale value along with fulfillment of statutory requirements of regulatory bodies. Proper quality control ensures the most effective utilization of available resources and a reduction in the cost of production ensuring:

- Lower running costs (less labor, rework, scrap)
- Reduced chances of non-quality product handling
- Motivated employees

- Improved market share
- High reputation
- International competitiveness
- Increased revenue generation

Philip Crosby's Idea of Quality

Philip Crosby defined quality as a "conformity to certain specifications set forth by management and not some vague concept of 'goodness.' These specifications are not arbitrary either; they must be set according to customer needs and wants." Crosby has developed 14 steps for an organization to follow in building an effective quality program which substantiates that management is primarily responsible for quality and workers only follow.

Crosby defined the four absolutes of quality management:

- Quality is conformance to requirements not as 'goodness' or 'elegance.'
- Quality prevention is preferable to quality inspection.
- Zero defects are the quality performance standard not " that is close enough."
- Quality is measured in monetary terms as the price of non-conformance.

Dr Joseph Juran's Idea of Quality

Dr. Joseph Juran defines quality as "fitness for use regarding design, conformance, availability, safety, and field use. "This concept more closely incorporates the viewpoint of the customer. The quality system should measure everything under the process and rely on problem-solving techniques. Unlike Deming, Juran focuses on top to down management and technical methods rather than worker pride and satisfaction.

BASIC CONCEPTS OF QUALITY

Quality of a service or product depends on the attributes like timeliness, competence, consistency, convenience, accessibility, accuracy and responsiveness.

The basic concept of quality works on (Fig. 4.1):
- Quality specifications
- Gradation
- Inspection
- Quality control
- Quality assurance
- Quality management
- Total quality management
- Quality standards

Quality definition: Quality depends on the producer's perspective and the consumer's perspective, but the ultimate determinant is fitness for consumers use.

Gradation: Category or rank given to different quality requirements for products, processes, or systems having the same functional use, e.g. ISO series.

Inspection: It is the sorting/segregation of non-conforming or defective items from the conforming items and to decide if rework is needed.

Quality control: Quality control is the amalgamation of operational techniques and activities that are adapted to achieve the quality confirmation requirements.

Quality assurance: Quality assurance is the systematic and planned actions necessary to provide adequate confidence that a product or service satisfies the given requirement for quality. Quality assurance covers the whole life cycle of the product including production, processing, and end customer use.

Quality management: Is a systematic set of documented operating procedures, implemented and maintained ensuring the production of quality products consistently.

Total quality management: This is a comprehensive approach towards quality management system. It is the process of individual and organizational efforts to install and make a permanent climate ensuring continuous improvement in its ability to deliver high quality products and services to customers and all the stakeholders.

Quality standards: These are set of documents assimilated to provide details of requirements, specifications, guidelines or characteristics that are used for consistency assurance of materials, products, processes, and services in accordance with specified purposes, i.e. ISO standards (Fig. 4.2).

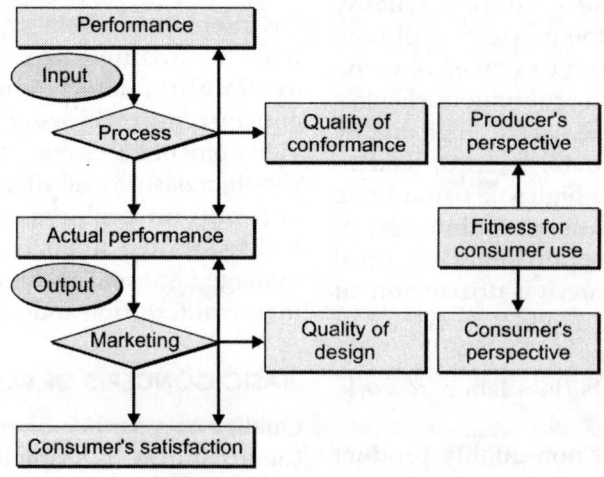

Fig. 4.1: Aspects of quality

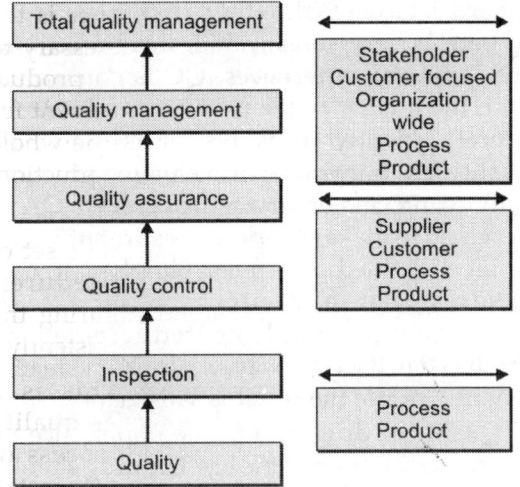

Fig. 4.2: Hierarchical process of quality

QUALITY CONTROL

Quality control (QC) is a comprehensive practice that aims to promote the performance of organizations through the cultivation of sound quality culture. QC is concerned with the development of ethical values and convictions to make every employee aware of the fact that quality is the primary goal of the organization. QC is a process employed to ensure a certain level of quality in a product or service. It includes all necessary actions the business model deemed necessary to provide control and verification of specific characteristics of a product or service. The fundamental goal of QC is to ensure that the products, services or processes provided by an enterprise meet specific requirements and are dependable, satisfactory and fiscally sound. Essentially, QC involves the examination of a product, service or process for certain minimum levels of quality.

Some Important Definitions of Quality Control

Alford and Beatty: "Quality control may be defined as that industrial management technique or group of techniques using which

products of uniform acceptable quality are manufactured."

J.A. Shubin: "Quality control means the recognition and removal of identifiable causes and defects and variables from the set standards."

K.G. Lockyer: "Quality control is used to connote all those activities which are directed for defining, controlling and maintaining quality."

H.N. Broom: "Quality control is systematic control by the management of the variables in the manufacturing process that affect goodness of the end-product."

Bethel, at water and Stackman: "Quality control is systematic control of these variables in the manufacturing process which affect the excellence of the end product. These variables result from the application of materials, men, machines and manufacturing condition. "

Tome, Simen, and McGill: "Quality control includes techniques and systems for the achievement of the required quality in the articles produced and for the elimination of substandard goods."

Joseph Manueb: "Quality control is a system of inspection, analysis and action applied to a manufacturing process so that, by inspecting a small portion of the product currently produced, an analysis of its quality can be made to determine what action is required on the operation in order to achieve and maintain the desired level of quality."

DJ Desmond: "Quality control is a technique of scientific management which has the object of improving industrial efficiency by concentrating on better standards of quality and on controls to ensure that these standards are always maintained. It is not intended to show what is wrong with current technology, but rather to establish what can be achieved with existing methods when they are operated correctly."

Objectives of Quality Control

The basic objective of the QC is to undertake activities and procedure that ensure achieving the desired qualities in the product. The critical objectives of the QC are:

- Develop a quality oriented company culture that values the characteristics of quality that the system follows and strives for continuous improvement.
- Establish the desired quality standards and specification for the pharmaceutical products which are acceptable to the regulatory authorities and customers.
- Develop, standardize and document the testing methods for the in-process and final products with determining the compliance with applicable standards.
- Draw out and document the role and responsibilities of the QC staffs. Detail the skills, training, and qualifications that are prerequisites for carrying out specific tasks. Generate the protocol and schedule for the additional training requirements of the QC staff.
- Identifies the flaws/variations in the raw materials and the manufacturing processes in order to ensure a product with a specified quality standard.
- Evaluate the product manufacturing processes and testing methods, and suggest further improvements in their functioning.
- Determination of the extent of quality deviation possibly can occur in the product during the manufacturing process.
- Analyze the root causes in detail that are responsible for any occurred deviation and document the recommended corrective action.

Requirement of Quality Control

The goal of a QC team is to identify products or services that do not meet the company's specified standards of quality. Often, quality control is confused with Quality Assurance (QA) though the difference between these two

is hard to be defined, as the working spectrum of both is very similar. Still, there are some fundamental differences. QC is concerned with the quality of the product, while QA is process oriented measures for assurance of quality. QC is involved in evaluation product, activity, process or service, by contrast, QA is designed to make sure processes are sufficient to meet defined objectives. Simply put, QA ensures that a product or service is manufactured, implemented, created or produced in the right way, while QC evaluates whether or not the result is satisfactory.

Quality of drug is of prime importance to ensure its safety and efficacy. The drug should have a specific, proven, identifiable chemical structure with minimum identifiable impurities and must be stable at various environmental conditions. In India especially the temperature and humidity vary drastically from season to season and from place to place, adversely affecting product quality. Maintaining the quality of the drug products not only mean the level of purity but also quantification of identifiable impurity that can lead to toxicity or reduce the effectiveness of the drug. QC department formally does testing, and use a series of analytical measurements to assess the quality of the manufactured product. For QC to be adequate, the system must test the same things, in the same way, every time repetitively. A test plan is merely a high-level summary of the areas (functionality, elements, regions, etc.) to be tested with an estimate of the duration of testing and statement of required resources.

QC department helps the production department to build quality rather than controlling quality. Building quality is not the only responsibility of QA or QC, but of every person working in the organization whether belonging to purchase, stores, production or maintenance departments as QA is the responsibility of every employee while QC becomes the supporting service. QC acceptance or rejection decisions are shared with personnel's from material purchase, production, and maintenance so that everybody comes to know about the causes so that the same mistake should not be repeated. QC department takes a final decision regarding the acceptance or rejection of the final product and reports to the factory manager or plant manager.

Quality Control Documentation Sections

- Product development
- Critical process control
- Facilities and equipment
- Building and premises
- Facility qualification
- Equipment selection
- Equipment control
- Equipment qualification
- Control of material
- Manufacturing control
- Batch production and control record
- Validation
- Packaging
- Laboratory control
- Quality system
- Personnel
- Contractors
- Storage and distribution
- Continuous monitoring and improvement

Quality System

- Change control system
- Deviation control
- Annual product review
- Trend analysis
- Stability
- Complaint handling
- Recall
- Audit

Control of Material

- Specification
- Vendor qualification

- Receiving control
- QC release
- Status labeling
- Shelf life control
- Storage control
- Dispensing control
- Inventory rotation system

Deviation Control

- Reporting
- Documentation
- Investigation of the root cause
- Corrective action and preventive action (CAPA)
- Review of quality unit
- Decision based on risk assessment

Recall Control

- Notification to the regulatory body
- Notification to customers
- Reconciliation
- Periodic testing
- Trend analysis
- Trend charts
- Trend values
- Find out causes of out of test [OOT]
- CAPA
- Risk assessment and decision on the batch

Requirements for Quality Control Laboratory

QC laboratories are developed independently of the production areas with required space as per FDA guidelines and designed appropriately for the testing operations to be carried out in different sections of wet and dry chemistry. The laboratory should have adequate area for basic installation and ancillary purposes. The designing of the QC laboratory essentially takes into account the suitability of construction materials and ventilation. The QC laboratories are provided with the regular supply of water of appropriate quality for cleaning and testing purposes.

Separate areas are required for physico-chemical, biological, microbiological or radio-isotope analysis. Adequate space is provided depending on the section wise requirements for logical placement of instruments and also to avoid mix-ups and cross-contamination. Sufficient and suitable storage space is to be provided for keeping the test samples, retained samples, reference standards, reagents, and records. Separate instrument room with adequate area is required for sensitive and sophisticated instruments employed for analysis. Separate air handling units and other requirements are installed for biological, microbiological and radioisotopes testing areas. The microbiology section is equipped with air lock arrangements, laminar air flow work station, and other necessary measures considered essential for maintaining area sterility.

RESPONSIBILITIES OF QUALITY CONTROL SECTION

All procedures and responsibility of QC department are written in the form of official document:

1. QC department has the responsibility for approving or rejecting all procedures or specifications which affect the strength, quality, identity, and purity of drug product.

2. All procedures and process of production department affecting quality are to be approved by QC or QA department with signature, e.g. standard operating procedure, validation, vendor certification protocols, handling of the complaint, process control procedures, and all design qualifications. These protocols and procedures can be changed from time to time but with written permission and signature of the QC department.

3. The establishment of required laboratory control mechanisms, including any changes made in due course are drafted by the concerned appropriate organizational unit, reviewed and approved by the QC unit. The written procedures are followed while performing any test and observations are documented. Any deviation from the written test procedure, standards, sampling plans, specifications or other laboratory control system is recorded and justified.

4. Laboratory controls encompass the establishment of scientifically sound and appropriate sampling plans and test procedures for raw material, drug product containers, closures, in-process materials, labeling, and the finished drug products. It is designed to assure that components conform to specifications, standards as appropriate for identity, strength, quality, and purity. Laboratory controls include:

   • Description of sampling and testing methods for raw, in-process and final processed materials to represent the whole batch and adequately identified by the coding system.

   • Determination of conformance to written testing procedures as described in standard operating procedures and manuals and appropriate following of all precautions.

   • Assurance of calibration of instruments, apparatus, gauges, and recording devices at suitable intervals following an established written program containing specific directions, schedules, limits for accuracy and precision. It also includes provisions for remedial action in the event accuracy and/or precision limits are not met. Instruments, apparatus, gauges, and recording devices not meeting established specifications should not be used.

   • Determination of conformance to approved written specifications for acceptance decision of components, containers, closures, drug product and labels used in the manufacturing, processing, packing or holding of drug products. The specifications include a description of the sampling and testing procedures used. Procedures are also required for appropriate retesting of any component, drug product container, or closure that is subject to deterioration.

5. Contract manufacturer should have adequate facilities to analyze drug formulations and for individual tests outsourcing to public testing laboratory is permitted. Frequent audit of contract manufacturer unit is must to be done.

6. When a product is given on contract basis to be manufactured by another company, it is not mandatory to analyze the samples again which are analyzed by the contract company, but QC department compares data for a batch to batch trend analysis of the manufacturing process (Fig. 4.3).

QUALITY ASSURANCE

Quality assurance (QA) is an overall management plan to guarantee the integrity of the quality management process. QA department is the asset of any pharmaceutical company as it builds the brand value of a company and increases market share by delivering quality medicinal products. QA is a broad range concept covering all affairs that individually or collectively influence the quality of a product. QA responsibility is to ensure that products manufactured are having the defined quality characteristics as required for their intended use. QA department continuously monitors the process of manufacturing, data evaluation and suggests the best methods to increase quality, productivity and economy. The responsibilities of the QA department are extended from raw material purchase to final consumption of the pharmaceutical product.

Quality of drug product is tested and documented at all the stages of manufacturing and packaging continually. QA practices following the cGMP guidelines to build quality in the final product. During product development, all the standards and specifications are developed for materials, process and machines to minimize the chances of rejection undertakes regular review of the manufacturing process along with periodic quality audit. During the inspection and testing of products, acceptance or rejection depends on the decision of the QC department. QA department has two primary quality functions to perform:

1. In-process control
2. Customer complaint handling

REQUIREMENTS OF QUALITY ASSURANCE SECTION

QA department work in coordination with the QC, having authority to accept or reject any

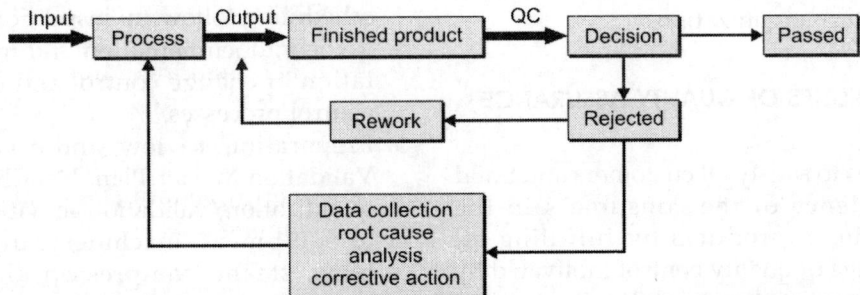

Fig. 4.3: The working process of quality control for product appraisal

material, process or finished product and to inspect production records and investigate any deviation. In case products are manufactured in another company by loan license the QA department has the authority to inspect the facility, accept or reject any material or finished product. QA set up must have adequate laboratory facilities to test and approve the in-process materials utilized in the manufacturing of medicines. The system of QA in the appropriation of pharmaceutical products manufacturing ensures that:

1. The pharmaceutical products are designed and developed following the requirements of GMP and other associated regulatory codes such as those of GLP.
2. Adequate controls are exercised for starting materials, intermediate, bulk, and in-process product quality controls.
3. Adequate systems are being developed of supply and use of the correct starting and packaging materials.
4. Arrangements are made for the manufacturing of products following standardized process and instrument calibrations, and validations are carried out.
5. The finished product is correctly processed, and quality checked following established procedures.
6. The finished products are released for sale or supplied after authorization of QC and QA department that batch has been produced and quality controlled as per the requirements of the label claim and any other provisions relevant to drug regulatory organization.

RESPONSIBILITIES OF QUALITY ASSURANCE SECTION

QA's goal is to satisfy all customers and build the confidence of the consumers in the organization's products by fulfilling all requirements of quality control motivated by stakeholders and especially customers external to the organization. QA efforts are directed towards the development of ethics and positive attitude in the employees. The Personnel's working in the organization should be motivated to invent new process and methods to improve quality and efficiency. QA is responsible for the development of a globally competent regulatory system in the pharmaceutical manufacturing facility. Responsibilities in general are:

1. Implementation of GMP/GLP regulations as specified by regulatory organizations like USFDA, WHO, ICH, MHRA, ANVISA, TGA requirements of cGMP guidelines and various other regulatory agencies. Active participation in various international regulatory inspections (USFDA/MHRA/ANVISA/WHO/Health Canada, etc).
2. Regulatory review and filing of various dossiers in US/EU/China/MCC/Brazil/Nordic countries and other regulatory agencies across the globe. Preparation of the supplements, annual reports, and other amendments as required. Review of stability data/trends/impurity profiles.
3. Handling the regulatory inspections, conduction of project specific inspections of laboratory procedures to evaluate compliance with analytical methods, standard operating procedures, and report filing: Conduction of manufacturing and other general facility inspections as assigned and identifying issues requiring follow-up inspection and consulting with supervisor for the scheduling follow-up inspection.
4. Review, documentation and implementation of change control and deviation control processes.
5. Preparation, review, and execution of Validation Master Plan. Handling of the qualification/validation activities related to equipment/machinery, utility systems, steam, compressed air, HVAC system, water system, cleaning, and other facilities.

6. Development of written procedures for production and process control targeted to product identity, strength, quality, and purity assurance. Performance validation for the manufacturing processes are conducted for output quality control measures following established procedures, and also by internal and external audits.

7. Assessment for any possible occurrence of variation in the in-process material and final product characteristics. Initiate, implement and control written manufacturing specifications and processing procedures to assure conformance to the original design or any approved changes in that design.

8. Preparation of laboratory data for compliance with methods and standard operating procedures. Result table preparation for analytical reports of samples relating to completeness and accurate representation of the data and report filing.

9. Handling of internal audit of the QA system and external audit by a consultant for improving systems efficacy. Conduction of audits for vendors and subcontractors as assigned. Evaluate audit and inspection findings and consulting with supervisor regarding the appropriate course of action and reporting requirements.

10. QA collects information from the market regarding product quality, efficacy, potency, adverse reactions, complaints, and customer satisfaction, called post-marketing quality assurance or phase VI pharmacovigilance.

11. Built quality systems, review/rewrote SOPs, design and implement the new batch record system, direct validation group, and develop and implement the training program. QA also plays an active role in simplifying procedures while maintaining regulatory compliance.

12. Introduction and generation of statistical tools, training information management system, Quality Management System modules, and Document Management Systems (software).

13. QA is responsible for discerning counterfeit products and complaints management (Fig. 4.4).

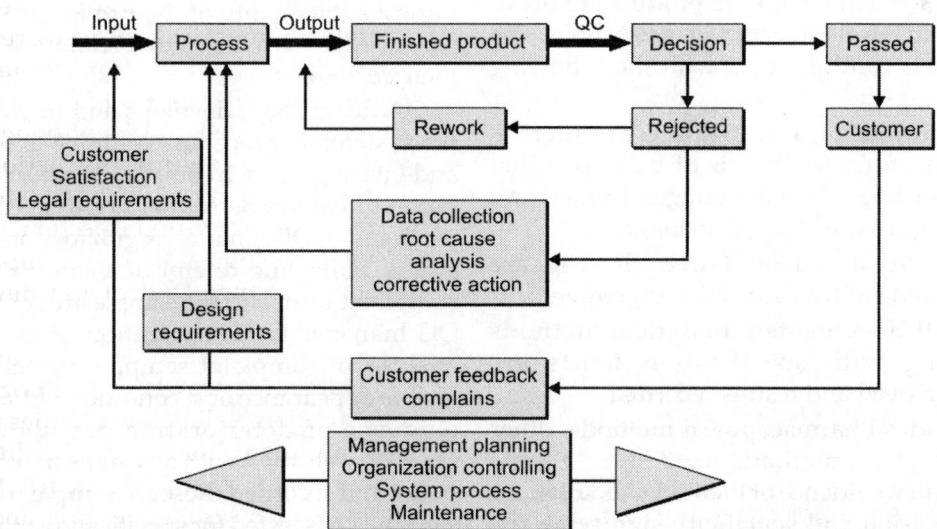

Fig. 4.4: The working process of quality assurance for overall quality management

IN-PROCESS CONTROL

In-process controls are the checks carried out during the ongoing manufacturing process before its completion. The objectives of in-process control measures are not only to control the product but also verify process control efficiency. The function of in-process controls is to monitor the compliance of the manufacturing process with the defined specifications including control of equipment and environment. In-process materials are sampled at predefined schedules and tested for identity, strength, quality, and purity as appropriate and approved by the QC unit during the production process. In-process controls are performed at regular intervals during a manufacturing process step, e.g. granulation, blending, tableting, encapsulation of tablet formulation. These in-process testing functions are performed according to methods approved by QC and the results recorded following documented parameters usually, by the production personnel. The responsibility distribution and task assignment for the in-process control must be laid down in organizational instructions. The detailed in-process control requirements specific for particular type product are documented in the manufacturing instructions. The in-process control works with the following objectives:

1. Sampling of intermediate products is done for each batch of each product according to the documented procedure authorized by the QC manager.
2. Identity and assay (strength) tests are carried out for each active ingredient.
3. Well-documented analytical methods along with specification limits are employed and results recorded.
4. Besides Pharmacopoeial methods, other analytical methods used should have written evidence of method validation for precision and specificity signifying the official use.

5. Batch fulfilling the requirement defined by QC are approved and released by QA manager.
6. QA department has the list of approved people who have the authority to release the batches.
7. If deviation is found in yield or product fail to comply with the specification, it is investigated carefully and documented.
8. Batch failed, can be reprocessed according to approved and documented procedures and only after ensuring that reprocessed material meets appropriate standards, specifications, and QA released any other relevant criteria.

CUSTOMER COMPLAINTS HANDLING

Complaints indicate customer dissatisfaction related to the quality of a product or service. Despite the mandatory regulatory obligation of pharmaceutical companies to produce products with strict quality parameters still, there are frequent cases of a customer complaint. The manufacturer should thoroughly investigate any complaint regarding the product. A good complaint handling system also gives the company an opportunity to improve the quality of the products and in a way to establish a committed relationship with their customers.

QA department develops and implements the systematic procedure in order to register and investigate each complaint received. This process involves personnel's from marketing, production, QC, finance, regulatory and legal affairs. Following receipt of a complaint, the complaint form and the sample are sent to the QC manager for investigation. A complete analysis of complaint samples are made for visible appearance and condition of the pack, evidence of deterioration are identified. Quantity returned with any signs of misuse is noted and recorded. Reserve sample from the same batch is tested for specification matching requirements. If the complaint is related to the toxic or adverse reaction, the relevant biological tests are carried out. In case the batch number of raw material used in the complaint specific batch is the same for other batches, reserve samples of those particular batches are also tested. The test results are recorded and evaluated by the QC manager to recommend the corrective actions needed to be taken. The QA manager sends the reply to the complainer regarding investigation findings. If a batch fails to comply with the defined specifications, the batch is recalled from the market and complaint records are reviewed for corrective action. Details of complaint information are sent to the concerned manufacturing department to take preventive action to avoid these situations in the future. Complaint records are maintained up to one year to product expiry or one year after the date of receiving the complaint. Complaint handling system is carefully developed by QA department taking concern about the following issues:

- Any complaint concerning a product defect is to be recorded with all the original details.
- Personnel responsible for handling the complaints and deciding the measures to be taken are designated together with sufficient supporting staff. Written procedures describing actions to be taken are followed. This should specially mention the need to consider a product recall initiative in the case the complaint concerned about a possible product defect.
- All complaints concerning potentially defective products are to be reviewed carefully according to written procedures. Personnel from QC are usually involved in the review of such investigations.
- Special attention is given to establish whether a complaint was because of counterfeiting.
- If product defect beyond acceptance limit is discovered or suspected in a batch, consideration are also given whether other

batches also to be checked in order to determine the root cause and ascertain required changes to be implemented. In particular, the batches that contain reprocessed product from the defective batch must be investigated.

- Corrective measures related decisions undertaken following a complaint investigation is recorded and referenced to the corresponding batch records.
- Complaints records are regularly reviewed for indication of specific or recurring problems that require attention and might justify the recall of marketed products.
- Competent authorities are informed while considering action following possible faulty manufacture, product deterioration, counterfeiting or any other serious quality problems with a product.

A Customer Feedback System is maintained by QA using the input from the Technical and Customer Service Department. All customer complaints are logged and classified depending on the type of complaint (performance or physical appearance related). All complaints are numbered and tracked by QA from receipt of the initial call until closure.

Product Recall Procedure

Pharmaceutical companies have a system to recall the defective or suspected of the defective products from the market promptly and effectively. These are the critical factors considered while developing a product recall system:

- Authorized persons are designated to be responsible for the execution and coordination of recalls with sufficient supporting staff to handle all aspects of the recalls with the appropriate degree of urgency.
- The distribution records are readily made available to the authorized person containing sufficient information of wholesalers and directly supplied customers (including, exported products, samples for clinical

tests and promotional samples) to permit an effective recall.

- Established written recall procedures are needed to be regularly reviewed and updated, enabling the organization recall activity. Recall operations are such designated to be capable of being initiated promptly down to the required level in the distribution chain.
- Instructions are made in the written procedures regarding storage of recalled products in a secure segregated area while their fate is decided.
- All competent authorities are promptly informed about the recall of a product following it is expected to be or is suspected of being defective.
- The progress of the recall process is monitored and recorded including the disposition details of the product. A final report is issued mentioning reconciliation between the delivered and recovered quantities of the products.
- The effectiveness of the arrangements for recalls is tested and evaluated from time to time through mock drills.

COST OF QUALITY

Quality is of utmost importance for ensuring excellent performance and success of any organization. To ensure effective quality organization must pay attention to quality control in all its actions. Focus on quality helps the organization to improve and maintain a high level of customer satisfaction as well as to all stakeholders.

In earlier days quality functions were limited to inspection of finished goods to segregate good quality of product from the defective ones. Subsequently, the function was expanded to include control of overall aspects in the manufacturing process to ensure that production of defective products is minimized at all stages, and was named QC. However, the quality management functions nowadays encompass all the activities in the organization and aim to ensure quality in everything that an organization does. The total amount spent in efforts and maintenance related to product quality deficiencies is quantified as Cost of Quality. It is a general perception that higher quality requires higher costs, either for buying better materials and machines or for hiring more skilled labor. Proper management and quality planning, based on an evaluation of critical quality issues, eventually results in cost reduction and profit enhancement.

Most of the consumer products possess a level of quality so that it could be easily sold in the market, but the pharmaceutical products must possess a maximum defined level of quality as they are related to the health of consumers. In order to measure the quality of pharmaceutical products, accurate standard measurement and specification levels are established. Batch to batch production deviation from the pre-determined standards are not permitted and continuously looked out. Mandatorily highest level of quality standard maintenance of pharmaceutical products needs investment of enormous amount. Cost of Quality are the costs associated with finding, preventing and correcting defective work. The quality costs are a considerable burden ranging from 20 to 40% of the total sales value, but these costs can be significantly reduced with the implementation of a proper management system. One of the critical functions of the QA manager is to reduce the total cost associated with quality functions in the pharmaceutical company.

Costs of Quality is referred to as the costs incurred to prevent defects and remove defective products. The term Cost of Quality is a measure to quantify the total cost of quality-related efforts and deficiencies. The two main components of Cost of Quality is the cost of good quality or the cost incurred for assuring quality conformance and cost of poor quality or the cost incurred to bear the consequences of non-conformance. This total quality cost can be split into two fundamental areas.

COST OF CONFORMANCE

Cost of conformance is the total expense of ensuring good quality of the manufactured product. It includes costs of QA activities such as planning, setting standards, training of personnel, developing pilot processes, etc. and costs of QC activities like testing, documentation, reviews, inspections, and audits:

- Planning: Planning to do the right thing the first time and at the right time. The quality related mission and vision development, and planning for systematic supervision of compliance.
- Standards: Following related quality standards for products like Pharmacopoeial, and national and international guidelines.
- Training: On the job training, quality training, workshops, and seminars, etc.
- Pilot process: The processes followed in the company for various activities, *viz.* manufacturing, testing and analytical, storekeeping, cleaning and housekeeping, maintenance, etc. are developed and tested in pilot scale for specification compliance.
- Testing: Testing of the raw material, in-process and final products are done continuously on every batch of the product following standard procedure to check the compliance to quality standards.
- Documentation: Writing working instructions, technical instructions, SOPs, manuals and other related paperwork done to assure compliance.
- Reviews: Review of all activities done regularly in predetermined schedules to find out if any deviation to specification or standard procedures.
- Inspection: Regular supervision and inspection of equipment, instrument, buildings and staff performance.

- Auditing: Internal, external and extrinsic auditing done for a systematic and independent examination of data, documents, records, operations, and performances to assure quality to regulatory bodies and customers.

The price paid for assurance to conformance of quality guidelines is the cost of conformance.

COST OF NON-CONFORMANCE

Cost of non-conformance is the cost incurred by the organization due to a failure to achieve a good quality product. It includes both in-process costs generated by quality failures or scraps, cost of rework, re-performance of lost work (for products used internally), and possible loss of business due to waiting time for rework, downtime due to non-working machinery, possible legal redress and potential costs of recall and return of complaint product:

- Scrap: Throwing away the in-process or final product of a batch as it is not up to the required standard or out of specification and cannot be reprocessed.
- Rework: Doing the job over again as it was not correctly done in the first time. When a batch of materials with unacceptable quality is reprocessed to make it acceptable following a method other than that used to produce the original material is reworked.
- Re-processing: As per the guidelines the pharmaceutical manufacturing process is such designed to have the ability to do 'right first time.' In case a batch of the final product fails to meet its release specifications, it is complicated to justify putting this back into manufacturing to produce the new final product. Reprocessing is the treatment of a batch of materials with unacceptable quality by repeating the same process steps from a defined stage of production.

- Waiting time: Time wasted while waiting for a processing area or equipment engaged in rework or reprocessing to be free for the regular work.
- Downtime: Not being able to do a job because of a machine broke down or not in proper order.
- Recall: A defective or suspected of the defective products in case of any quality or safety related complaint, the entire batch of the particular product is recalled from the market promptly and effectively.
- Return: Products returned from the market are tested for quality compliance, and if found satisfactory may be considered for resale/relabelling or any suitable alternative action. The products are destroyed following a written procedure when they fail to comply with the quality specification.
- Legal redress: Pharmaceuticals are highly regulated industry and consumer rights are adequately safeguarded by legal provisions guaranteeing the quality, safety, and efficacy of the products. In the pharmaceutical industry, specific provisions provide for patient information claims. Product liability suits have become a considerable problem for the drug manufacturer.

The price paid for not having a well-qualified quality system or a quality product is the cost of non-conformance.

SEGMENTS OF QUALITY COST

Preparation of cost estimates for pharmaceutical companies should always consider the cost of quality. Not investing in building a proper quality system can cost more than that costs for developing and maintaining a quality framework. Cost of conformance and non-conformance further has four segments in quality costs. The costs for appraising a product or service for conformance to requirements or the cost of good quality is divided into prevention cost and appraisal cost. Costs directed towards prevention of non-conformance or the cost incurred for poor quality has segments of internal and external failure costs resulting from failing to meet requirements. Examples of 'poor quality' include labeling errors, design errors, mistakes in user manuals and leaflets, as well as lousy documentation.

Prevention Costs

This is the cost incurred on system and methods employed for minimizing and avoiding defects and preventing failure. Prevention area covers quality management areas like planning, preparation, review, training, preventative maintenance, avoiding defects and evaluation. It is the costs of activities that are specifically designed to prevent the occurrence of inferior quality products. Prevention costs are directed to minimize the chances of having defective products by applying statistical process control, quality engineering, staff training and implementation of quality management tools like strategies.

Appraisal Costs

Appraisal costs are the costs that a company incurs to detect defective products before delivering to the customers. Appraisal cost is a part of the quality control process to ensure that products and services meet customer expectations and regulatory requirements. It is the cost involved in assuring quality standard conformity of products. Appraisal cost covers expense in activities designed to find quality standard implementation related problems such as calibration, validation, testing, inspection, and audit.

Internal Failure Costs

Failure costs are the cost that is incurred to remove defects from the products before shipping them to customers. This area covers the costs that are borne by the organization for handling scrap, rework, redesign, retesting, modifications, corrective actions, downtime, concessions, shortage, and overtime. Along with the costs of finding and fixing problems, there are many forms of internal failure costs borne by companies. The costs of material reprocessing due to deviations, any missed milestones, under-utilization of equipment, under-utilization of personnel and time lag to get back to the schedule after quality failure are the issues related to internal failure costs.

External Failure Costs

This covers the costs spent towards the compensatory actions if in case defective products are being shipped to customers. Failure costs arise after the supply of defective product to the customer which includes the customer service costs, penalty cost due to insufficient and untimely customer service, the cost incurred for recalling batch due to customer complaints or cost of patching a released product, and other administrative costs in dealing with failure and loss of goodwill.

TOTAL COST OF QUALITY

The total cost of quality is the sum total of the above four segments of quality costs. This represents the difference between the actual production cost of a product and what would be the projected cost if there were no possibility of any substandard product or products failure due to defects.

Total Cost of Quality= Cost of good quality (Prevention cost + Appraisal cost) + Cost of poor quality (Internal failure cost + External failure cost).

Some of the above costs are hidden or indirect cost, and most of the classical costing methods do not consider them while calculating the product cost. Money invested in design, development, manufacturing facility, analysis, and distribution, etc. are the direct cost, but unavoidable as they, in turn, reduce the indirect cost. Quality related certification achievement many times gives the idea of the cost incurred in developing quality (Fig. 4.5).

With highly defective products, prevention and appraisal costs are very low, but failure

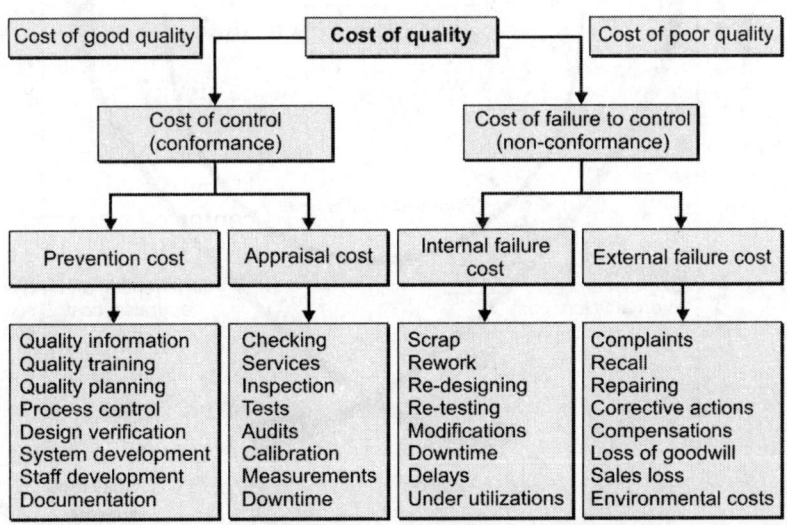

Fig. 4.5: Different aspects of cost of quality

costs are very high, yielding a high total quality cost. With zero defect products, likewise, failure costs are meager, but prevention and appraisal costs are very high. The total cost of quality oscillates between the four segments of cost of quality on a revolving basis with an outcome of little or no overall reduction in the total cost of quality.

TROUBLE SHOOTING WITH COST OF QUALITY DATA

A better understanding of product quality aspects which help to manage the costs in a better way is the solution for overcoming the problem of high cost of quality. Prevention and appraisal costs help in finding errors that can be corrected while they are still internal failures, but it is cheaper to deal compared to becoming them external failures. Understanding quality costs hopefully help to shift some of the test efforts to the most cost-effective places. Understanding quality costs are actually to analyze where to spend time and money to get the best out of it. It is a common practice to find and fix a defect during unit testing early in the development cycle. There are many limitations to unit testing still though getting a better unit test effort helps in releasing a better product sooner.

Optimization of total quality costs shuffles between these extremes at the bottom of the concave curve (Fig. 4.6):

- Cost of quality aspect must be taken into consideration during project approval decisions, as changes or supposed 'improvements' can shift cost of quality from one category to another, with little net effect. For example, a new machine purchased to reduce scrap can cause higher setup, inspection and maintenance costs of setting the scrap savings with no net improvement in cost of quality instantly but lately, it will pay off.
- Complete and clear cost of quality input data results in proper interpretation and implementation over a time frame. Variability in quality cost data add significant noise to the cost of quality data, clouding

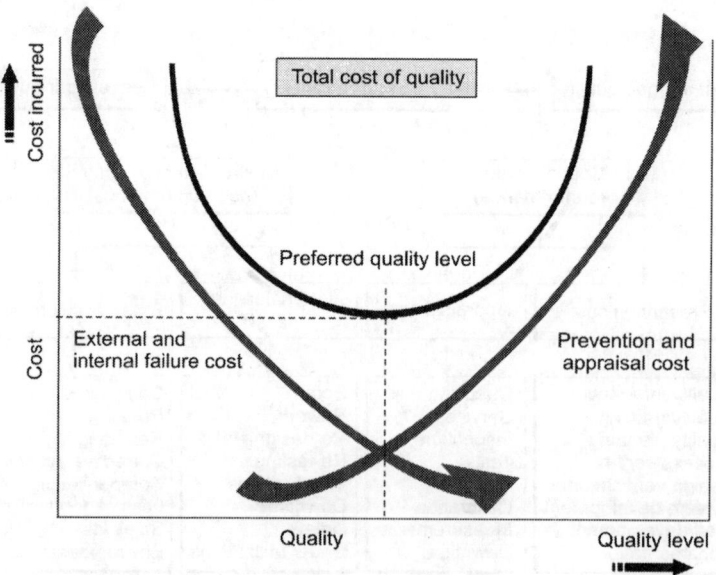

Fig. 4.6: The oscillating nature of the total cost of quality

the interpretation and hiding significant trends for extended periods.

- Instead of focusing on the more significant cost category and quality variations, efforts should be directed at easy way data collection and stepwise implement of changes.
- Loosen down, or superficial implement-ation of cost of quality data increases the work exercises with little or no benefit.
- Cost of quality data when used relevantly in an effective manner gives the best results. Decisions are often made without realizing or considering the impact on cost of quality, thereby resulting in the irrelevancy of the cost of the quality system.
- Cost of quality data collection becomes increasingly costly and bureaucratic over time, making it slow responding towards significant changes and less worthy.
- Statistical analysis of cost of quality data must be performed before implementation. In the absence of which early recognition of trends can be missed, and random variations are mistaken for significant signals. It causes

wasting of time and resources distracting everyone from the real issues.

- Cost of the quality system is evaluated closely with other key performance indicators systems, which ensured a more in-depth understanding of cause–effect relationships.
- The cost of quality cost data generation and measurement system must be ideally less than ~1% of the apparent savings expected to be generated by the use of the data.

Pharmaceutical companies have to reduce product defects but this, in turn, increases the cost of good quality involving higher investments in testing, evaluation, training of operators, inspection, audits, etc. In an ideal zero defect world, failure costs would also be zero, but full elimination of appraisal and prevention costs is not possible but can be significantly reduced by adaptation of better process performance. Six Sigma concepts emphasize building quality into a process and doing things 'right first time' (Fig. 4.7). Sigma philosophy while striving for zero defect performance can smooth out an increase in the

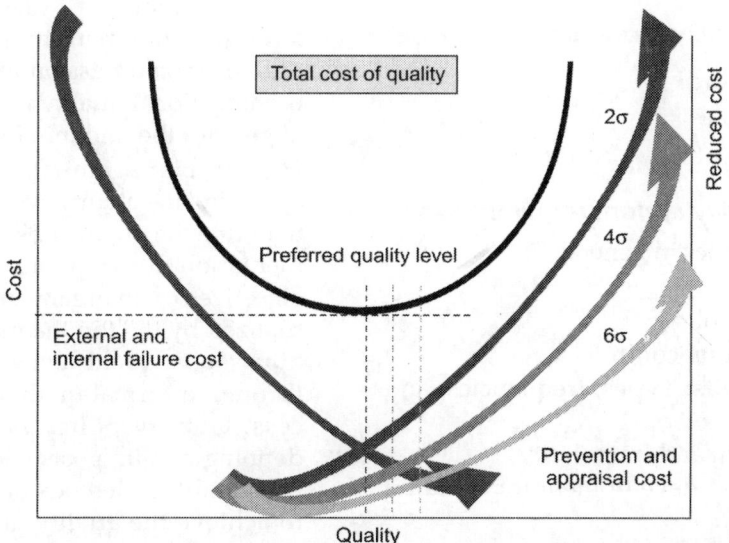

Fig. 4.7: Reduction in cost of good quality by adopting 6σ concept

cost of good quality by implementing better process control. Processes with better sigma adaptation can significantly lower prevention and appraisal costs ranging from more than 40 to less than 1%.

QUALITY MANUAL

Pharmaceutical companies prepare quality manual in simple, easy to understand and readily available form focusing on aspects of quality requirements. The quality policy is provided to every employee and displayed at various places. The entire administration works according to quality policy. Managing Director of the company or other supreme authority signs and authorize before it is published. Periodic revision of quality policy and quality manual are done as specified in the protocol. The quality manual must be practical, easy to implement, legible and free of confusions. Individual training sessions related to quality policy and quality manual are conducted to ensure proper implementation. The specific timeline is decided to revise manual without affecting regular work which is ideally 8–12 months.

Contents of Quality Manual

Section 1: General
1. Quality policy
2. Company profile

Section 2: Quality system requirements
3. Responsibilities in general
4. Personnel
5. Design control
6. Documentation control
7. Quality audits: Types, frequencies, and findings
8. Identification and traceability
9. Research and development for building quality
10. Vendor selection process and development

11. Purchase controls
12. Sampling equipment and procedures
13. Testing and release of finished products
14. Material handling storage and distribution
15. Labels, cartons, inserts and other printed material controls
16. Stability studies programmes and procedures
17. Statistical techniques
18. Manufacturing operations and in-process controls

1. **Quality Policy:** Pharmaceuticals are committed to maintaining the highest level of quality in the manufacturing and sale of products. Product quality compliance for all applicable regulatory requirements, continuous improvement and customer satisfaction underlie the efforts directed in the development, manufacturing, advertising, and sales of medicines. In the modern quality system the policies, objectives, and plans are the means by which senior managers articulate their vision of quality applicable to all levels of the organization. To achieve this management must incorporate a strong commitment to quality as in the organizational mission in developing an organizational quality policy that should align with the said mission.

Higher management responsible for operating the quality system are expected to define the quality objectives for implementation of the quality policy. Quality objectives of an organization are conceptualized by the top the management and other subsequent levels as responsible through a formal quality planning process. Quality policy is the statement defining quality goals and quality objectives and the methods or strategies used to achieve the quality goals. Objectives are typically aligned with the manufacturer's strategic plans. The quality system functions effectively provided the management supports the objectives with the necessary resources and has measurable goals that are monitored regularly. Management uses quality planning to identify resources and define methods achieving quality objectives. Quality plans are documented and communicated to all personnel at different levels to ensure awareness of operational activities aligned with strategic and quality goals.

Quality policy enumerates the organizational structure, responsibilities, procedures, processes, and resources for implementing quality management system.

2. **Company Profile:** Company profile is a short introduction on the initiation and progress of the company from its inception to the till date along with subsidiaries and supporting divisions, working stations and certification details. A short profile of its sales and distribution network, warehouses and employees are also included.

3. **Responsibilities in general:** Quality compliance is the moral responsibility of every employee working in the organization. Management is responsible for communicating quality policy to all the employees and for ensuring full understanding and commitment to quality. Proper implementation of quality assurance principles and integrity of function between concerned departments of the organization are the responsibility of:

- The President and Vice Presidents have executive level responsibility for quality policy implementation and are responsible for creating a positive atmosphere where quality has the highest priority.
- The Managing Director is responsible for overseeing the development,

implementation, and maintenance of the quality policy.

- The Directors, Managers, and Supervisors are charged with the development and implementation of quality policy.
- The QA and QC staffs are responsible for ensuring the quality system is adequately maintained and implemented. Each supervisor is responsible for assuring that quality systems are followed in his or her area.
- Each employee is responsible for quality in his or her work and for suggesting improvements in quality.

Groups of executives from both QA and QC are expected to be dedicated exclusively to quality management system. QA department assists in the development of quality systems and conducts periodic audits to assure faithful and effective implementation. The QA has the following responsibilities regarding quality policy management:

- Establish quality goals and objectives and develop plans to meet those goals and objectives.
- Evaluation and identification of quality related problems.
- Corrective action recommendation for solutions to quality problems.
- Initiation of corrective action for the prevention of quality related problem occurrence and proper implementation of preventive actions.
- Control of non-conforming products.
- Report quality related issues to the management.

The QA department is responsible for quality systems management, but the implementation of these systems and quality *per se* is the responsibility of the QC department. Regarding quality policy implementation the responsibilities of QC are:

- The QC departments test products at all stages of the manufacturing process, from raw materials to finished goods.
- Release product against predetermined specifications.

4. **Personnel:** Qualified and experienced personnel is hired for specific jobs, and conduction of regular training assured that staff is skilled to perform all aspects of their jobs. Copies of job descriptions, job applications, resumes and annual performance reviews are kept on the respective personnel files in the Human Resources (HR) department. QA and HR department conduct regular training program (including the applicable regulations) for employees of all sections. Upon satisfactory completion of the training certificate of completion is given to the employee. QA usually maintains a master log of all certificates issued for completion of training. Ongoing training is necessary to assure that all personnel working is familiar with the applicable requirements of the company. The pharmaceuticals are also required to provide risk analysis training to managers and supervisors responsible for the manufacture and testing of products. Experience and trained employees are in a way responsible for assuring that the new employees became familiar with the pertinent aspects of these regulations. QA keeps an up-to-date record of the latest version of regulations and standards. Each department should maintain job-specific training records for all the employees. Supervisors are responsible for conducting job-specific training, training on new or revised documents, and for assuring that training is effective by maintaining training records.

5. **Design control:** Different design control parameters are adapted for different types of products:
   - Approval of the design goals (Design Input)
   - Review of feasibility studies (Design Review)
   - Approval of the product description (Design Output)
   - Review of process development activities and preparation of manufacturing related documents (Design Verification Review)
   - Review and approval of product validation data and transfer to manufacturing (Final Design Review/Data Review)
   - Development of testing protocol
   - Definition of product design goals for assay development
   - Risk analysis and management

6. **Documentation control:** All operations are required to be written and approved to assure consistent quality. The QA department is responsible for controlling the issue, distribution, revision and archiving of documentation control procedures.

The documents that must be controlled include:
   - The Quality Manual and Quality Policy
   - Quality System documentation
   - Design Control Records
   - Master Records
   - Standard Operating Procedures
   - Vendor Qualifications
   - Purchase Orders
   - Manufacturing Procedures
   - Testing Procedures
   - Calibration and Maintenance Records
   - Validation Data
   - Internal Audit Reports and Management Reviews
   - Different Forms
   - Document Change Requests
   - Customer Complaints
   - Customer Orders and Contracts

- Personnel Records/Training records
- Notifications and Recalls

A formal Document Change Request (DCR) procedure is adopted for revising existing documents and creating the new one. Review and approval by the department in which it is to be implemented. QA department or other concerned technical departments are involved in the document change process. The QA Supervisor reviews a draft with assistance from designated individuals. The other related document control adopted with DCR procedures are:

- Preparation and maintenance of document master files
- The master document replacement procedure
- Data management: General procedures and definitions

7. **Quality audits types, frequencies, and findings.** Quality audits are periodic, documented examination and verification of functional procedures, records and other elements of the quality system to assess conformity with the quality standard requirements. Quality audit is carried out by an internal or external quality auditor or an audit team at predefined time intervals. Quality audits involve procedural or result-based assessment criteria to determine compliance with the defined quality system processes and specifications. Quality Management undertakes quality system review usually at least twice a year for suitability and effectiveness of operations. During the pre-audit meeting, actions are allocated and minutes are recorded regarding the system development.

The prime objectives of quality audits are:

- Ascertain compliance of the quality management system in achieving the expected results meeting the pre-established requirements.
- Reassure that the quality management system continues to conform to the standards and functioning as per the established operating procedures.
- Detect irregularities or defects in the quality system and to identify weaknesses.
- Assure adequacy and suitability of the management system for current and future operations.
- Review the effectiveness of previous corrective actions taken against audit observations.
- Review the actions taken against complaints received, root cause identification and corrective action recommendation.
- To review the finding of audits and identify any areas of recurring problems or requiring potential improvements.
- To review trend analysis reports of nonconforming items to identify the possible improvements to be implemented.

Internal audits are mostly done by personnel not directly responsible for the functions being audited within that company, and external audits are outsourced recruiting trained auditors. Internal quality system audits are usually done once per annum to satisfy conformance of all concerned activities with the approved procedures. Comprehensive audit programmes are compiled at least a year in advance by the QA manager. Whenever a particular need arises the frequency of the audit may be increased at the discretion of the QA manager. Nonconformance if observed is recorded, documented and is brought to the attention of the person responsible, and subjected to timely corrective action to ensure full rectification in the audit the corrective actions are reviewed for effectiveness.

8. **Identification and traceability:** This is the ability to trace a batch of the product back to all the raw materials used in its manufacturing. Tracing most of the raw materials up to its finished products stage is also an essential feature of quality system. A unique identification number and a lot number (or receiving number) are given to all materials used to manufacture products. Store department is responsible for assigning receiving numbers to incoming raw materials. This provides complete traceability from receipt of raw materials to final shipment to the customer. Batch numbers for all finished products are sequentially assigned from the batch number database at the time of manufacturing and packaging.

9. **Research and development (R&D) for building quality:** Advances in science have directed the focus of scientific community on the safety and efficacy of pharmaceuticals, medical devices, biologicals, agrochemicals, and chemicals used on human and animals along with the effects on the environment. Quality management in scientific R&D has become an essential tool for ensuring the implementation of developments within a rigorous and robust quality framework. Pharmaceutical industries develop, manufacture and market drug products obeying a variety of laws and regulations ensuring safety and efficacy following licensing/marketing authorization to be used as medications. Testing the purity of medicinal products are done ensuring accuracy, precision, reliability, and repeatability of the method in conformance to the measurements with legal specifications. All critical factors related to safety, efficacy, and purity of drug products are considered as the pharmaceuticals work in a regulated environment. The R & D department performed all activities related to early drug development research, i.e. analytical method development and validation for new products, formulation development, pre-clinical and clinical studies, comprehensive testing of API and finished dosages form and generation of regulatory submission documentation.

The major working areas of pharmaceutical R&D department are:

- Drug discovery: This is the process of potential new drug discovery and designing. Modern drug discovery involves the identification of potential new drug by the screening of optimized compounds to increase the efficacy, potency, stability, and bioavailability and to decrease side effects. Drug discovery is a lengthy, expensive and complicated process with a low success rate. Once an understudy compound fulfils all of the requirements to be a potential therapeutic agent, it is progressed for the process of drug development before preclinical and clinical trials.

- Drug development: This refers to activities undertaken after a new compound is identified to have potential therapeutic value to be developed as a suitable medication. Objectives of drug development are to validate dosing feasibly of new drug entity and develop appropriate formulation.

- Pre-clinical and clinical studies: These are studies done to establish the safety and efficacy of a drug compound in animals and humans. These studies include a combination of *in vitro* and *in vivo* animal studies and clinical trials. These studies require massive capital investment and are lengthy procedures making it difficult for small and medium scale pharmaceuticals but a strength of the large pharmaceutical companies.

- Formulation development: Pharmaceutical formulations are developed mostly as oral, topical or injectable dosage forms. Comprehensive preformulation studies are required to develop suitable formulations and optimize dosage forms to carry forward for preclinical or clinical applications. Preformulation involves the characterization of a drug's physical, chemical, and mechanical properties in order to choose optimal excipients. Most of pharmaceutical R&Ds develop new formulations for an API as per the market need to cater patient requirements and eventually to increase the sale value. Formulation studies involve developing a preparation of the APIs which is both stable and acceptable to the patient possibly with some new advantages.

- Analytical method development: Analytical methods play essential roles in the discovery, development, and manufacture of pharmaceuticals. A number of new drug entities with partial structural modification of the existing one are introduced in the market every year. Mostly new drugs are included in the pharmacopeias after a time lag from the date of introduction of the drug in the market when standard analytical procedures for testing these drugs are not available in the respective pharmacopeias. Identification and quantification of impurities is a time consuming crucial task undertaken during pharmaceutical process development. Presence of any unwanted chemical compound even in small amounts can influence the efficacy and safety of pharmaceutical products. Various analytical methodologies are developed and employed for the determination of impurity related components in pharmaceuticals. R & D department develops test methods for the new drugs and impurities, and validate available official test methods that are used by quality control laboratories to ensure the identity, purity, and quality of drug products. Pharmaceutical combination products containing more than one drug are formulated to meet previously unmet patients need by providing combination therapeutic effects with two or more drugs. These combination products present challenges to the R & D scientists and analytical chemists in the development and validation of simultaneous analytical assay methods.

10. **Vendor selection process and development:** Supplier selection and evaluation process primarily consider supplier profile, regulatory compliance, quality, cost, services, and risk bearing ability of the vendor. The selection and evaluation criteria are described below:

- Supplier profile: This criterion encompasses a detailed evaluation of the supplier's market reputation, flexibility, capacity, financial health, and production facility.

- Regulatory compliance: In the vendor selection process it is essential to take into consideration the regulatory track record history of the supplier. The following documentation aspects are taken into consideration to obtain a comprehensive picture of the supplier's compliance status,
  - Production facilities and equipment
  - Materials controls
  - Quality management systems
  - Process validation approach
  - Documentation standard
  - Product quality review
  - cGMP compliance and regulatory track record

- Change/deviation management
- Recalls and complaints
- Availability of drug master filing (DMF) in different countries

- Quality: Quality requirement of raw material and component is of vital importance in vendor selection as the pharmaceutical industry is the most regulated one. Regulatory bodies mandatorily demand quality products from drug manufacturers; it behooves the pharmaceutical firms to select suppliers with quality certification and proven record of world class services to ensure supply of quality raw materials.
- Cost: Cost is traditionally considered as one of the most critical aspects of supplier selection criteria in the purchasing and supply management philosophy.
- Services: The level of services expected to be provided by a vendor, adherence to delivery time, value added services and ease of communication are mainly considered.
- Risk: The ability to manage predictable and unpredictable risks that may occur is also important.

11. **Purchase controls:** The functions of the purchasing department are to procure materials, machines, and tools at the most favorable terms and conditions essentially maintaining the quality. Purchase department decides on the quality, quantity, items, price and time of purchase of materials. Purchase control is concerned with the purchase of raw and packaging materials having the right quality in required quantity at a reasonable price and at the right time. The purchase control system is used to manage the purchasing activity of a company by providing a link between the inventory and the accounts. Critical attention is required to be paid regarding purchase procedures of materials with emphasis to cost, quality, volume, time, and delivery conditions. Purchase control process initiates with the issue of materials requisition and ends with the receipt of materials and payment of the materials cost. Purchase control system records the purchase orders placed with vendors and track the orders in different phases of the product receiving and invoicing.

Purchasing control covers the following areas:

- Contract and supply agreements: Purchasing and Sales (Store) department is responsible for the development of policy regarding the assurance of customer contracts and supply agreements are in place when required. The Corporate Legal department manages intellectual property contracts, customer contracts, and supply agreements.
- Specifications: Written specifications are made available to all personnel's responsible for purchasing and receiving activities for raw materials and packaging material. The store department generates the requirement of materials as per the material requisition made by the production, R & D and QC department matching with the availability of materials in the inventory.
- Vendor control: Qualified vendors are listed on each raw material specification. Vendor qualification describes how to qualify new vendors including outsourced services and processes. Audit and inspections track the vendor performance. The qualified and validated vendor audit procedure is developed and maintained. Vendors who do not perform well may be disqualified and replaced.
- Purchase management: All materials used in product manufacturing are

verified against the purchase order. The purchase orders are placed to the vendors for specific materials which includes an order acceptance number and a request for a Certificate of Analysis where appropriate. Purchase orders contain information, i.e. vendor ID, description of the material, quantity ordered, unit cost and total cost with the location, dates ordered.

- Receiving: Receiving and quarantined procedure of the incoming material are maintained according to the regulatory requirements. Incoming materials should be received following documented procedures. All deliveries are inspected against the purchase order for type, quantity and external transit damage. The quantity ordered and eventually received is matched with the purchase order, and inventory labels are affixed. Additional inspection may include verification against Certificates of Analysis, in-house material specifications or incoming testing procedures. In the case of non-conforming or damaged material, purchase department communicate with suppliers regarding return and compensation.

12. **Sampling equipment and procedures:** Starting from receipt of material in store through the manufacturing to packaging of final product sampling is done to ensure compliance with its defined specifications. During all the steps of the manufacturing process through bulk intermediates up to finally packed finished product are sampled as described in the SOP.

The sampling instructions for raw material, packaging material, intermediate product, bulk product, and finished product include:

- The sampling plan
- Method of sampling
- Sampling equipment to be used
- Specific sampling area
- Quantity to be sampled
- Sampling container to be used
- Precautions to be observed for sterile and hazardous materials
- Instructions if any required for subdivision or pooling of sampled material
- The cleaning method of sampling equipment

13. **Testing and release of finished products:** A finished product is a product in the retail pack or a transportable pack. Final inspection and testing are completed before any batch of the product are released for sale. Finished products are held in the quarantine area of manufacturing until finally released by QA when the batch satisfactorily shows confirmance to specifications. Guidance document/SOP is maintained describing the control tests to be done on finished products along with specifications. Development of well-qualified acceptance criteria for finished products after test/inspection activities is critical for maintaining the quality of the manufactured products.

- Sampling: As 100% inspection of the finished product is not possible to do, sampling is done following the statistical process. Part of the sample is kept as retention samples and others are subjected to after packing QC testing.
- Testing: Finished products are tested following standard test method against the approval material specification and details entered in finished product specification and test report.
- QA inspection sheet: The test results are entered in the QA inspection sheet, and QA authorized personnel enters the final evaluation of the product as released or rejected and signs.

- Finished product register: All the details of the finished product are entered in finished product register before shipment.
- Finished product trend card: All the details of the finished product test results are entered in finished product trend card maintained for particular products.
- Finished product shipping form: Shipping and transportation details of the finished product are filled in finished product shipping form.
- All documentation, *viz.* completed batch production and control report (BPCR), the test report of IPQC, the test report of finished product, any other report like deviation if any or sterility is reviewed and the product is physically inspected before release, stickers are placed on the product and batch record. A formal report/certificate of analysis is prepared and maintained in BPCR.

All inspections and testing are supported by completed documentation. Release by exception must be documented and approved by the QA manager. The part batch release is generally not acceptable, can only be done under a justified exceptional condition or deviation control system.

14. **Material handling, storage, and distribution:** It is of prime importance to store material in the same condition as required for their stability and also to minimize damage or deterioration of products in delivery and distribution to the customer. Storage conditions for different raw materials, in-process and finished goods, are specified in the appropriate documents with specifications. Materials are handled in a manner to ensure first in-first out (FIFO) with proper quarantine management. All materials are marked with a status label (quarantine, under test, approved, rejected), expiration date or retest date whichever appropriate. The expiration date is monitored, and the outdated product is removed from stock for appropriate disposal or retesting. Designated and appropriate storage areas are maintained to protect product integrity of susceptible products like an antibiotic, steroids, β-lactams, anticancer and heat labile drugs and are regularly environmentally monitored. Power back-up must be available in case of a power outage. Stability studies are conducted during product development and also routinely to validate recommended storage conditions for a particular product category.

QC personnel test and inspect finished products using statistically valid sampling plans and release product for distribution only after it meets acceptance criteria. Finished products are assembled according to written procedures and adequately identified with a part number, lot or receiving number and acceptance status before they are placed in the warehouse. Finished products should be packaged and labeled for distribution in such a manner to assure physical and functional integrity during transportation. The mode of transportation and conditions are chosen to protect the quality of the product.

15. **Labels, cartons, inserts and other printed material controls:** Product packaging is designed to protect the product from environmental stress and physical damage during shipping. The effectiveness of the packaging in protecting the product should be monitored for every lot by analyzing data received through the internal QC testing. Label control is the responsibility of both of the QA and manufacturing departments. Documented printed material Literature

Approval system is maintained, through which new labels and literature copy is circulated for approval before printing. All labels, literature, and packaging are subjected to incoming inspection. Each label is assigned a unique number and is revision controlled. The variable information (batch no., manufacturing date or expiry date) subjected to be printed on labels during manufacturing and packaging should be in password secured files. All labeling operations require label inspection and reconciliation. Pre-printed labeling materials must be stored in locked cabinets or access controlled areas. Finished products are labeled according to written procedures. The final product is processed for packaging after proper line clearance by QA before the start of the next operation. QC personnel inspect finished products using statistically valid sampling plans. The relevant procedures for labeling controls are contained in:

- Labeling guidelines
- Labeling control
- Labeling review form
- Instruction sheets—revising
- Printing and inspecting
- Line clearance and
- Inspection of assembled labeling kits

16. **Stability study programmes and procedures:** Stability study guidelines provide the core stability study plan and data generation requirements for registration of active pharmaceutical ingredients (API) and finished pharmaceutical products (FPP). Stability testing provides evidence about the quality consistency of API or FPP when exposed to a variety of unfavorable environmental factors such as temperature, humidity, and light. Stability programme also includes the study of product related factors that influence its quality, for example, the interaction of API with excipients,

container closure systems or with the packaging materials. In general, the drug products are evaluated under designated storage conditions with appropriate tolerances. The stability tests are designed predominantly to check the thermal stability and sensitivity to moisture. Stability study duration and specific storage conditions chosen for a product should be sufficient to cover the storage and shipment period and shelf life of a particular API or EPP.

The equipment used for stability studies is custom designed stability chamber capable of controlling the storage conditions within the ranges defined in guidelines (ICH, WHO, ASEAN, etc.). The long-term testing usually takes place over a minimum of 12 months period and are continued for a period sufficient to cover the proposed re-test period or shelf-life. Data from the accelerated storage condition and the intermediate storage condition are used to evaluate the effect of short-term excursions outside the labeled storage conditions (like during shipping). In case 'significant change' occurs any time during six months accelerated storage testing condition, additional testing at the intermediate storage condition is conducted and evaluated against 'significant change' criteria. 'Significant change' for a drug product is defined as failure to meet its defined specification. The storage condition in stability studies (temperature and humidity) for long term, intermediate and accelerated studies depends on recommended/intended storage condition of the drug product (room temperature, refrigerator, and freezer) and climatic/temperature zone of the country which is under consideration for marketing authorization. The testing frequency and test parameters depend on the type of stability study and type of formulation respectively. The commonly followed stability testing conditions followed for solid dosage form are:

Study duration	Storage condition	The minimum period covered for data submission
Long-term	25° ± 2°C/60% ± 5% RH or 30° ± 2°C/65% ± 5% RH 30° ± 2°C/75% ± 5% RH	6 to 12 months
Intermediate	30° ± 2°C/65% ± 5% RH	6 months
Accelerated	40°± 2°C/75% ± 5% RH	6 months

This specified storage condition is for general case products recommended for storage at room temperature. The long-term stability studies are conducted at conditions 25° ± 2°C/60% ± 5% RH or 30° ± 2°C/65% ± 5% RH or 30° ± 2°C/75% ± 5% RH which is determined by the climatic condition under which the drug product is intended to be stored. Testing in more severe long term storage conditions 30° ± 2°C/75% ± 5% RH works as an alternative to testing conditions 25°C/60% RH or 30°C/65% RH. When the long-term testing conditions are 30° ± 2°C / 65% ± 5% RH or 30°± 2°C/75% ± 5% RH intermediate testing conditions are not required.

17. **Statistical techniques:** Statistical methods are used wherever applicable to ensure product quality consistency. Statistical methods are compelling tools regularly used nowadays in the quality process. Statistical methods are selected with care to assure suitability with the required application for an objective based output. Application of statistical methods assists in elimination or minimization of the variation in the quality system, which is subjected to variations due to variability in design, equipment, and components. Statistical techniques are mostly applied to assess the design input (determining requirements to fulfil quality expectations), design control (for periodic evaluation to provide assurance of acceptable quality products), shelf life (to determine appropriate storage conditions for products), process control (to determine the capabilities of machine and process), defect analysis (understanding problems related to implementation) and data analysis (review of process and products).

Statistical tools used are:
* Statistical sampling and inspection
* Flowcharts: Pictorial diagrams of processes or systems
* Histograms: Plot frequency of events
* Analysis of variance
* Regression analysis
* Level of significance
* Consistency table
* Risk analysis
* Root cause analysis
* Pareto diagrams—assist with sorting crucial problems

18. **Manufacturing operations and in-process controls**
Production and process control: In the product development stage, the manufacturing process that requires strict controls for a particular product is identified, and the effects of variables and appropriate limits are established. This process control encompasses details of product planning, written manufacturing procedures, calibration, supervision, inspection, training of employee for process awareness. Documentations are done for the following procedures:
* Product and process control
* Engineering and maintenance
* Master formula record

- Validation of equipment, machines, process, personnel
- Weighing and dispensing of material
- In-process QA at various stages
- Acceptance activities
- Calibration programme
- Specific instructions for sterile products
- Reserve samples
- Training programme and details of various modules
- Non-conforming products
- Corrective actions and preventive actions
- Complaints and handling system
- Product recalls
- Returned goods and disposal system

When a change in the manufacturing process is required, it is strictly managed by change control procedure which is developed, adequately qualified and validated as per regulatory requirements.

- Written procedures contain details of raw and packaging materials, instructions for the production process, equipment required, working environment, filling and labeling instructions, record sheets, expiration dating, in-process testing and acceptance criteria.
- Monitoring of product manufacturing is done by a review of batch records containing the current revisions of the documents required for the manufacturing of a particular product. The batch record for every product is assembled under the document control system, and QC department keeps the official copies of these documents and matches specifications as per the master formula record. QA monitors compliance through review and approval of completed batch records before the final product release.
- The deviation control procedure handles deviations from the approved manufacturing procedures as per the prequalified specifications. A deviation specification is issued for any deviation in the manufacturing procedure even if the final product ultimately meets final release specifications.
- All new inclusions in manufacturing, measuring and test equipment are inspected and validated, against manufacturer's specifications and identified with a permanent identification number. Pieces of equipment are calibrated regularly as perscheduled following the specifications of individual equipment. Improperly maintained or calibrated equipment must not be used. The QC maintains records of calibration and maintenance and/or QA Department. QA audits equipment periodically to ensure compliance of the calibration proceeding according to schedule.
- The manufacturing supervisor/ chemist /lead personnel contributes to quality system improvement through training and assisting employees with new and specialized processes, interpreting instructions and communicating process changes. An internal Notification Procedure is adapted to circulate the inter-departmental message upon receipt of new process or equipment.

Documentation of quality related records are necessary for assurance of conformance to the regulations and also to aid management in reviewing the effectiveness of the quality system and making decisions on improvement proposals. Records are maintained to assure compliance with specifications and standards. All records are stored in conditions to facilitate their preservation and ready access by appropriate personnel. The records are retained for at least four years, or as specified in individual SOPs or customer contracts.

Non-conforming product: The system for non-conforming materials works under the administration of QA with the participation of the QC department. Quality System develops a procedure for the identification, evaluation, segregation, documentation, and disposition of non-conforming product. Appropriate technical personnel review the non-conforming material and make decisions concerning the disposition of that material in Review Board (RB) meeting called upon by employees with knowledge of non-conforming materials. Minutes of the RB meetings are maintained in master control documents of the product. A summary of RB meetings is distributed quarterly to managers for review.

All non-conforming materials are marked with quarantine stickers or labeled appropriately. Also, physically separated from conforming material until final disposition. QC can release minor non-conformities after corrective actions with adequate documentation. All corrective actions must be approved appropriately and adequately documented. A reworked product must undergo all required inspections and tests as well as any additional inspection or testing required by the RB. Reworked material must pass the same release criteria as the original product.

Disposition of major non-conformities lies with the QC and QA. The related procedures are:

- Review Board responsibility
- Deviation specification
- Corrective action and preventive action
- Rework procedure
- Reprocessing procedure
- Procedure for quarantine of rejecting product
- Procedure for disposition of rejected products

Corrective action and preventive action: Preventive and corrective actions are undertaken to tackle any identified product or procedure non-conformity. Corrective action is adopted to remedy identified non-conformities. Preventive action is adopted to eliminate the cause of a potential non-conformance and to prevent future recurrences. Whenever appropriate, a root cause analysis is done to identify the underlying cause of the non-conformity. An action plan is put together by QA as being responsible for monitoring and documenting the progress of corrective and preventive action and to ensure its completion. Corrective or preventive action that results in adaptation of changes is approved and documented through the document change request system or department level document control.

Staff training: Pharmaceutical regulatory emphasize regular training of employees to ensure that all personnel are trained and skilled to undertake their assigned activities and responsibilities effectively. The HR department procures and recruits employees capable of meeting the technical skill, experience and educational requirements as per the company's activities, but continual upgradation is of utmost importance.

The managerial personnel is responsible for recommending the training needs of all the staff. Ensuring that all employees allocated with specific tasks are suitably qualified and experienced to execute those tasks is the responsibility of QA and QC managers. Once training needs are identified, the Directors arrange experts and facilities for in-house training. Full records along with evaluation details are maintained of all training undertaken by the employees.

Management Review: Management reviews are scheduled twice in a year to ensure continuity in assessment, efficiency, and effectiveness of the whole quality system. The management review committee is constituted with appropriate personnel from all the key functional areas like Managing Director, management representative and all department heads. This review includes an assessment of opportunities, change needs, possibilities for improvement, along with quality policy aim, and objectives. It focuses on the improvement of product quality as per the needs of the customer and regulatory requirements. The proceeding is recorded and maintained.

The inputs for management review are:
- Process performance
- Audit data and results
- Factors affecting the quality management system
- Customer feedback and complaints
- Review of corrective and preventive action
- Review of the previous management review meeting
- Compliance after a previous management review meeting
- Recommendations of previous management review

The outputs of the management review are:
- Meeting quality needs (resource, equipment, finance, etc)
- Resolving customer complaints
- Improvement of the quality management process
- Improvement of product acceptability
- Compliance of previous management review meeting shortcomings

For continuous improvement of the quality system, the company management needs to utilize the tools like the quality policy, quality objective, audit results, corrective action, preventive action, management review, data analysis, resource management, quality risk management, and change management.

QUALITY MANAGEMENT PROGRAMME AND SYSTEMS

Introduction

Quality Systems Approach to Pharmaceutical cGMP Regulations guidance is intended to help manufacturers implementing modern quality system and risk management approaches to fulfil the requirements of the current good manufacturing practice (cGMP) regulations as per 21 CFR. The guideline delineates the comprehensive *quality systems (QS) model highlighting* consistency with the cGMP regulatory requirements for manufacturing human and veterinary drugs, and biological drug products. The guideline also explains how manufacturers can implement such quality systems in full compliance with cGMP.

Background and Purpose of QMP

The pharmaceutical companies implement Quality Management system (QMS) with an aim to integrate quality system and risk management approaches into existing programs in encouraging adoption of modern and innovative manufacturing technologies. The cGMP initiative is spurred by the fact that despite the regular major revision of the cGMP regulations time to time, many advances in manufacturing technologies took place continuously upgrading understanding of quality systems. Nowadays pharmaceutical manufacturers are implementing comprehensive quality systems along with risk management approaches in manufacturing practices.

A Quality System Guidance Development working group (QS working group) was created by the cGMPs for the 21st Century Initiative steering committee to compare the current cGMP regulations with other existing quality management systems. The QS working group is intended to map the relationship between cGMP regulations and various quality system models, such as the Drug Manufacturing Inspections Program (i.e. systems-based inspectional program), ISO Quality Standards, and other quality related Publications. The QS working group determined that the cGMP regulations do not consider all of the elements that constitute the most current quality management systems. Recently developed QS guidelines stress on the practice of quality management, quality assurance, and risk management tools in addition to quality control. The QS working group examined precisely compatibility of the cGMP regulations with the elements of the modern quality system in current drug manufacturing perspectives. Quality has been identified as a key strategy by WHO to ensure availability of safe drugs for all patients. The WHO and ICH have developed the QMP as an innovative initiative designed to build capacity in quality management for drugs at the global level.

Objectives of QMP

This focuses on promoting the principles of quality systems and assisting drug services and national authorities to implement effective quality systems through:

- Development of capacity in quality management.
- Identifications and strengthening of quality training.
- Development of advocacy and training materials on quality management.
- Establishment of External Quality Assessment Schemes for drugs.

- Development of a monitoring and evaluation system for the provision of post-training support and follow-up
- Creation of effective quality networks.

Goal of Guidance

The guidance provides a comprehensive quality systems model, that when implemented enabled the manufacturers to achieve a robust, modern quality system fully compliant with cGMP regulations. The guidance demonstrates the compatibility of the requirements of the cGMP regulations with the comprehensive quality system model. The inherent flexibility of the cGMP regulations enables manufacturers to implement the quality system appropriate for specific operations. The over arching philosophy articulated by both quality system and the cGMP regulations orchestrated the mission 'Quality should be built into product and testing alone cannot be relied on to ensure product quality (Fig. 4.8).'

This guidance aimed to serve as a bridge between the old regulations and current understanding of quality systems. In addition to being part of the FDA's cGMP initiative, the guidelines are useful for various other reasons:

- The mutual goal of the quality system is to provide high-quality drug product to the consumer. A well-built quality system will prevent or reduce the number of recalls, returned or salvaged products, and defective products entering the marketplace.
- Harmonization of the cGMPs with other widely used quality management systems including ISO 9000 will improve pharmaceutical quality management requirements. The convergence of quality management principles across different regions and among various product types have made it desirable in the era of globalization with the increasing prevalence of drug and biological device combination products.

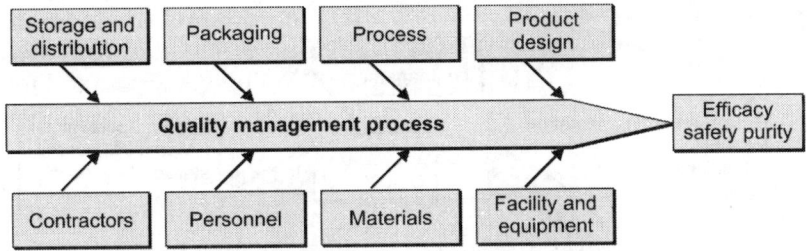

Fig. 4.8: Aspects of the quality management process

- The modern quality systems coupled with the knowledge of manufacturing process and product attributes can handle different categories of changes in facilities, equipment, and processes without the need for regulatory submission. Manufactures with appropriate process knowledge employing a robust quality system can implement various types of improvements without the need for a prior regulatory filing. Also, an effective quality system will lower the risk of manufacturing problems.
- A quality system provides the necessary framework for implementation of quality by design (building in quality form the development phase and throughout a product' life-cycle), continuous improvement, and risk management in the drug manufacturing processes, and appropriate use of finite resources.

This guidance applies to manufacturers of the drug (APIs), drug product (finished pharmaceuticals), veterinary products, biological products and components used in the manufacture of all these products. The guideline aims at:
- Performance with the intended results that satisfy the quality requirements.
- Motivated by stakeholders internal to the organization, especially the organization's management.
- Implementation of an effective, efficient, and continually improving quality system.
- Scope covers all activities that affect the total quality related business results of the organization.

The important quality management programme and systems applicable to handle pharmaceutical production and manufacturing discussed herewith are:
1. Total quality management
2. Product complaint management
3. Pharmaceutical Quality System (ICH Q10)
4. Guidance for Industry: Quality Systems Approach to Pharmaceutical cGMP Regulation
5. Quality Risk Management (ICH Q9)

TOTAL QUALITY MANAGEMENT

Introduction

Perfect quality pharmaceutical products need higher financial resources and human efforts. Total quality control is the description of the culture, attitude and organization structure of a company that aims to provide continual quality products to its customers to satisfy their needs. Total Quality Management (TQM) is an approach and art of management to control quality in an organized and cost-effective manner. TQM concept was first proposed by Dr. W. Edwards Deming in the late 1950s which was heartily endorsed by Japan in their recovery from World War II. Making a product perfect form the first trial is one of the principal objectives of TQM. Implementing a successful TQM program cost is reduced instead of increasing. TQM is the application of quantitative methods and human resource to improve all the process

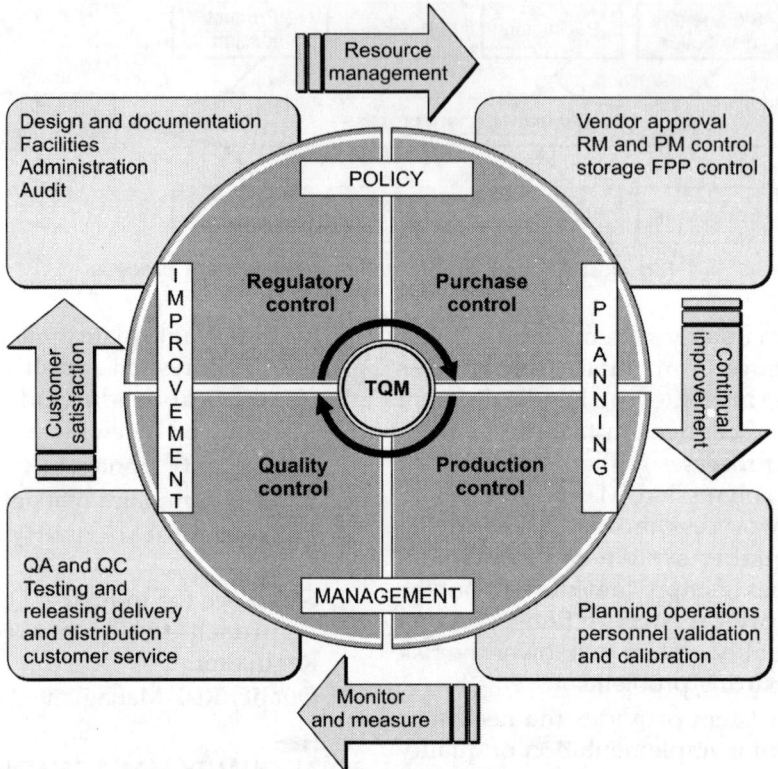

Fig. 4.9: Quality system management process

within the organization on a long-term outcome basis (Fig. 4.9).

TQM is an essential practice in the pharmaceutical manufacturing sector. TQM is a management technique and a process by which an organization ensures that all its operations are carried on in accordance with the set standards of quality. TQM not only take into account the manufacturing processes but also includes the quality management at all levels and stages of operations, *viz.* from the purchase of raw materials to the final distribution of the finished products. In the competitive highly regulated global market place the major factor that helps in withstanding regulatory compliance pressure by the organizations are systems of successful implementation of quality in leadership, management, employees, work processes,

product, and system. Pharmaceutical products should meet not only regulatory constraints but also customer and community needs. Continuous improvement helps in providing timely, cost-effective and innovative products.

The Primary Elements of TQM

TQM is a management system in a customer focused organization that involves all employees in continual improvement of all aspects of the organization. TQM uses strategy, data and effective communication to integrate the quality principles into the culture and activities of the organization. TQM is a structured system for meeting the quality needs and standards by creating organization wide participation in the planning and implementation of continuous improvement in all processes (Fig. 4.10).

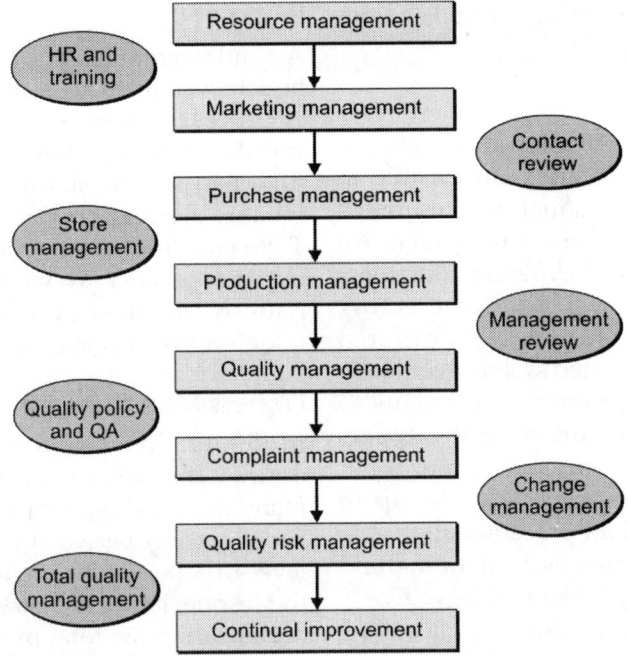

Fig. 4.10: Interaction between different stages of quality management process

Total Employee Involvement

Participation of all employees toward achieving the common goal of quality is the most crucial element of TQM. High-performance work systems integrate continuous improvement efforts within regular operations. Well-controlled system managed work teams are one of the most important forms of empowerment towards implementing TQM.

Personnel Communication

In day-to-day operations, effective communication plays a vital role in maintaining morale and in motivating employees at all levels. Regular interaction and communications should involve strategies issues, method development tactics and adherence to timeline. Communication at all levels and between different sections like QA and QC, production, store and management representative helps in improvement of transparency, cooperation, and teamwork capability.

Strategic Approach

A critical part of quality management is the strategic and systematic approach to achieve the organization's vision, mission, and goals. The strategic planning includes the conception of a strategic plan for execution of the goal that integrates quality as a core component.

Continual Improvement

A major thrust factor contributing achievement of TQM is continual process improvement. The implemented systems and process require regular review for detection of deviation and failures. Continual improvement in the process by corrective and preventive measures reduces the chances of deviation, in turn, reducing the rejection and disapproval ultimately ensuing high quality cost-effective products. Organizations applying both analytical and creative ways for continual improvement become more competitive and efficient in minimizing quality failure, thus meeting the stakeholder expectations.

System Integration

Although every organization has a unique work culture, it is virtually impossible to achieve excellence in product services unless a good quality culture has been fostered. All organizations consist of different functional specialties processing interconnecting functions, organized into vertically structured departments. An integrated system eventually connects quality improvement elements to continually improve and cater the expectations of customers, employees, and other stakeholders. Micro-processes add up to larger processes, and all processes aggregate into the managerial processes defining and implementing the quality strategy. Every employee of the organization must understand the vision, mission, and guiding principles that govern the quality policies and objectives (Fig. 4.11).

Process Focus

A fundamental part of TQM integration can be achieved by focusing on process execution. A process is a series of activities drawing inputs from suppliers (external) or staffs (internal) and transforming them into outputs (quality products) delivered to the customers. TQM ensures that the sequential steps carried out in a process are well defined and continuously monitored to measure performance to detect unexpected variation rapidly.

Process Management

In the quality system, policy management defines the process in a specified way as manuals and directives with integration and coordination between employees at every level in a particular organization. Quality is the responsibility of every one working in an organization, as total quality control can be achieved when quality is maintained at each and every step of a process which involves staffs from all the departments starting from

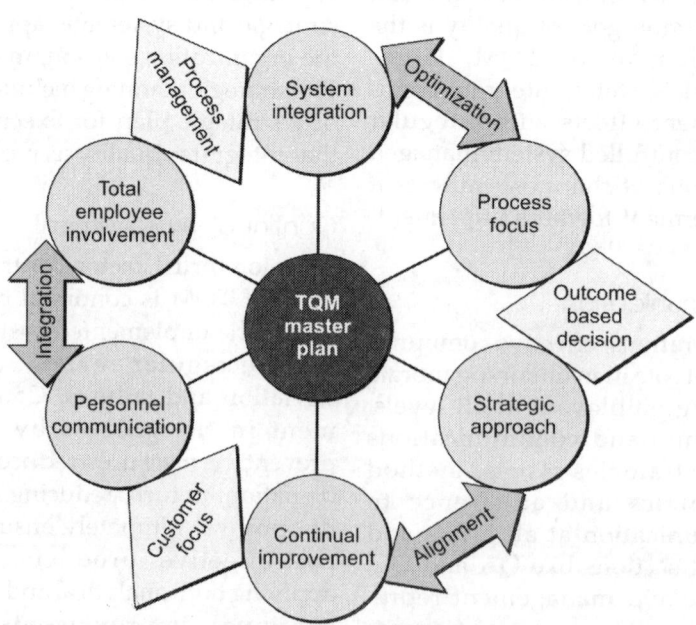

Fig. 4.11: Contributing elements to total quality management master plan

purchase, store, production, QC, QA along with sales and distribution personnel.

Outcome Based Decision

Data analysis for performance measurement are necessary in order to assess the compliance status of the quality specification and guideline in an organization. Periodic internal or external audits measure performance. TQM requires that an organization should continually collect and analyze data in order to improve decision making accuracy in corrective and preventive measures.

Customer Focus

The customers who determine the level of quality are the ultimate end user of pharmaceutical products like all other products, but the quality of pharmaceutical products is the mandatory requirement for regulatory compliance and marketing authorization. Integrating quality into the design process of pharmaceutical formulations and continuous upgrading of formulations meeting the changing requirements of the customer determines the market sustain of the companies.

Practice of TQM

Effective integration between functions and activities of employees can be developed with the help of regular communication which contributes to process management. Optimization between system integration and focus on process helps to make correct outcome based decision. Strategic approach aligned with continual improvement delivers customer focused products. Coordination between these three systems with an aim to produce and maintain quality products is the concept called TQM.

These elements are considered so essential to TQM goal achievement that organizations define them as a set of core values and principles on which the organization is to operate. TQM is a dynamic management system, which continuously evolved over the last half of the 20th century. Currently, two of the most effective and popular "new" management models are Lean, and Six Sigma models which utilize the basic TQM elements and add on some extra refinements to achieve a more robust and powerful system for cost-effective customer focused products with quality excellence. Overall implementation of TQM depends on adoption of a quality improvement culture having commitment and cooperation from employees. Continuous improvement in process and effective control focusing on customer need can be conceptualized as fulfilling needs of the regulatory bodies in case of pharmaceutical products.

PRODUCT COMPLAINT MANAGEMENT

Product complaints management is essential from the regulatory compliance perspective. Many pharmaceutical companies view complaint management as a process not related to the overall management of customer relationships, but is a vital part of consumer management. Product failure can be fatal for customers and have severe legal implications for manufacturers. Uniform and secure platform to manage product complaints right from initiation through the review requires an immediate and real-time response system. The dynamic and stringent regulatory landscape is making it mandatory for organizations to track, record and report all complaints concerning product quality and safety, and to take appropriate follow-up actions to prevent reoccurrence of such incidents. Regulatory and competitive pressures are compelling pharmaceutical manufacturing organizations to change the product complaint management strategy. A properly executed complaints management programme can decrease customer complaint maintenance and compensation costs, increase revenues, and improve company's ability to track historical customer and product trends, which is useful to forecast the future market, product and customer needs. In pharmaceuticals, effective complaints management is hard to achieve, and it can also be difficult to ensure compliance with government regulations.

Functionality of the Complaint Management System

The complaint management should provide an integrated approach to the complaint with the interaction of various stakeholders, such as manufacturers, patients, doctors, and regulatory authorities. The core functionality should be integrated with ADR reporting processes and peripheral applications. The complaint management process covers various functions in stages:

- Receipt: Consolidation of different channels of complaint receipt such as web, email, fax, telephone, sales team and so on is done into one uniform platform. Customers should have either a web portal to log complaints online or a toll-free number to submit complaints.
- Routing and escalation: Automatic routing of complaints is done depending on the severity and type of complaint about further investigations, i.e. forwarding quality problems to QC, production related issues to production control or safety problems to QA. This ensures automatic escalation of the non-completed actions in the workflow including an automated trigger for internal corrective and preventive action.
- Data and complaint management: Critical information related to a product complaint to final sign-off is automatically tracked by the capturing data from online product complaints system. This system is able to trace all data related to storage, archival and retrieval of all the product compliant-related documents. Data uploading is an important requirement of the receipt functionality where investigational data about the complaint can be uploaded during the complaint life cycle.

- Task management: Automatic task management features are developed for different consequences related to complain processing.
- Processing and reporting: Compliant are managed via processing across the various cross-functional departments of the company as required in a collaborative framework. The system should also include an option to view compliant summaries, in-process complaints, investigational outcome and performance trend analysis as per type, product and department.
- User management: This system is intended to track actual users and take appropriate compensatory action as per the complaint processing requirement.

A Step-by-step Solution to Complaint Management

Some of the salient features of good complaint management solutions are:

1. **Functionality:**
   - Single complaint enabled with multiple processing (parent-child notifications)
   - Web-based application integrated with workflow for easy understanding
   - Multiple language capability
   - Report generation
   - Escalation management
   - Reminders as required
   - Complaint closure form
   - Document management system integrated to record all attachments and reports with an individual complaint
   - Electronic signatures
   - Integration with sales and distribution processes
   - Integration with adverse event handling processes.
2. **Standardized and automated:** The system needs to have a standardized integrated, centralized process to report the complaint related events to the

regulatory authorities in the required time frame (typically 3 days).

3. **Safety and security:** The solution will interface with multiple systems in sales, customer relationship, production, material management, design, drug development, and regulatory requirements.

4. **Performance:** The technical solution is enabled with multiple integration points, workflows and data elements. The proposed solution for the complaint management should encompass clear business rules, SOPs, and workflows in a simple architectural form. An efficient and easy to use notification as well as a high-performance reporting system is also linked for solution implementation.

Benefits

A robust complaint management solution should provide with processes and technologies for gathering, classifying and preserving product information in order to diagnose the problem, anticipate the outcome and resolve the issue. It should offer direct access to specific product details required for quick problem resolution, along with a web-based entry and status reporting system for efficient customer service. A quick alert system for quality personnel should be there for critical and recurring customer reports related to a specific product. The alert system is invaluable for the management enabling quick defect-correction and customer notification before it can become a widespread issue. The solution should also result in reduced costs of compliance through minimum time and costs of processing complaints, uniform compliance, and high-quality content among all partners.

This solution can provide companies to look forward to the following benefits:
• Standardized, consistent and complete complaint handling and data collection process.
• Increased data consistency and enhanced reporting capability.
• Increased customer loyalty through quicker response time.
• All complaints captured in one single database.
• The standardized process can be rolled out globally, within a short time frame.

PHARMACEUTICAL QUALITY SYSTEM (ICH Q10)

International Conference on Harmonisation of Technical Requirements for Registration of Pharmaceuticals for Human Use
ICH Harmonised Tripartite Guideline Current Step 4 version dated 4 June 2008

(Courtesy: https://www.ich.org/fileadmin/Public_Web_Site/ICH_Products/
Guidelines/Quality/Q10/Step4/Q10_Guideline.pdf)

ICH harmonized tripartite guideline describes the requirements of the respective section in detail that is recommended to be followed by the pharmaceutical companies. Regional GMP requirements, the ICH Q7 Guideline, "Good Manufacturing Practice Guide for Active Pharmaceutical Ingredients," and ISO quality management system guidelines constitute the foundation for ICH Q10. ICH Q10 provides a harmonized model for a pharmaceutical quality system throughout the life cycle of a product and is intended to be used together with regional GMP requirements. The responsibilities for management described in this guideline are intended to encourage the use of science and risk based approaches at each life cycle stage, thereby promoting continual improvement across the entire

CUSTOMER PRODUCT COMPLAINT REPORT FORM

Product details

Product name:	Strength:
Manufacturer:	Pack size:
Batch no.:	Expiry date:

Product storage condition (protection from sunlight, heat, moisture, etc.):

Complaint details

Complainant name:	Date:
Address:	Contact No.:

Type of Complaint	**Complaint concern**
Product Appearance:	Product elegance:
Odour:	Package condition:
Packaging:	Product stability:
Labeling:	Product efficacy:
Break in cold chain:	Product integrity:
Storage condition:	Product safety:
Any other:	

Detail description of complaint

Additional information

Integrity of package and sealing at the time of product receipt by the customer:

Overall appearance and condition of product:

Product complaint submitted to

Name:	Department:
Date:	Sign:

PRODUCT COMPLAINT PROCESSING REPORT

Product details

Product name: Strength:

Batch no.:   Pack size: Expiry date:

Product recommended storage condition:

Product description

Sample receipt: Quantity:

Product condition:

Product condition in accordance with complaint: Yes   No

Detailed description of complaint:

Classification of complaint pertaining to quality

Minor   Major   Critical

Assessment of complaint

Complaint on product quality (refer to production dept.):

Ref. no.:... Date:....................................

Complaint on adverse drug reactions (refer to clinical dept.):

Ref. no.:... Date:....................................

Complaint not clearly defined (investigate and make recommendation):

Ref. no.::... Date:....................................

Corrective action taken (Ref. no.:................................. Date:....................................)

Name of reporter:

Designation:

Department:

Sign: Date:

product life cycle. When implemented, the effectiveness of the pharmaceutical quality system can generally be evaluated during a regulatory inspection at the manufacturing site. Potential opportunities to enhance science and risk based regulatory approaches are identified in Annexure 1.

1. INTRODUCTION

This document establishes a new ICH tripartite guideline describing a model for an effective quality management system for the pharmaceutical industry, referred to as the Pharmaceutical Quality System. Throughout this guideline, the term "pharmaceutical quality system" refers to the ICH Q10 model. ICH Q10 describes one comprehensive model for an effective pharmaceutical quality system that is based on International Standards Organisation (ISO) quality concepts, includes applicable Good Manufacturing Practice (GMP) regulations and complements ICH Q8 "Pharmaceutical Development" and ICH Q9 "Quality Risk Management." ICH Q10 is a model for a pharmaceutical quality system that can be implemented throughout the different stages of a product life cycle. Regional GMP requirements currently specify much of the content of ICH Q10 applicable to manufacturing sites. ICH Q10 is not intended to create any new expectations beyond current regulatory requirements. Consequently, the content of ICH Q10 is additional to current regional GMP requirements.

ICH Q10 demonstrates an effective pharmaceutical quality system to enhance the quality and availability of medicines around the world in the interest of the public health industry and regulatory authorities. Implementation of ICH Q10 throughout the product life cycle facilitate innovation and continual improvement and strengthen the link between pharmaceutical development and manufacturing activities.

2. SCOPE

This guideline applies to the systems supporting the development and manufacture of pharmaceutical drug substances (i.e. API) and drug products, including biotechnological and biological products. The elements of ICH Q10 should be applied in a manner that is appropriate and proportionate to each of the product lifecycle stages, recognizing the differences among, and the different goals of each stage. For the purposes of this guideline, the product lifecycle includes the following technical activities for new and existing products:

- Pharmaceutical Development
  - Drug substance development;
  - Formulation development (including container/closure system);
  - Manufacture of investigational products;
  - Delivery system development;
  - Manufacturing process development and scale-up;
  - Analytical method development.
- Technology transfer
  - Analytical method development. New product transfers during development through manufacturing;
  - Analytical method development. Transfers within or between manufacturing and testing sites for marketed products.
- Commercial manufacturing
  - Analytical method development. Acquisition and control of materials;
  - Analytical method development. Provision of facilities, utilities, and equipment;
  - Analytical method development. Production (including packaging and labeling);
  - Analytical method development. Quality control and assurance;
  - Analytical method development. Release;

– Analytical method development. Storage;
– Analytical method development. Distribution (excluding wholesaler activities).
• Product discontinuation
  – Retention of documentation;
  – Sample retention;
  – Continued product assessment and reporting.

Regulatory approaches for a specific product or manufacturing facility should be commensurate with the level of product and process understanding, the results of quality risk management, and the effectiveness of the pharmaceutical quality system.

3. OBJECTIVES

Implementation of the Q10 model results in the achievement of three main objectives which complement or enhance regional GMP requirements.

3.1. Achieve Product Realization

To establish, implement and maintain a system that allows the delivery of products within the quality attributes appropriate to meet the needs of patients, health care professionals, regulatory authorities and other internal and external customers.

3.2. Establish and Maintain a State of Control

To develop and use effective monitoring and control systems for process performance and product quality, thereby assuring continued suitability and capability of processes. Quality risk management is useful in identifying the effectiveness of monitoring system control.

3.3. Facilitate Continual Improvement

To identify and implement appropriate product quality improvements, process improvements, variability reduction, innovations, and pharmaceutical quality system enhancements, thereby increasing the ability to fulfil quality needs consistently. Quality risk management is useful for identifying the prioritized areas needing continual improvement.

3.4. Enablers: Knowledge Management and Quality Risk Management

Use of knowledge management and quality risk management enable a company to implement ICH Q10 effectively and successfully. These enablers facilitate achievement of the quality objectives by providing the means for risk-based decisions related to product quality.

4. DESIGN AND CONTENT CONSIDERATIONS

a. The design, organization, and documentation of the pharmaceutical quality system should be well structured and clear to facilitate common understanding and consistent application.
b. The elements of ICH Q10 are applied in a manner that is appropriate and proportionate to each of the product life cycle stages, recognizing the different goals and knowledge available for each stage.
c. The size and complexity of the company's activities are taken into consideration when developing a new pharmaceutical quality system or modifying an existing one. The design of the pharmaceutical quality system should incorporate appropriate risk management principles.
d. The pharmaceutical quality system includes appropriate processes, resources, and responsibilities to assure the quality of outsourced activities and purchased materials.
e. Management responsibilities, are to be identified within the pharmaceutical quality system.
f. The pharmaceutical quality system includes elements like process performance and product quality monitoring, corrective and preventive action, change management and management review.

g. Performance indicators, are to be identified and used to monitor the effectiveness of processes within the pharmaceutical quality system.

5. QUALITY MANUAL

A Quality Manual or equivalent documentation approach is to be established that contains the description of the pharmaceutical quality system. The description should include:

a. The quality policy;
b. The scope of the pharmaceutical quality system;
c. Identification of the pharmaceutical quality system processes, as well as their sequences, linkages, and interdependencies. Process maps and flow charts are useful tools for visually depicting pharmaceutical quality system processes;
d. Management responsibilities within the pharmaceutical quality system.

6. MANAGEMENT RESPONSIBILITY

Leadership is essential to establish and maintain a company-wide commitment to quality and for the performance of the pharmaceutical quality system.

a. Senior management has the ultimate responsibility to ensure an effective pharmaceutical quality system is in place to achieve the quality objectives, and that roles, responsibilities, and authorities are defined, communicated and implemented throughout the company.
b. Management should:
  1. Participate in the design, implementation, monitoring, and maintenance for an effective pharmaceutical quality system;
  2. Demonstrate strong and visible support for the pharmaceutical quality system and ensure its implementation throughout their organization;

3. Ensure timely and effective communication, and escalation process exists to raise quality issues to the appropriate levels of management;
4. Define individual and collective roles, responsibilities, authorities, and interrelationships of all organizational units related to the pharmaceutical quality system. Ensure these interactions are communicated and understood at all levels of the organization.
5. Conduct management reviews for process performance and product quality;
6. Advocate continual improvement;
7. Commit appropriate resources.

6.1 Quality Policy

a. Senior management establishes a quality policy that describes the overall intentions and direction of the company related to quality.
b. The quality policy includes an expectation to comply with applicable regulatory requirements and should facilitate continual improvement of the pharmaceutical quality system.
c. The quality policy should be communicated to and understood by personnel at all levels in the company.
d. The quality policy is to be reviewed periodically for continuing effectiveness.

6.2 Quality Planning

a. Senior management ensures that the quality objectives needed to implement the quality policy are defined and communicated.
b. All relevant levels of the company should support quality objectives.
c. Quality objectives should align with the company's strategies and be consistent with the quality policy.
d. Management provides the appropriate resources and training to achieve quality objectives.

e. Performance indicators that measure progress against quality objectives are established, monitored, communicated regularly and acted upon as appropriate.

6.3 Resource Management

a. Management determines and provides adequate and appropriate resources (human, financial, materials, facilities and equipment) to implement and maintain the pharmaceutical quality system and continually improve its effectiveness.

b. Management also ensures that resources are appropriately applied to a specific product, process or site.

6.4 Internal Communication

a. Management ensures that appropriate communication processes are established and implemented within the organization.

b. Communications processes should ensure the flow of appropriate information between all levels of the company.

c. Communication processes ensure the appropriate and timely escalation of certain product quality and pharmaceutical quality system issues.

6.5 Management Review

a. Senior management is responsible for pharmaceutical quality system governance through management review to ensure its continuing suitability and effectiveness.

b. Management assesses the conclusions of periodic reviews of process performance and product quality and the pharmaceutical quality system.

6.6 Management of Outsourced Activities and Purchased Materials

The pharmaceutical company is ultimately responsible for ensuring processes which are in place to assure the control of outsourced activities and quality of purchased materials. These processes should incorporate quality risk management and include:

a. Assessing before outsourcing operations or selecting material suppliers, the suitability and competence of the other party is checked for providing the material using a defined supply chain (e.g. audits, material evaluations, qualification);

b. Defining the responsibilities and communication processes for quality-related activities of the involved parties. For outsourced activities, this should be included in a written agreement between the contract giver and contract acceptor;

c. Monitoring and review of the performance of the contract acceptor or the quality of the material from the provider, and the identification and implementation of any needed improvements;

d. Monitoring of incoming ingredients and materials to ensure that they are from approved sources delivered by the agreed supply chain.

7. CONTINUAL IMPROVEMENT OF PROCESS PERFORMANCE AND PRODUCT QUALITY

This section describes the life cycle stage goals and the four specific pharmaceutical quality system elements that augment regional requirements to achieve the ICH Q10 objectives.

7.1 Pharmaceutical Development

The goal of pharmaceutical development activities is to design a product and its manufacturing process to consistently deliver the intended performance and meet the needs of patients and healthcare professionals and regulatory authorities. The results of exploratory and clinical development studies, while outside the scope of this guidance, are inputs to pharmaceutical development.

7.2 Technology Transfer

The goal of technology transfer activities is to transfer product and process knowledge between development and manufacturing, and within or between manufacturing sites to achieve product realization. This knowledge forms the basis for the manufacturing process, control strategy, process validation approach and ongoing continual improvement.

7.3 Commercial Manufacturing

The goals of manufacturing activities include achieving product realization, establishing and maintaining a state of control and facilitating continual improvement. The pharmaceutical quality system should assure that the desired product quality is routinely met, suitable process performance is achieved, the set of controls are appropriate, improvement opportunities are identified and evaluated.

7.4 Product Discontinuation

The goal of product discontinuation activities is to manage the terminal stage of the product life cycle effectively. For product discontinuation, a pre-defined approach is used to manage activities such as retention of documentation and samples and continued product assessment (e.g. complaint handling and stability) and reporting in accordance with regulatory requirements.

8. PHARMACEUTICAL QUALITY SYSTEM ELEMENTS

The elements described below are required in part under regional GMP regulations. However, the Q10 model intends to enhance these elements in order to promote the life cycle approach to product quality. These four elements are:
- Process performance and product quality monitoring system;
- Corrective action and preventive action (CAPA) system;
- Change management system;

- Management review of process performance and product quality.

These elements should be applied in a manner that is appropriate and proportionate to each of the product life cycle stages, recognizing the differences among, and the different goals of, each stage. Throughout the product life cycle, companies are encouraged to evaluate opportunities for innovative approaches to improve product quality.

8.1 Process Performance and Product Quality Monitoring System

Pharmaceutical companies should plan and execute a system for the monitoring of process performance and product quality to ensure a state of control is maintained. An effective monitoring system assures the continued capability of processes and controls to produce a product of desired quality and to identify areas for continual improvement. The process performance and product quality monitoring system should include:

a. Quality risk management policy is used to establish a control strategy. This can include parameters and attributes related to drug substance and drug product materials and components, facility and equipment operating conditions, in-process controls, finished product specifications, and the associated methods. The control strategy facilitates timely feedback/feed-forward and appropriate corrective action and preventive action;

b. Provide the tools for measurement and analysis of parameters and attributes identified in the control strategy (e.g. data management and statistical tools);

c. Analyze parameters and attributes identified in the control strategy to verify continued operation within a state of control;

d. Identify sources of variation affecting process performance and product quality for potential continual improvement activities to reduce or control variation;

e. Include feedback on product quality from both internal and external sources, e.g. complaints, product rejections, non-conformances, recalls, deviations, audits, and regulatory inspections and findings;

f. Provide knowledge to enhance process understanding, enrich the design space (where established), and enable innovative approaches to process validation.

8.2 Corrective Action and Preventive Action (CAPA) System

A pharmaceutical company must have a system for implementing corrective actions and preventive actions resulting from the investigation of complaints, product rejections, non-conformances, recalls, deviations, audits, regulatory inspections and findings, and trends from process performance and product quality monitoring. A structured approach to the investigation process should be used with the objective of determining the root cause. The level of effort, formality, and documentation of the investigation should be commensurate with the level of risk, in line with ICH Q9. CAPA methodology results in product and process improvements and enhanced product and process understanding.

8.3 Change Management System

Innovation, continual improvement, outputs of process performance, product quality monitoring and CAPA drive implementation of change management. In order to evaluate, approve and implement these changes correctly, a company should have an effective change management system. There is generally a difference in the formality of change management processes before the initial regulatory submission and after submission, where changes to the regulatory filing might be required under regional requirements.

Change management system ensures that continual improvement has been undertaken in a timely and effective manner. It should provide a high degree of assurance there are no unintended consequences of the change.

The change management system should include the following, as appropriate for the stage of the life cycle:

a. Quality risk management should be utilized to evaluate the proposed changes. The level of effort and formality of the evaluation should be commensurate with the level of risk;

b. Proposed changes should be evaluated relative to the marketing authorization, including design space, where established, and/or current product and process understanding. There should be an assessment to determine whether a change to the regulatory filing is required under regional requirements. Working within the design space is not considered

Table 4.1: Application of process performance and product quality monitoring system throughout the product life cycle

Pharmaceutical development	Technology transfer	Commercial manufacturing	Product discontinuation
Process and product knowledge generated and process and product monitoring conducted throughout development can be used to establish a control strategy for manufacturing.	Monitoring during scale-up activities can provide a preliminary indication of process performance and the successful integration into manufacturing. Knowledge obtained during transfer and scale up activities can be useful in further developing the control strategy.	A well-defined system for process performance and product quality monitoring should be applied to assure performance within a state of control and to identify improvement areas.	Once manufacturing ceases, monitoring such as stability testing should continue to completion of the studies. Appropriate action on the marketed product should continue to be executed according to regional regulations.

a change from a regulatory filing perspective, however, from a pharmaceutical quality system standpoint, all changes should be evaluated by the change management system;

c. Proposed changes should be evaluated by expert teams contributing the appropriate expertise and knowledge from relevant areas (e.g. Pharmaceutical Development, Manufacturing, Quality, Regulatory Affairs, and Medical), to ensure that changes are technically justified.

d. After implementation, an evaluation of the change is to be undertaken to confirm the change objectives were achieved and that there was no deleterious impact on product quality.

8.4 Management Review of Process Performance and Product Quality

Management review should assure that process performance, and product quality is managed over the life cycle. Depending on the size and complexity of the company, management review can be a series of reviews at various levels of management and should include a timely and effective communication and escalation process to raise relevant quality issues to senior levels of management for review.

a. The management review system should include:
1. The results of regulatory inspections and findings, audits and other assessments, and commitments made to regulatory authorities;

2. Periodic quality reviews include:
   i. Measures of customer satisfaction such as product quality complaints and recalls;
   ii. Conclusions of process performance and product quality monitoring;
   iii. The effectiveness of the process and product changes including those arising from corrective action and preventive actions.
3. Any follow-up actions from previous management reviews.

b. The management review system should identify appropriate actions, such as:
1. Improvements to manufacturing processes;
2. The provision, training and/or realignment of resources;
3. Capture and dissemination of knowledge.

9. CONTINUAL IMPROVEMENT OF THE PHARMACEUTICAL QUALITY SYSTEM

This section describes activities that should be conducted to manage and continually improve the pharmaceutical quality system.

9.1 Management Review of the Pharmaceutical Quality System

Management should have a formal process for reviewing the pharmaceutical quality system on a periodic basis. The review should include:

Table 4.2: Application of corrective action and preventive action system throughout the product life cycle

Pharmaceutical development	Technology transfer	Commercial manufacturing	Product discontinuation
Product or process variability is explored. CAPA methodology is useful where corrective actions and preventive actions are incorporated into the iterative design and development process.	CAPA can be used as an effective system for feedback, feed-forward and continual improvement.	CAPA should be used, and the effectiveness of the actions should be evaluated.	CAPA should continue after the product is discontinued. The impact on product remaining on the market should be considered as well as other products which might be impacted.

Table 4.3: Application of change management system throughout the pharmaceutical product life cycle

Pharmaceutical development	Technology transfer	Commercial manufacturing	Product discontinuation
Change is an inherent part of the development process and should be documented; the formality of the change management process should be consistent with the stage of pharmaceutical development.	The change management system should provide management and documentation of adjustments made to the process during technology transfer activities.	A formal change management system should be in place for commercial manufacturing. Oversight by the quality unit should assure appropriate science and quality risk based assessments.	Any changes after product discontinuation should go through an appropriate change management system.

a. Measurement of achievements of pharmaceutical quality system objectives;
b. Assessment of performance indicators that can be used to monitor the effectiveness of processes within the pharmaceutical quality system, such as:
  1. Complaint, deviation, CAPA and change management processes;
  2. Feedback on outsourced activities;
  3. Self-assessment processes including risk assessments, trending, and audits;
  4. External assessments such as regulatory inspections, findings, and customer audits.

9.2 Monitoring of Internal and External Factors Impacting the Pharmaceutical Quality System

Factors monitored by management can include:
a. Emerging regulations, guidance and quality issues that can impact the Pharmaceutical Quality System;

b. Innovations that might enhance the pharmaceutical quality system;
c. Changes in the business environment and objectives;
d. Changes in product ownership.

9.3 Outcomes of Management Review and Monitoring

The outcome of a management review of the pharmaceutical quality system and monitoring of internal and external factors can include:
a. Improvements of the pharmaceutical quality system and related processes;
b. Allocation or reallocation of resources and/or personnel training;
c. Revisions of quality policy and quality objectives;
d. Proper documentation, timely and effective communication of the results of the management review and actions, including escalation of relevant issues to senior management.

Table 4.4: Application of management—review and monitoring throughout the pharmaceutical product life cycle

Pharmaceutical development	Technology transfer	Commercial manufacturing	Product discontinuation
Aspects of management review can be performed to ensure the adequacy of the product and process design.	Aspects of management review should be performed to ensure the developed product and process can be manufactured at commercial scale.	Management review should be a structured system, as described above, and should support continual improvement.	Management review should include such items as product stability and product quality complaints.

ANNEXURE 1

Scenario	Potential opportunity
1. Comply with GMPs	Compliance—status quo
2. Demonstrate an effective pharmaceutical quality system, including effective use of quality risk management principles (e.g. ICH Q9 and ICH Q10).	Opportunity to: • Increase the use of risk-based approaches for regulatory inspections.
3. Demonstrate product and process understanding, including effective use of quality risk management principles (e.g. ICH Q8 and ICH Q9).	Opportunity to: • Facilitate science based pharmaceutical quality assessment; • Enable innovative approaches to process validation; • Establish real-time release mechanisms.
4. Demonstrate effective pharmaceutical quality system and product and process understanding, including the use of quality risk management principles (e.g. ICH Q8, ICH Q9, and ICH Q10).	Opportunity to: • Increase use of risk based approaches for regulatory inspections; • Facilitate science based pharmaceutical quality assessment; • Optimize science and risk based post-approval change processes to maximize benefits from innovation and continual improvement; • Enable innovative approaches to process validation; • Establish real-time release mechanisms.

ANNEXURE 2

ICH Q10 Pharmaceutical Quality System Model

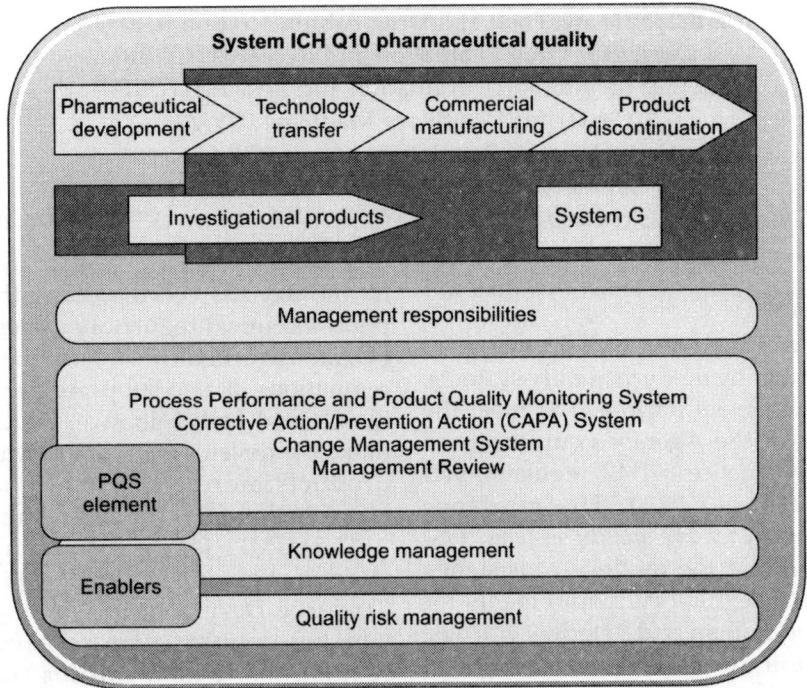

Fig. 4.12: Diagram of the ICH Q10 pharmaceutical quality system model*

This diagram illustrates the major features of the ICH Q10 Pharmaceutical Quality System (PQS) model. The PQS covers the entire lifecycle of a product including pharmaceutical development, technology transfer, commercial manufacturing, and product discontinuation. The PQS augments regional GMPs as illustrated in Fig. 4.12. The diagram illustrates that regional GMPs apply to the manufacturer of investigational products.

The next horizontal bar illustrates the importance of management responsibilities at all stages of the product life cycle. The

following horizontal bar lists the PQS elements which serve as the major pillars under the PQS model. These elements should be applied appropriately and proportionally to each life cycle stage cognizing opportunities to identify areas for continual improvement.

The bottom set of horizontal bars illustrates the enablers: Knowledge management and quality risk management, which are applicable throughout the lifecycle stages. These enablers support the PQS goals of achieving product realization, establishing and maintaining a state of control, and facilitating continual improvement.

---

* Pharmaceutical Quality System (ICH Q10)
EMA/INS/GMP/79818/2011

GUIDANCE FOR INDUSTRY: QUALITY SYSTEMS APPROACH TO PHARMACEUTICAL CGMP REGULATIONS

Contains Nonbinding Recommendations of U.S. Department of Health and Human Services
Participants are: Food and Drug Administration (USFDA)
Center for Drug Evaluation and Research (CDER)
Center for Biologics Evaluation and Research (CBER)
Center for Veterinary Medicine (CVM)
Office of Regulatory Affairs (ORA)
September 2006, Pharmaceutical CGMPs
(*Courtesy*: *https://www.fda.gov/downloads/Drugs/Guidances/UCM070337.pdf*)

1. INTRODUCTION

This guidance is intended to help manufacturers implementing modern quality systems, and risk management approach to meet the requirements of the Agency's current good manufacturing practice (cGMP) regulations (21 CFR parts 210 and 211). The guidance describes a *comprehensive quality systems (QS) model*, highlighting the model's consistency with the cGMP regulatory requirements for manufacturing human and veterinary drugs, including biological drug products. The guidance also explains how manufacturers implementing such quality systems can be in full compliance with parts 210 and 211.

1.1. Background of the Guidance

In August 2002, the FDA announced the Pharmaceutical cGMPs as an intent to integrate *quality systems* and *risk management* approaches into its existing programs with the goal of encouraging industry to adopt modern and innovative manufacturing technologies. The cGMP initiative was spurred by the fact that since 1978, when the last major revision of the cGMP regulations was published, there have been many advances in manufacturing science and the understanding of quality systems. This guidance is intended to help manufacturers implementing modern quality systems and risk management approaches to meet the requirements of the Agency's cGMP regulations. The Agency also saw a need to

harmonize the cGMPs with other non-U.S. pharmaceutical regulatory systems and with FDA's own medical device quality systems regulations. It also supports the objectives of the Critical Path Initiative, which intends to make the development of innovative medical products more efficient so that safe and effective therapies can reach patients sooner.

The cGMPs for the 21st Century Initiative steering committee created a Quality System Guidance Development working group (QS working group) to compare the current cGMP regulations, which call for some specific quality management elements, to other existing quality management systems. The QS working group mapped the relationship between cGMP regulations (parts 210 and 211 and the 1978 Preamble to the cGMP regulations) and various quality system models, such as the Drug Manufacturing Inspections Program (i.e. systems-based inspectional program), the Environmental Protection Agency's Guidance for Developing Quality Systems for Environmental Programs, ISO Quality Standards, other quality publications, and experience from regulatory cases. The QS working group determined that although the cGMP regulations do provide great flexibility, they do not incorporate explicitly all of the elements that today constitute most quality management systems.

The cGMP regulations and other quality management systems differ somewhat in the organization and certain constituent elements;

however, they are very similar and share underlying principles. For example, the cGMP regulations stress quality control. More recently developed quality systems stress quality management, quality assurance, and the use of risk management tools, in addition to quality control. The QS working group decided that it would be instrumental to examine precisely how the cGMP regulations and the elements of a modern, comprehensive quality system fit together in today's manufacturing world.

1.2 The Goal of the Guidance

This guidance describes a comprehensive quality systems model, which, if implemented, will allow manufacturers to support and sustain robust, modern quality systems that are consistent with cGMP regulations. The guidance demonstrates how and where the elements of this comprehensive model can fit within the requirements of the cGMP regulations. The inherent flexibility of the cGMP regulations should enable manufacturers to implement a quality system in a form that is appropriate for their specific operations.

The overarching philosophy articulated in both the cGMP regulations *and* in robust modern quality systems is: *Quality should be built into the product, and testing alone cannot be relied on to ensure product quality.*

This guidance is intended to serve as a bridge between the 1978 regulations and our current understanding of quality systems. In addition to being part of the FDA's cGMP initiative, this guidance is being issued for a number of reasons:

- A quality system addresses the public and private sectors' mutual goal of providing a high-quality drug product to patients and prescribers. A well-built quality system should reduce the number of (or prevent) recalls, returned or salvaged products, and defective products are entering the marketplace.

- It is essential that the cGMP regulations are harmonized to the extent possible with other widely used quality management systems, including ISO 9000, non-U.S. pharmaceutical quality management requirements, and FDA's medical device quality system regulations. This guidance serves as a first step to highlight common elements between the cGMP regulations and Quality Management Systems. With the globalization of pharmaceutical manufacturing and the increasing prevalence of drug- and biologic-device combination products, the convergence of quality management principles across different regions and among various product types is very desirable.

- The FDA has concluded that modern quality systems, when coupled with the manufacturing process and product knowledge and the use of effective risk management practices, can handle many types of changes to facilities, equipment, and processes without the need for prior approval of regulatory submissions. Manufacturers with a robust quality system and appropriate process knowledge can implement many types of improvements. In addition, an effective quality system may result in shorter and fewer FDA inspections by lowering the risk of manufacturing problems.

- A quality system can provide the necessary framework for implementing *quality by design* (building in quality from the development phase and throughout a product's life cycle), continual improvement, and risk management in the drug manufacturing process. A quality system adopted by a manufacturer can be tailored to fit the specific environment, taking into account factors such as the scope of operations, the complexity of processes and the appropriate use of finite resources.

1.3 The Scope of the Guidance

This guidance applies to manufacturers of drug products (finished pharmaceuticals), including products regulated by the Center for Biologics Evaluation and Research (CBER), the Center for Drug Evaluation and Research (CDER), and the Center for Veterinary Medicine (CVM). It may also be useful to manufacturers of components (including active pharmaceutical ingredients) used in the manufacture of these products. Instead, the document explains how implementing comprehensive quality systems can help manufacturers achieve compliance with 21 CFR parts 210 and 211.

1.4 Organization of this Guidance

To provide a reference familiar to the industry, the quality systems model described in section IV of this guidance is organized, in its major sections according to the structure of international quality standards. Major sections of the model include the following:
- Management responsibilities
- Resources
- Manufacturing operations
- Evaluation activities

Under each of these sections, the key elements found in modern quality systems are discussed. When an element correlates with a cGMP regulatory requirement, that correlation is noted. In some cases, a specific cGMP regulation is discussed in more detail as it relates to a quality system element. At the end of each section, a table is included listing the quality system elements of that section and the specific cGMP regulations with which they correlate. A glossary is included at the end of the document.

2. SIX-SYSTEM INSPECTION MODEL

The FDA's Drug Manufacturing Inspection Compliance Program, which contains instructions to FDA personnel for conducting inspections, is a system-based approach to inspection and is very consistent with the robust quality system model presented in this guidance. Figure 4.13 shows the relationship between the six systems: The quality system and the five manufacturing systems. The quality system provides the foundation for the manufacturing systems that are linked and function within it. The quality system model described in this guidance does not consider the five manufacturing systems as discrete entities but instead integrates them into appropriate sections of the model. One of the important themes of the systems based inspection compliance program is that one can assess whether each of the systems is in a state of control or not (Fig. 4.13).

2.1 The Quality System Model

Implementation of an effective quality system in a manufacturing organization requires a significant investment of time and resources. However, the long-term benefits of implementing a quality system outweigh the costs. A robust quality systems model when properly implemented, can provide the controls to produce a product of acceptable quality consistently. The specific cGMP regulations correlate to the elements in the quality system model. Many of the quality system elements correlate closely with the cGMP regulations. The model is described according to four major factors:
- Management responsibilities
- Resources
- Manufacturing operations
- Evaluation activities

2.2 Management Responsibilities

Modern, robust quality systems models call for management to play a key role in the design, implementation, and management of the quality system. Management is responsible for establishing the quality system structure appropriate for the specific organization. Management has the ultimate responsibility

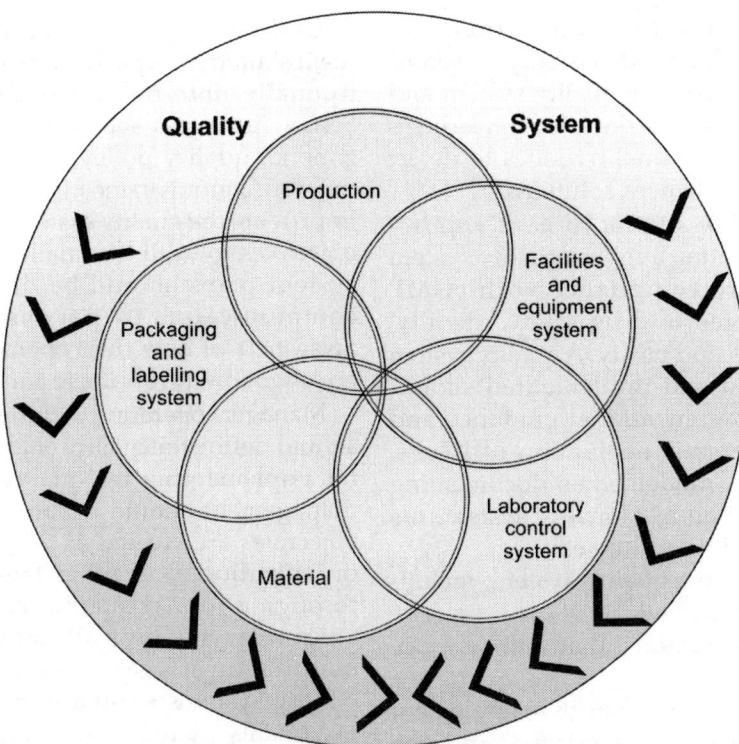

Fig. 4.13: The six sigma inspection model

to provide the leadership needed for the successful functioning of a quality system.

Provide leadership: In a robust, modern quality system, senior management should demonstrate a commitment to developing and maintaining their quality system. Quality system plans should be aligned with a manufacturer's strategic plans to ensure that the system is part of the manufacturer's mission and quality strategies. Senior managers set implementation priorities and develop action plans. All levels of management should provide support to the quality system by:

- Actively participating in system design, implementation, and monitoring, including system review
- Advocating continual improvement of operations of the quality system
- Committing necessary resources

Quality systems environment, all managers should demonstrate visible and robust support for the quality system and ensure its implementation throughout the organization (e.g. across multiple sites). All managers should encourage internal communication on quality issues among research and development, regulatory affairs, manufacturing and QU personnel.

Structure the organization: When designing a robust quality system, management has the responsibility to *structure* the organization and ensure that assigned authorities support the production, quality and management activities needed to produce quality products. Senior managers have the responsibility to ensure that the organization's structure is documented. All managers have the responsibility to communicate employee roles, responsibilities, and authorities within the system and ensure that interactions are defined and understood. Usually, a senior manager administers the quality system and can, thus, ensure that the organization receives prompt feedback on quality issues to detect problems and implement solutions.

Build a quality system to meet requirements: Implementing a robust quality system can help ensure compliance with cGMP regulations related to drug safety, identity, strength, quality, and purity. A quality system that is designed and implemented should provide clear organizational guidance and facilitates systematic evaluation of issues. According to the model, when documenting the implementation of a quality system, the following should be addressed:

- The scope of the quality system, including any outsourcing
- The quality standard that will be followed
- The manufacturer's policies to implement the quality systems criteria and the supporting objectives
- The procedures needed to establish and maintain the quality system

It is recommended under a modern quality systems approach that a formal process is established to change procedures in a controlled manner. Manufacturers develop and document control procedures to complete, secure, protect, and archive records, including data, which provide evidence of operational and quality system activities. Manufacturers to establish and follow scientifically sound and appropriate written controls for specifications, plans and procedures that direct operational and quality system activities and to ensure that these directives are accurate, appropriately reviewed, approved and available for use.

Establish policies, objectives, and plans: Policies, objectives, and plans under a modern quality system provide the means by which senior managers articulate their vision and commitment to quality.

Under a quality system, senior management should incorporate a strong commitment to quality into the organizational mission. Senior managers should develop an organizational quality policy that aligns with this mission; commit to meeting requirements and improving the quality system and propose the objectives to fulfil the quality policy. Quality system plans should be documented and communicated to personnel to ensure awareness of how their operational activities are aligned with strategic and quality goals.

Managers operating within a quality system should define the quality objectives identified for implementing the quality policy. Senior management should ensure that the quality objectives are created at the top level of the organization (and other levels as needed) through a formal quality planning process. Objectives are typically aligned with the manufacturer's strategic plans. Under a quality systems approach, managers would use quality planning to identify and allocate resources and define methods to achieve quality objectives.

Review the system: System review is a crucial component in any robust quality system to ensure its continuing suitability, adequacy, and effectiveness. Under a quality system, senior managers should conduct reviews of the quality system's performance according to a planned schedule. Such a review typically includes assessments of the process, product and customer needs (*customer* is defined as the recipient of the product, and the product is the goods or services provided). Under a quality systems approach, a review considers the following:

- The appropriateness of the quality policy and objectives
- The results of audits and other assessments
- Customer feedback, including complaints
- The analysis of data trending results
- The status of actions to prevent a potential problem or a recurrence

- Any follow-up actions from previous management reviews
- Any changes in business practices or environment that may affect the quality system (such as the volume or type of operations)
- Product characteristics meeting the customer's needs

When developing and implementing new quality systems, the review should take place more frequently than when the system has matured. Periodic reviews are performed by a qualified source, external to the organization, may also be useful in assessing the suitability and effectiveness of the system. Review outcomes typically include:

- Improvements to the quality system and related quality processes
- Improvements to manufacturing processes and products
- Realignment of resources

Under a quality system, the results of a management review would typically be recorded. Planned actions should be implemented using effective corrective and preventive action and change control procedures.

2.3 Resources

Appropriate allocation of resources is the key to creating a robust quality system and complying with the cGMP regulations. Under a robust quality system, sufficient resources should be allocated for the quality system and operational activities. Under the model, senior management, or a designee, should be responsible for providing adequate resources for the following:

- To supply and maintain the appropriate facilities and equipment to manufacture a quality product consistently
- To acquire and receive materials that are suitable for their intended purpose
- For processing the materials to produce the finished drug product

- For laboratory analysis of the finished drug product, including collection, storage, and examination of in-process, stability, and reserve samples

Personnel development: Under a quality system, senior management should support a problem-solving and communicative organizational culture. Managers should encourage communication by creating an environment that values employee suggestions and acts on suggestions for improvement. Management should also develop cross-functional groups to share ideas to improve procedures and processes.

In a quality system, personnel should be qualified to do the operations that are assigned to them in accordance with the nature and potential risk of their operational activities. Managers define appropriate qualifications for each position to help ensure that individuals are assigned with appropriate responsibilities. Personnel should also understand the effect of their activities on product quality and customer satisfaction. Personnel should be selected based on their scientific and technical understanding, product knowledge, process knowledge and/or risk assessment abilities to appropriately execute certain quality functions with identifying educational qualification, training, and experience or any combination thereof.

Under a quality system, continued training is critical to ensure that the employees remain proficient in their operational functions and their understanding of cGMP regulations. Typical quality systems training should address the policies, processes, procedures, and written instructions related to operational activities, the product/service, the quality system, and the desired work culture (e.g. team building, communication, change, behavior). Training should focus on both the employees' specific job functions and the related cGMP regulatory requirements.

Managers establish training programs goals as:

- Evaluation of training needs
- Provision of training to satisfy these needs
- Evaluation of the effectiveness of training
- Documentation of training and/or re-training

When operating in a robust quality system environment, it is important to verify that skills gained from training are implemented in day-to-day performance.

Facilities and equipment: Under a quality system, the technical experts (e.g. engineers, development scientists), who have an understanding of pharmaceutical science, risk factors, and manufacturing processes related to the product, are responsible for defining specific facility and equipment requirements. Under the cGMP regulations, the quality unit (QU) has the responsibility of reviewing and approving all initial design criteria and procedures about facilities and equipment and any subsequent changes. Equipment must be qualified, calibrated, cleaned, and maintained to prevent contamination and mix-ups. The cGMP regulations strongly emphasis on process equipment while other quality systems focus only on testing equipment.

Control outsourced operations: Outsourcing involves hiring a second party under a contract to perform the operational processes that are part of a manufacturer's inherent responsibilities. For example, a manufacturer may hire another firm for packaging and labeling or perform cGMP regulatory training. Quality systems call for contracts (quality agreements) that clearly describe the materials or service, quality specification responsibilities, and communication mechanisms. Under a quality system, the manufacturer should ensure that a contract firm is qualified before signing a contract with that firm. The contract firm's personnel should be adequately trained and monitored for performance according to their quality system, and the contract firm's and contracting manufacturer's quality standards should not conflict. It is critical in a quality system to ensure that the management of the contractor is familiar with the specific requirements of the contract. However, under the cGMP requirements, the manufacturer's QU is responsible for approving or rejecting products or services provided under a contract.

2.4 Manufacturing

Significant overlap exists between the elements of a quality system and the cGMP regulation requirements for manufacturing operations.

Design, develop, and document the product and processes: Significant characteristics of the product being manufactured should be defined from design to delivery, and control should be exercised overall changes. Manufacturing processes, procedures, and changes must be defined, approved and controlled. It is important to establish responsibility for designing or changing products. Documenting processes, associated controls, and changes to these processes help ensure that sources of variability are identified. Documentation includes:

- Resources and facilities used
- Procedures to carry out the process
- Identification of the process owner who will maintain and update the process as needed
- Identification and control of important variables
- Quality control measures, necessary data collection, monitoring, and appropriate controls for the product and process
- Any validation activities, including operating ranges and acceptance criteria
- Effects on related process, functions, or personnel

Managers to ensure that the appropriate technical experts determine product specifications and process parameters (e.g. development scientists). Experts would have an understanding of pharmaceutical science, equipment, facilities and process and how variations in materials and processes can ultimately affect the finished product. Packaging and labeling controls with critical stages in the pharmaceutical manufacturing process should be as per approved procedures. As part of the design process, before commercial production, the controls for all processes within the packaging and labeling system be planned and documented in written procedures. Distinct labels with discriminating features for different products, such as different strengths, should be included to prevent mislabeling and resulting recalls.

Examine inputs: The term *input* includes any material that goes into a final product, no matter whether the manufacturer purchases the material or produced for the purpose of processing. *Materials* include items such as components (e.g. ingredients, process water, and gas), containers, and closures. A robust quality system should ensure that all inputs to the manufacturing process are reliable as per control procedures that have been established for the receipt, production, storage and use of all inputs. The cGMP regulations require either testing or use of a certificate of analysis (COA) plus an identity analysis for the release of materials for manufacturing. Reliability can be validated by conducting tests and comparing the results to the supplier's COA. Sufficient initial tests should be done to establish reliability and to determine a schedule for periodic reassessment. As an essential element of purchasing controls, it is recommended that data trends for acceptance and rejection of materials be analyzed for information on supplier performance.

The quality systems approach also calls for periodic auditing of suppliers based on risk assessment. An audit should also include a systematic examination of the supplier's quality system to ensure that reliability is maintained. It is recommended that a combination approach is used (i.e. verify the suppliers' COA through analysis *and* audits of the supplier). Procedures should also be established to encompass the acceptance, use, or the rejection and disposition of materials produced by the facility (e.g. purified water). Systems that produce these in-house materials should be designed, maintained, qualified, and validated where appropriate to ensure that the materials meet their acceptance criteria. Also, it is recommended that changes to materials (e.g. specification, supplier, or materials handling) be implemented through a change control system (certain changes require review and approval by the QU). It is also important to have a system in place to respond to changes in materials from suppliers so that necessary adjustments to the process can be made and unintended consequences avoided.

Perform and monitor operations: An important purpose of implementing a quality systems approach is to enable a manufacturer to more efficiently and effectively validate, perform, and monitor operations and ensure that the controls are scientifically sound and appropriate. The goal of establishing, adhering to, measuring, and documenting specifications and process parameters are to objectively assess whether an operation is meeting its design and product performance objectives. A design concept established during product development typically matures into a commercial design after process experimentation and progressive modification.

Risk management helps to identify areas of process weakness or higher risk and factors that can influence critical quality attributes that should receive increased scrutiny. The FDA recommends that scale-up studies be used to help demonstrate that fundamentally sound design has been fully realized. With proper design and reliable mechanisms to transfer process knowledge from development to commercial production, a manufacturer should be able to validate the manufacturing process. Conformance batches provide initial proof that the design of the process produces the intended product quality. Sufficient testing data will provide essential information on the performance of the new process, as well as a mechanism for continual improvement. Modern equipment with the potential for continual monitoring and control can further enhance this knowledge base. Although initial commercial batches can provide evidence to support the validity and consistency of the process, the *entire product life cycle* should be addressed by the establishment of continual improvement mechanisms in the quality system. Thus, in accordance with the quality systems approach, process validation is not a one-time event, but an activity that continues throughout a product's life.

Data and information recorded by the production department provide insight into the product's state of control. Change control systems should provide a dependable mechanism to prompt implementation of technically sound manufacturing improvements. Under a quality system, written procedures are followed, and deviations from them are justified and documented to ensure that the manufacturer can trace the history of the product, as appropriate, concerning personnel, materials, equipment and product release records. Both the cGMP regulations and quality systems models call for the monitoring of critical processes that may be responsible for causing variability during production. For example:

·Process steps must be verified by a second person or a validated computer system. Batch production records must be prepared contemporaneously with each phase of production. Time limits for production are established when they are important to the quality of the finished product; the manufacturer should have the ability to establish production controls using in-process parameters that are based on desired process endpoints measured using real-time testing or monitoring apparatus (e.g. blend until mixed vs. blend for 10 minutes).

Procedures must be in place to prevent the growth of objectionable microorganisms in finished products that are not required to be sterile and to prevent microbial contamination of finished products purported to be sterile. Sterilization processes must be validated for sterile drugs.

Manufacturing processes must consistently meet their parameters, and in-process materials must meet acceptance criteria or limits so that, ultimately, finished pharmaceutical products will meet their acceptance criteria. Collected data are used to evaluate the quality of a process, product, and analysis for potential suggestions for improvement. A quality systems approach calls for the manufacturer to develop procedures that monitor, measure, and analyze the operations (including analytical methods and/or statistical techniques). Monitoring of the process is important due to the limitations of testing. A well-managed quality system can significantly detect the unanticipated variables. Procedures should be revisited as needed to refine operational design based on new knowledge. Data collection procedures, consider the following:

- Are the data collection methods documented?
- When the product life cycle data will be collected?
- How and to whom the measurement and monitoring activities will be assigned?
- When analysis and evaluation (e.g. trending) of laboratory data be performed?
- What records should be collected?

Change control is warranted when data analysis or other information reveals an area for improvement. Changes to an established process must be controlled and documented to ensure that desired attributes for the finished product are met. When developing a process change, it is important to keep in mind the process design and scientific knowledge of the product. If major design issues are encountered through process experience, a firm may want to revisit the adequacy of the design of the manufacturing facility, the design of the manufacturing equipment, the design of the production and control procedures, or the design of laboratory controls. When implementing a change, its effect should be determined by monitoring and evaluating those specific elements that may be affected based on an understanding of the process. Application of risk analysis may facilitate evaluating the potential effect of the change in the process. Evaluating the effects of a change can entail additional tests or examinations of subsequent batches (e.g. additional in-process testing or additional stability studies).

Under a quality systems approach, procedures should be in place to ensure the accuracy of test results. Any invalidation of a test result should be scientifically sound and justified. The manufacturer should consider storage and shipment requirements to meet special handling needs (in the case of pharmaceuticals, one example might be refrigeration). Trends should be continually identified and evaluated. One way of accomplishing this is the use of statistical process control. The information from trend analyses can be used to continually monitor quality, identify potential variances before they become problems, bolster data already collected for the annual review, and facilitate improvement throughout the product life cycle.

Address nonconformities: A key component in any quality system is handling nonconformities and/or deviations. The investigation, conclusion, and follow-up must be documented. It is important to measure the working efficiency of the process, and the product attributes (e.g. specified control parameters, strength) for confirmatory to the predecided planned. Discrepancies must be detected from all stages of the process and quality control activities. As not all discrepancies result in product defects; however, it is important to document and handle discrepancies appropriately. A discrepancy investigation process is critical when a discrepancy is found to affect the product quality.

In a quality system, it is crucial to develop and document procedures that define who is responsible for halting and resuming operations, recording non-conformities, investigating discrepancies, and taking remedial action. Whenever a product or process does not meet requirements, it is essential to identify and/or segregate the product so that it is not distributed to the customer. Remedial action includes the following:

- Correct the non-conformity
- With proper authorization, allow the product to proceed with the justification of the conclusions regarding the problem's impact
- Use the product for another application where the deficiency does not affect the products' quality
- Reject the product

The corrected product or process should also be re-examined for conformance and assessed for the significance of the nonconformity. If the non-conformity is significant, based on consequences to process control, process efficiency, product quality, safety, efficacy, and product availability, it is important to evaluate how to prevent recurrence. If an individual product that does not meet requirements has been released, the product must be recalled. Customer complaints must be reviewed and then investigated if a discrepancy is identified. Manufacturers should always refer to the specific regulations to ensure that they are complying with all regulations.

2.4 Evaluation Activities

As in the previous section, the elements of a quality system correlate closely with the requirements in the cGMP regulations.

Analyze data for trends: Quality systems call for continuous monitoring of trends and improving systems. This can be achieved by monitoring data and information, identifying and resolving problems, and anticipating and preventing problems. Quality systems procedures involve collecting data from monitoring, measurement, complaint handling, or other activities, and tracking this data over time. The information generated is essential for achieving problem resolution or problem prevention. Although the cGMP regulations require product review on at least an annual basis, quality systems approach calls for trending on a more frequent basis as determined by risk. Trending enables the detection of potential problems as early as possible to plan corrective and preventive actions. Trending information is used to examine processes, and trend analyses help focus internal audits.

Conduct internal audits: A quality systems approach calls for audits to be conducted at planned intervals to evaluate effective implementation and maintenance of the quality system and to determine if processes and products meet established parameters and specifications. Audit procedures should be developed and documented to ensure that the planned audit schedule takes into account the relative risks of the various quality system activities, the results of previous audits and corrective actions. Procedures also define auditing activities such as the scope and methodology of the audit, selection of auditors, and audit conduct (audit plans, opening meetings, interviews, closing meeting, and reports). Procedures should describe how auditors are trained in objective evidence gathering, their responsibilities, and auditing procedures. It is critical to maintain records of audit findings and assign responsibility for follow-up to prevent problems recurring.

Management is responsible for taking timely action to resolve audit findings and ensure that follow-up actions are completed, verified, and recorded.

Quality risk management: Effective decision-making in a quality systems environment is based on an informed understanding of quality issues. Elements of risk should be considered relative to the intended use of a product, and in the case of pharmaceuticals, patient safety is of utmost importance. Management should assign priorities to activities or actions based on an assessment of the risk including both the probability of occurrence of harm and of the severity of that harm. Implementation of quality risk management includes assessing the risks, selecting and implementing risk management controls commensurate with the level of risk, and evaluating the results of the risk management efforts. Since risk management is an iterative process, it should be repeated if new information is developed that changes the need for, or nature of, risk management. Risk management is used as a tool in the development of product specifications and critical process parameters.

Corrective actions: Corrective action is a reactive tool for system improvement to ensure that significant problems do not recur. Both quality systems and the cGMP regulations emphasize corrective actions. Quality systems approach call for procedures to be developed and documented to ensure that the need for action is evaluated relevant to the possible consequences, the root cause of the problem is investigated, possible actions are determined, a selected action is taken within a defined time frame, and the effectiveness of the action taken is evaluated. Documenting corrective actions taken is essential. It is essential to determine what actions will reduce the likelihood of a problem recurring. Following are the sources that can be used to gather such information:

- Non-conformance reports and rejections
- Returns
- Complaints
- Internal and external audits
- Data risk assessment related to operations and quality system processes
- Management review decisions

Preventive actions: Being proactive is an essential tool in quality systems management. Succession planning, training, capturing institutional knowledge, and planning for personnel, policy, and process changes are preventive actions that help ensure that potential problems and root causes are identified, possible consequences assessed, and appropriate actions considered. The selected preventive actions should be evaluated and recorded, and the system should be monitored for the effectiveness of the action. Problems can be anticipated, and their occurrence can be prevented by reviewing data and analyzing risks associated with operational and quality system processes, and by keeping abreast of changes in scientific developments and regulatory requirements.

Promote improvement: The effectiveness and efficiency of a quality system can be improved through the quality activities described in this guidance. Management may choose to use other improvement activities as appropriate. It is critical that senior management is involved in the evaluation of this improvement process.

3. CONCLUSION

Good intentions alone are not sufficient to ensure good products. A robust quality system can promote process consistency by integrating effective knowledge-building mechanisms into daily operational decisions. Implementation of a *comprehensive quality systems model* for human and veterinary pharmaceutical products, including biological products, will facilitate compliance with the regulation. The central goal of a quality system is the consistent production of safe and effective products and ensuring that these activities are sustainable. Specifically, successful quality systems share the following characteristics:

- Science-based approaches
- Decisions based on an understanding of the intended use of a product
- Proper identification and control of areas of potential process weakness
- Responsive deviation and investigation systems that lead to timely remediation
- Sound methods for assessing and reducing risk
- Well-defined processes and products, starting from development and extending throughout the product life cycle
- Systems for careful analysis of product quality
- Supportive management (philosophically and financially)

Both good manufacturing practice and good business practice require a robust quality system. When fully developed and effectively managed, a quality system leads to consistent, predictable processes that ensure that pharmaceuticals are safe and effective.

QUALITY RISK MANAGEMENT (ICH Q9)

International Conference on Harmonisation of Technical Requirements
for Registration of Pharmaceuticals for Human Use
ICH Harmonised Tripartite Guideline Current Step 4 version dated 9 November 2005
(Courtesy: https://www.ich.org/fileadmin/Public_Web_Site/ICH_Products/Guidelines/Quality/Q9/Step4/
Q9_Guideline.pdf)

1. INTRODUCTION

Risk management principles are effectively utilized in many areas of business and government including finance, insurance, occupational safety, public health, pharmacovigilance, and by agencies regulating these industries. Although there are some examples of the use of *quality risk management* in the pharmaceutical industry today, they are limited and do not represent the full contributions that risk management has to offer. The importance of *quality systems* has been recognized in the pharmaceutical industry, and it is becoming evident that quality risk management is a valuable component of an effective quality system.

It is commonly understood that *risk* is defined as the combination of the probability of occurrence of *harm* and the *severity* of that harm. However, achieving a shared understanding of the application of risk management among diverse *stakeholders* is difficult because each stakeholder might perceive different potential harms, place a different probability on each harm occurring and attribute different severities to each harm. In context to pharmaceuticals, there are a variety of stakeholders, including patients, medical practitioners, government and industry, but the protection of the patient by managing the risk to quality is considered to be of prime importance.

The manufacturing and use of drug products, including its components, necessarily entail some degree of risk. The risk to its quality is just one component of the overall risk. It is important to understand that product *quality* should be maintained throughout the *product lifecycle* such that the attributes that are important to the quality of the drug products remain consistent with those used in the clinical studies. An effective quality risk management approach ensures high quality of the drug products to be delivered to the patients by providing a proactive means to identify and control potential quality issues during development and manufacturing. Additionally, the use of quality risk management can improve decision-making effectiveness when a quality problem arises. Effective quality risk management can facilitate better and more informed decisions, provide regulators with greater assurance of a company's ability to deal with potential risks and beneficially affect the extent and level of direct regulatory oversight.

The purpose of this document is to offer a systematic approach to quality risk management. It serves as a foundation or resource document in support with other ICH Quality documents and complements existing quality practices, requirements, standards, and guidelines within the pharmaceutical industry and regulatory environment. It specifically provides guidance on the principles and some of the tools of quality risk management that can enable more effective and consistent risk-based decisions, both by regulators and industry.

1.1 Scope

This guideline provides principles and examples of tools for quality risk management that can be applied to different aspects of pharmaceutical quality. These aspects include development, manufacturing, distribution, and the inspection and submission/review processes throughout the life cycle of drug substances, drug products, biological and biotechnological products (including the use of raw materials, solvents, recipients, packaging and labeling materials.

1.2 Principles

Two primary principles of quality risk management are:

- The evaluation of the risk to quality should be based on scientific knowledge and ultimately link to the protection of the patient; and
- The level of effort, formality, and documentation of the quality risk management process should be commensurate with the level of risk.

2. QUALITY RISK MANAGEMENT PROCESS

Quality risk management is a systematic process for the assessment, control, communication and review of risks to the quality of the drug products across the product life cycle. A model for quality risk management is outlined in the diagram (Fig. 4.14). The emphasis on each component of the framework might differ from case to case, but a robust process will incorporate consideration of all the elements at a level of detail that is commensurate with the specific risk.

Decision nodes are not shown in the diagram because decisions can occur at any point in the process. These decisions might be return to the previous step and seek further information, to adjust the risk models or even to terminate the risk management process based upon information that supports such a decision. Note: "Unacceptable" in the flowchart does not only refer to statutory, legislative or regulatory requirements, but also to the need to revisit the risk assessment process (Fig. 4.14).

2.1 Responsibilities

Quality risk management activities are usually, but not always, undertaken by interdisciplinary teams, that include experts from the appropriate areas (e.g. quality unit, business development, engineering, regulatory affairs, production operations, sales and marketing, legal, statistics and clinical) in addition to individuals who are knowledgeable about the quality risk management process. Decision makers are:

- Take responsibility for coordinating quality risk management across various functions and departments of their organization; and
- Assure that a quality risk management process is defined, deployed and reviewed and that adequate resources are available.

2.2 Initiating a Quality Risk Management Process

Quality risk management should include systematic processes designed to coordinate, facilitate and improve science-based decision making with respect to risk. Possible steps used to initiate and plan a quality risk management process might include the following:

- Define the problem and/or risk question, including pertinent assumptions identifying the potential for risk;
- Assemble background information and/or data on the potential hazard, harm or human health impact relevant to the risk assessment;
- Identify a leader and necessary resources;
- Specify a timeline, deliverables and appropriate level of decision making for the risk management process.

2.3 Risk Assessment

Risk assessment consists of the identification of hazards and the analysis and evaluation of risks associated with exposure to those

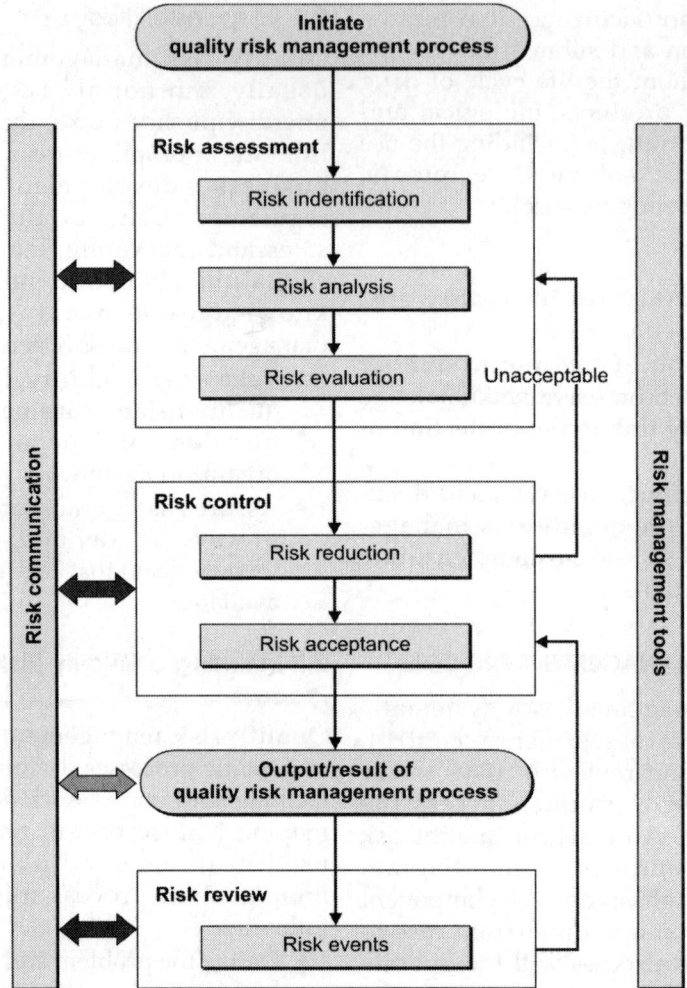

Fig. 4.14: Overview of a typical quality risk management process

hazards. Quality risk assessments begin with a well-defined problem description or risk question. When the risk in question is well defined, an appropriate risk management tool and the types of information needed to address the risk question will be more readily identifiable. As an aid to clearly defining the risk(s) for risk assessment purposes, three fundamental questions are often helpful:

1. What might go wrong?
2. What is the likelihood (probability) it will go wrong?
3. What are the consequences (severity)?

Risk identification: Risk identification is a systematic use of information to identify hazards referring to the risk question or problem description. Information can include historical data, theoretical analysis, informed opinions and the concerns of stakeholders. Risk identification addresses the "What might go wrong?" question, including identifying the possible consequences. This provides the basis for further steps in the quality risk management process.

Risk analysis: Risk analysis is the estimation of the risk associated with the identified hazards. It is the qualitative or quantitative process of linking the likelihood of occurrence and severity of harms. In some risk management tools, the ability to detect the harm (detectability) also affects the estimation of risk.

Risk evaluation: Risk evaluation compares the identified and analyzed risk against given risk criteria. Risk evaluations consider the strength of evidence for all three of the fundamental questions. In an effective risk assessment, the robustness of the data set is important because it determines the quality of the output. Revealing assumptions and reasonable sources of uncertainty in this output help to identify its limitations. Uncertainty is due to a combination of incomplete knowledge about a process and its expected or unexpected variability. Typical sources of uncertainty include knowledge gaps in pharmaceutical science and process understanding, sources of harm (e.g. failure modes of a process, sources of variability) and the probability of detection of problems.

The output of a risk assessment is either a quantitative estimate of risk or a qualitative description of a range of risk. When risk is expressed quantitatively, a numerical probability is used. Alternatively, risk can be expressed using qualitative descriptors, such as "high," "medium," or "low," which should be defined in as much detail as possible. Sometimes a "risk score" is used to define descriptors in risk ranking further. In quantitative risk assessments, a risk estimate provides the likelihood of a specific consequence, given a set of risk-generating circumstances. Thus, quantitative risk estimation is useful for one particular consequence at a time. Alternatively, some risk management tools use a relative risk measure to combine multiple levels of severity and probability into an overall estimate of relative risk. The intermediate steps within a scoring process can sometimes employ quantitative risk estimation.

2.4 Risk Control

Risk control includes decision making to reduce and/or accept risks. The purpose of risk control is to reduce the risk to an acceptable level. The amount of effort used for risk control should be proportional to the significance of the risk. Decision makers might use different processes, including benefit cost analysis, for understanding the optimal level of risk control.

Risk control might focus on the following questions:

- Is the risk at an acceptable level?
- What can be done to reduce or eliminate risks?
- What is the appropriate balance among benefits, risks, and resources?
- Are new risks introduced as a result of the identified risks being controlled?

Risk reduction: Risk reduction focuses on processes for mitigation or avoidance of quality risk when it exceeds a specified (acceptable) level. Risk reduction might include actions taken to mitigate the severity and probability of harm. Processes that improve the detectability of hazards and quality risks might also be used as part of a risk control strategy. The implementation of risk reduction measures can introduce new risks into the system or increase the significance of other existing risks. Hence, it might be appropriate to revisit the risk assessment to identify and evaluate any possible change in risk after implementing a risk reduction process.

Risk acceptance: Risk acceptance is a decision to accept the risk. Risk acceptance can be a formal decision to accept the residual risk, or it can be a passive decision in which residual risks are not specified. For some types of harms, even the best quality risk management practices might not eliminate risk. In these circumstances, it might be agreed that an appropriate quality risk management strategy has been applied and that quality risk is reduced to a specified (acceptable) level. This (specified) acceptable level depends on many parameters and should be decided on a case-by-case basis.

2.5 Risk Communication

Risk communication is the sharing of information about risk and risk management between the decision makers and others. Parties can communicate at any stage of the risk management process. The output/result of the quality risk management process should be appropriately communicated and documented. Communications occur among interested parties, e.g. regulators and industry, industry and the patient and within a company or regulatory authority, etc. The included information might relate to the existence, nature, form, probability, severity, acceptability, control, treatment, detectability or other aspects of risks to quality. Between the industry and regulatory authorities, communication concerning quality risk management decisions might be affected through existing channels as specified in regulations and guidance.

2.6 Risk Review

Risk management is an ongoing part of the quality management process with a mechanism implemented to review or monitor events. The output/results of the risk management process should be reviewed to take into account new knowledge and experience. Once a quality risk management process has been initiated, that process should continue to be utilized for events that might impact the original quality risk management decision, whether these events are planned (e.g. results of product review, inspections, audits, change control) or unplanned (e.g. root cause from failure investigations, recall). The

frequency of any review should be based upon the level of risk. Risk review might include reconsideration of risk acceptance decisions.

3. RISK MANAGEMENT METHODOLOGY

Quality risk management provides documented, transparent and reproducible methods to accomplish steps of the quality risk management process based on current knowledge about assessing the probability, severity and sometimes detectability of the risk. Traditionally, risks to quality have been assessed and managed in a variety of informal ways (empirical and/ or internal procedures) based on, for example, a compilation of observations, trends, and other information. Such approaches continue to provide useful information that might support topics such as handling of complaints, quality defects, deviations and allocation of resources.

Additionally, the pharmaceutical industry and regulators also assess and manage risk using recognized risk management tools and/ or internal procedures (e.g. standard operating procedures). Below is a non-exhaustive list of some of these tools:
- Basic risk management facilitation methods (flowcharts, check sheets, etc.);
- Failure mode effects analysis (FMEA);
- Failure mode, effects and criticality analysis (FMECA);
- Fault tree analysis (FTA);
- Hazard analysis and critical control points (HACCP);
- Hazard operability analysis (HAZOP);
- Preliminary hazard analysis (PHA);
- Risk ranking and filtering;
- Supporting statistical tools.

It might be appropriate to adapt these tools for use in specific areas about drug substance and drug products quality. Quality risk management methods and the supporting statistical tools can be used in combination (e.g. Probabilistic Risk Assessment). Combined use provides the flexibility that facilitates the application of quality risk management principles.

4. CONCLUSION

Quality risk management process supports science-based and practical decisions making when integrated into quality systems (*see* Annexure II). Effective quality risk management facilitates better and more informed decisions, and provide regulators with greater assurance of a company's ability to deal with potential risks, that affect the extent and level of direct regulatory oversight. In addition, quality risk management can facilitate better use of resources by all parties.

Training of both industry and regulatory personnel in quality risk management processes helps in better understanding of decision-making processes and builds confidence in quality risk management outcomes. Quality risk management should be integrated into existing operations and documented appropriately. Annexure II provides examples of situations in which the use of the quality risk management process might provide information that could then be used in a variety of pharmaceutical operations.

These examples are provided for illustrative purposes only and are not a definitive or exhaustive list. Examples of industry and regulatory operations (*see* Annexure II):

- Quality management.

Examples of industry operations and activities (*see* Annexure II):

- Development;
- Facility, equipment, and utilities;
- Materials management;
- Production;
- Laboratory control and stability testing;
- Packaging and labeling.

Examples for regulatory operations

- Inspection and assessment activities.
  While regulatory decisions will continue to be taken on a regional basis, a common understanding and application of quality risk management principles could facilitate confidence and promote more consistent decisions among regulators by the same information. This collaboration could be important in the development of policies and guidelines that integrate and support quality risk management practices.

ANNEXURES

ANNEXURE I: RISK MANAGEMENT METHODS AND TOOLS

The purpose of this annex is to provide a general overview of and references for some of the primary tools that might be used in quality risk management by industry and regulators.

I.1 Basic Risk Management Facilitation Methods

Some of the simple techniques that are commonly used to structure risk management by organizing data and facilitating decision-making are:
- Flow charts;
- Check sheets;
- Process mapping;
- Cause and effect diagrams (also called an Ishikawa diagram or fishbone diagram).

I.2 Failure Mode Effects Analysis (FMEA)

FMEA provides an evaluation of potential failure modes for processes and their likely effect on outcomes and/or product performance. Once failure modes are established, risk reduction can be used to eliminate, contain, reduce or control the potential failures. FMEA relies on product and process understanding. FMEA methodically breaks down the analysis of complex processes into manageable steps. It is a powerful tool for summarizing the important modes of failure, factors causing these failures and the likely effects of these failures.

Potential areas of use(s)

FMEA can be used to prioritize risks and monitor the effectiveness of risk control activities. FMEA can be applied to equipment and facilities and might be used to analyze a manufacturing operation and its effect on the product or process. It identifies elements/operations within the system that render it vulnerable. The output/results of FMEA is used as a basis for design or further analysis or to guide resource deployment.

I.3 Failure Mode, Effects and Criticality Analysis (FMECA)

FMECA is extended to incorporate an investigation of the degree of severity of the consequences, their respective probabilities of

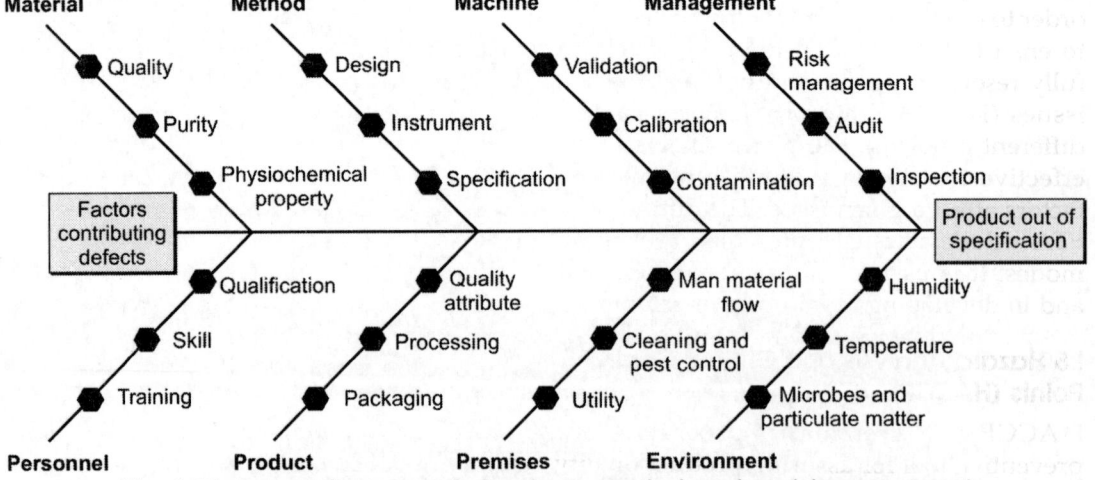

Fig. 4.15: Cause effect analysis for pharmaceutical product risk management

occurrence, and their detectability, thereby becoming a Failure Mode Effect and Criticality Analysis. FMECA can identify places where additional preventive actions might be appropriate to minimize risks.

Potential areas of use(s)

FMECA application in the pharmaceutical industry should mostly be utilized for failures and risks associated with manufacturing processes; however, it is not limited to this application. The output of an FMECA is a relative risk "score" for each failure mode, which is used to rank the modes on a relative risk basis.

I.4 Fault Tree Analysis (FTA)

The FTA tool is an approach that assumes failure of the functionality of a product or process. This tool evaluates system (or subsystem) failures one at a time but can combine multiple causes of failure by identifying causal chains. The results are represented pictorially in the form of a tree of fault modes. FTA relies on the experts' process understanding to identify causal factors.

Potential areas of use(s)

FTA can be used to establish the pathway to the root cause of the failure. FTA can be used to investigate complaints or deviations in order to fully understand their root cause and to ensure that intended improvements will fully resolve the issue and not lead to other issues (i.e. solve one problem yet cause a different problem). Fault Tree Analysis is an effective tool for evaluating how multiple factors affect a given issue. The output of an FTA includes a visual representation of failure modes. It is useful both for risk assessment and in developing monitoring programs.

I.5 Hazard Analysis and Critical Control Points (HACCP)

HACCP is a systematic, proactive, and preventive tool for assuring product quality, reliability, and safety (WHO Technical Report Series No 908, 2003 Annex 7). It is a structured approach that applies technical and scientific principles to analyze, evaluate, prevent, and control the risk or adverse consequence(s) of hazard(s) due to the design, development, production, and use of products. HACCP consists of the following seven steps:

1. Conduct a hazard analysis and identify preventive measures for each step of the process;
2. Determine the critical control points;
3. Establish critical limits;
4. Establish a system to monitor the critical control points;
5. Establish the corrective action to be taken when monitoring indicates that the critical control points are not in a state of control;
6. Establish a system to verify that the HACCP system is working effectively;
7. Establish a record-keeping system.

Potential areas of use(s)

HACCP might be used to identify and manage risks associated with physical, chemical and biological hazards (including microbiological contamination). HACCP is most useful when product and process understanding is sufficiently comprehensive to support the identification of critical control points. The output of a HACCP analysis is risk management information that facilitates monitoring of critical points not only in the manufacturing process but also other life cycle phases.

I.6 Hazard Operability Analysis (HAZOP)

HAZOP is based on a theory that assumes that risk events are caused by deviations from the design or operating intentions. It is a systematic brain storming technique for identifying hazards using so-called "guide-words." "Guide-words" (e.g. No, More, Other Than, Part of, etc.) are applied to relevant parameters (e.g. contamination, temperature) to help identify potential deviations from regular use or design intentions. It often uses a team of people with expertise covering the design of the process or product and its application.

Potential areas of use(s)

HAZOP can be applied to manufacturing processes, including outsourced production and formulation as well as the upstream suppliers, equipment and facilities for drug substances and drug products. It has also been used for evaluating process safety hazards. As is the case with HACCP, the output of a HAZOP analysis is a list of critical operations for risk management. This facilitates regular monitoring of critical points in the manufacturing process.

I.7 Preliminary Hazard Analysis (PHA)

PHA is a tool of analysis based on applying prior experience or knowledge of a hazard or failure to identify future hazards, hazardous situations, and events that might cause harm, as well as to estimate their probability of occurrence for a given activity, facility, product or system. The tool consists of:

1. The identification of the possibilities that the risk event happens,
2. The qualitative evaluation of the extent of possible injury or damage to health that could result,
3. A relative ranking of the hazard using a combination of severity and likelihood of occurrence, and
4. The identification of possible remedial measures.

Potential Areas of Use(s)

PHA might be useful when analyzing existing systems or prioritizing hazards where circumstances prevent a more extensive technique from being used. It can be used for the product, process, and facility design as well as to evaluate the types of hazards for the general product type, then the product class, and finally the specific product. PHA is most commonly used early in the development of a project when there is a little information on design details or operating procedures; thus, it will often be a precursor to further studies. Typically, hazards identified in the PHA are further assessed with other risk management tools.

I.8 Risk Ranking and Filtering

Risk ranking and filtering is a tool for comparing and ranking risks. Risk ranking of complex systems typically requires an evaluation of multiple diverse quantitative and qualitative factors for each risk. The tool involves breaking down a fundamental risk question into as many components as needed to capture factors involved in the risk. These factors are combined into a single relative risk score that can then be used for ranking risks. "Filters," in the form of weighting factors or cut-offs for risk scores, can be used to scale or fit the risk ranking to management or policy objectives.

Potential areas of use(s)

Risk ranking and filtering can be used to prioritize manufacturing sites for inspection/audit by regulators or industry. Risk ranking methods are particularly helpful in situations in which the portfolio of risks and the underlying consequences to be managed are diverse and difficult to compare using a single tool. Risk ranking is useful to evaluate both quantitatively-assessed and qualitatively-assessed risks within the same organizational framework.

I.9 Supporting Statistical Tools

Statistical tools can support and facilitate quality risk management. They can enable effective data assessment, aid in determining the significance of the data set(s), and facilitate more reliable decision making. A listing of some of the principal statistical tools commonly used in the pharmaceutical industry is provided:

- Control Charts, for example:
  - Acceptance Control Charts (ISO 7966);
  - Control Charts with Arithmetic Average and Warning Limits (ISO 7873);
  - Cumulative Sum Charts (ISO 7871);
  - Shewhart Control Charts (ISO 8258);
  - Weighted Moving Average.
- Design of Experiments (DOE);
- Histograms;
- Pareto Charts;
- Process Capability Analysis.

ANNEXURE II: POTENTIAL APPLICATIONS FOR QUALITY RISK MANAGEMENT

This Annexure is intended to identify potential uses of quality risk management principles and tools by industry and regulators.

II.1 Quality Risk Management as Part of Integrated Quality Management

Documentation

1. To review current interpretations and application of regulatory expectations;
2. To determine the desirability of and/or develop the content for SOPs, guidelines, etc.

Training and education

1. To determine the appropriateness of initial and/or ongoing training sessions based on education, experience and working habits of staff, as well as on a periodic assessment of previous training (e.g. its effectiveness);
2. To identify the training, experience, qualifications and physical abilities that allow personnel to operate reliably and with no adverse impact on the quality of the product.

Quality defects

1. To provide the basis for identifying, evaluating, and communicating the potential quality impact of a suspected quality defect, complaint, trend, deviation, investigation, out of specification result, etc;
2. To facilitate risk communications and determine the appropriate action to address significant product defects, in conjunction with regulatory authorities (e.g. recall).

Auditing/inspection

1. To define the frequency and scope of audits, both internal and external, taking into account factors such as:
   - Existing legal requirements;
   - Overall compliance status and history of the company or facility;
   - Robustness of quality risk management activities;
   - The complexity of the site;
   - The complexity of the manufacturing process;
   - The complexity of the product and its therapeutic significance;
   - Number and significance of quality defects (e.g. recall);
   - Results of previous audits/inspections;
   - Major changes in building, equipment, processes, key personnel;
   - Experience with manufacturing of a product (e.g. frequency, volume, number of batches);
   - Test results of official control laboratories.

Periodic review

1. To select, evaluate and interpret trend results of data within the product quality review;
2. To interpret monitoring data (e.g. to support an assessment of the appropriateness of revalidation or changes in sampling).

Change management/change control

1. To manage changes based on knowledge and information accumulated in pharmaceutical development and during manufacturing;
2. To evaluate the impact of the changes on the availability of the final product;
3. To evaluate the impact on product quality of changes to the facility, equipment, material, manufacturing process or technology transfers;
4. To determine appropriate actions preceding the implementation of a change, e.g. additional testing, (re)qualification, (re)validation or communication with regulators.

Continual improvement

1. To facilitate continual improvement in processes throughout the product life cycle.

II.2 Quality Risk Management as Part of Regulatory Operations

Inspection and assessment activities

1. To assist with resource allocation including, for example, inspection planning and frequency, and inspection and assessment intensity;
2. To evaluate the significance of, for example, quality defects, potential recalls, and inspectional findings;
3. To determine the appropriateness and type of post-inspection regulatory follow-up;
4. To evaluate the information submitted by industry including pharmaceutical development information;
5. To evaluate the impact of proposed variations or changes;
6. To identify risks which should be communicated between inspectors and assessors to facilitate a better understanding of how risks can be or are controlled (e.g. parametric release, process analytical technology (PAT)).

II.3 Quality Risk Management as Part of the development

1. To design a quality product and its manufacturing process to consistently deliver the intended performance of the product (ICH Q8);
2. To enhance knowledge of product performance over a wide range of material attributes (e.g. particle size distribution, moisture content, flow properties), processing options and process parameters;
3. To assess the critical attributes of raw materials, solvents, active pharmaceutical ingredient (API) starting materials, APIs, excipients, or packaging materials;
4. To establish appropriate specifications, identify critical process parameters and establish manufacturing controls (e.g. using information from pharmaceutical development studies regarding the clinical significance of quality attributes and the ability to control them during processing);
5. To decrease the variability of quality attributes:
   • Reduce product and material defects;
   • Reduce manufacturing defects.
6. To assess the need for additional studies (e.g. bioequivalence, stability) relating to scale up and technology transfer;
7. To make use of the "design space" concept (ICH Q8).

II.4 Quality Risk Management for Facilities, Equipment, and Utilities

Design of facility/equipment

1. To determine appropriate zones when designing buildings and facilities, e.g.
   • The flow of material and personnel;
   • Minimize contamination;
   • Pest control measures;
   • Prevention of mix-ups;
   • Open versus closed equipment;
   • Clean rooms versus isolator technologies;

- Dedicated or segregated facilities/equipment.
2. To determine appropriate product contact materials for equipment and containers (e.g. selection of stainless steel grade, gaskets, lubricants);
3. To determine appropriate utilities (e.g. steam, gases, power source, compressed air, heating, ventilation and air conditioning (HVAC), water);
4. To determine appropriate preventive maintenance for associated equipment (e.g. inventory of necessary spare parts).

Hygiene aspects in facilities

1. To protect the product from environmental hazards, including chemical, microbiological, and physical hazards (e.g. determining appropriate clothing and gowning, hygiene concerns);
2. To protect the environment (e.g. personnel, the potential for cross-contamination) from hazards related to the product being manufactured.

Qualification of facility/equipment/utilities

1. To determine the scope and extent of qualification of facilities, buildings, and production equipment and/or laboratory instruments (including proper calibration methods).

Cleaning of equipment and environmental control

1. To differentiate efforts and decisions based on the intended use (e.g. multi-versus single-purpose, batch versus continuous production);
2. To determine acceptable (specified) cleaning validation limits.

Calibration/preventive maintenance

1. To set appropriate calibration and maintenance schedules.

Computer systems and computer controlled equipment

1. To select the design of computer hardware and software (e.g. modular, structured, fault tolerance);
2. To determine the extent of validation, e.g.
   - Identification of critical performance parameters;
   - Selection of the requirements and design;
   - Code review;
   - The extent of testing and test methods;
   - Reliability of electronic records and signatures.

II.5 Quality Risk Management as Part of Materials Management

Assessment and evaluation of suppliers and contract manufacturers

1. To provide a comprehensive evaluation of suppliers and contract manufacturers (e.g. auditing, supplier quality agreements).

Starting material

1. To assess differences and possible quality risks associated with variability in starting materials (e.g. age, route of synthesis).

Use of materials

1. To determine whether it is appropriate to use material under quarantine (e.g. for further internal processing);
2. To determine the appropriateness of reprocessing, reworking, use of returned goods.

Storage, logistics and distribution conditions

1. To assess the adequacy of arrangements to ensure maintenance of appropriate storage and transport conditions (e.g. temperature, humidity, container design);
2. To determine the effect on product quality of discrepancies in storage or transport conditions (e.g. cold chain

management) in conjunction with other ICH guidelines;

3. To maintain infrastructure (e.g. capacity to ensure proper shipping conditions, interim storage, handling of hazardous materials and controlled substances, customs clearance);
4. To provide information for ensuring the availability of pharmaceuticals (e.g. ranking risks to the supply chain).

II.6 Quality Risk Management as Part of Production

Validation

1. To identify the scope and extent of verification, qualification and validation activities (e.g. analytical methods, processes, equipment and cleaning methods);
2. To determine the extent of follow-up activities (e.g. sampling, monitoring, and re-validation);
3. To distinguish between critical and non-critical process steps to facilitate the design of a validation study.

In-process sampling and testing

1. To evaluate the frequency and extent of in-process control testing (e.g. to justify reduced testing under conditions of proven control);
2. To evaluate and justify the use of process analytical technologies (PAT) in conjunction with parametric and real-time release.

Production planning

1. To determine appropriate production planning (e.g. dedicated, campaign and concurrent production process sequences).

II.7 Quality Risk Management as Part of Laboratory Control and Stability Studies

Out of specification results

1. To identify potential root causes and corrective actions during the investigation of out of specification results.

Retest period/expiration date

1. To evaluate the adequacy of storage and testing of intermediates, excipients and starting materials.

II.8 Quality Risk Management as Part of Packaging and Labeling

Design of packages

1. To design the secondary package for the protection of primary packaged product (e.g. to ensure product authenticity, label legibility).

Selection of container closure system

1. To determine the critical parameters of the container closure system.

Label controls

1. To design label control procedures based on the potential for mix-ups involving different product labels, including different versions of the same label.

BIBLIOGRAPHY

1. Ahmadvand S, Kazemi A. Familiarity with TQM. 2000. http://www.abkazemi.blogfa.com.
2. ANSI/ISO 17025-1999: General requirements for the competence of testing and calibration laboratories. American Society for Quality; 1999.
3. ANSI/ISO/ASQ Q9000-2000: Quality management systems: Fundamentals and vocabulary. American Society for Quality; 2000.
4. ANSI/ISO/ASQ Q9001-2000: Quality management systems: Requirements. American Society for Quality; 2000.
5. ANSI/ISO/ASQ Q9004-2000. Quality management systems: Guidelines for performance improvement. American Society for Quality; 2000.
6. Control Charts. Quality Risk Management Q9. ISO 7870; 1993.http://www.ich.org/fileadmin/Public_Web_Site/ICH_Products/Guidelines/Quality/Q9/Step4/Q9_Guideline.pdf.
7. CPGM 7356.002. Compliance Program – Drug Manufacturing Inspections. http://www.fda.gov/cder/dmpq/compliance_guide.htm.

8. Good Manufacturing Practices for Pharmaceutical Products: Main Principles. World Health Organization Technical Report Series, No. 908; 2003. http://www.who.int/medicines/library/qsm/trs908/trs908-4.pdf.

9. Guidance for Developing Quality Systems for Environmental Programs. EPA QA/G-1; 2002.http://www.epa.gov/quality/qs-docs/g1-final.pdf.

10. Guidance for Industry: Sterile Drug Products Produced by Aseptic Processing Current Good Manufacturing Practice. 2004. http://www.fda.gov/downloads/Drugs/.../Guidances/ucm070342.pdf.

11. Guidance for Industry for the Submission of Documentation for Sterilization Process Validation in Applications for Human and Veterinary Drug Products. Center for Drug Evaluation and Research (CDER and Center for Veterinary Medicine (CVM); 1994. http://www.fda.gov/cder/guidance/cmc2.pdf.

12. Guidance for Industry ICH Q8 Pharmaceutical Development. Revision 2; 2009.http://www.fda.gov/downloads/Drugs/.../Guidances/ucm 073507.pdf.

13. Guidance for Industry Q7A Good Manufacturing Practice Guidance for Active Pharmaceutical Ingredients. U.S. Department of Health and Human Services/ Food and Drug Administration; August 2001.

14. Guideline of General Principles of Process Validation. 1987: http://www.fda.gov/cder/guidance/pv.htm.

15. Guidelines for Failure Modes and Effects Analysis (FMEA) for Medical Devices. Dyadem Press, London; 2003: ISBN 0849319102.

16. ICH Q10 Pharmaceutical Quality System. http://www.ich.org/fileadmin/Public_Web_Site/ICH_Products/Guidelines/Quality/Q10/Step4/Q10_Guideline.pdf.

17. IEC 60812 Analysis Techniques for system reliability: Procedures for failure mode and effects analysis (FMEA). http://webstore.iec.ch/preview/info_iec60812%7Bed2.0%7Den_d.pdf.

18. IEC 61025 - Fault Tree Analysis (FTA). http://webstore.iec.ch/preview/info_iec61025%7Bed2.0%7Den_d.pdf.

19. Ishikawa K. (Translated by Liu DJ). What is Total Quality Control?; The Japanese Way.1985: ISBN 0139524339.

20. Juran JM, Gryna FM. Quality Planning and Analysis. 3rd Edition. McGraw-Hill, New York; 1993.

21. Kesmati M. The Effect of TQM on Efficiency. Oil Industry Research;2002.

22. Kesmati M. The Relationship between TQM and Organizations' Operation. Oil Industry Research; 2002.

23. McDermott R, Mikulak RJ, Beauregard MR. The Basics of FMEA. 1996: ISBN 0527763209.

24. Preamble to the Good Manufacturing Practice Final Regulations: Federal Register Docket No. 73N-0339]. 1978.http://www.fda.gov/cder/dmpq/preamble.txt.

25. Prince R. Quality Management in the American Pharmaceutical Industry: in Pharmaceutical Quality. Chapter 3, DHI Publishing, River Grove, IL; 2004.

26. Process Mapping by the American Productivity and Quality Center. 2002. ISBN 1928593739.

27. Risk Management Vocabulary: Guidelines for use in Standards. ISO/IEC Guide 73; 2002.http://www.iso.org/iso/catalogue_detail?csnumber=34998.

28. Safety Aspects - Guideline for their inclusion in standards. ISO/IEC Guide 51; 1999.http://webstore.iec.ch/preview/info_isoiecguide51%7Bed2.0%7Den.pdf.

29. Shim JK, Siegel GJ. Operation Management. Barron's Educational Series Inc., New York; 1999.

30. Stamatis DH. Failure Mode and Effect Analysis, FMEA from Theory to Execution, 2nd Edition, 2003: ISBN 0873895983.

31. Thornton AC. Variation Risk Management: Focusing Quality Improvement in Product Development. John Wiley and Sons, Inc., Hoboken, New Jersey; 2004.

32. WHO Technical Report Series No 908. Annex 7 Application of Hazard Analysis and Critical Control Point (HACCP) methodology to pharmaceuticals;2003.

Chapter 5

Source and Control of Quality Variation in Pharmaceuticals

CHAPTER OVERVIEW

- Quality variations in pharmaceutical product
- Source of quality variation
    Raw and Packaging Material
    Equipment
    Process
    Personnel
    Environment
    Laboratory
    Miscellaneous
- Quality variation in raw and packaging material
    Quality attributes of raw and packaging materials
    Receipt
    Good storage control practice
    Testing
    Sampling
    Release
- Control of quality variation in raw material
- Source and control of quality variation in container closure
    CGMP, CPSC and USP requirements on containers and closures
- Quality attributes of packaging components
    Description
    Suitability
    Quality control
    Stability
- Control of quality variation in pharmaceutical container closure
    Specifications
    Specification for different types of packaging material
    Sampling
    Testing
    Shipment

- Quality variation in pharmaceutical equipment
    Quality attributes of the pharmaceutical equipment system
    Equipment qualification
    Calibration and validation
- Control of quality variation in pharmaceutical equipment system
    Equipment placement and maintenance
    Equipment washing and cleaning facilities
    Automated or computerized systems
    General requirements of equipment
- Quality variation in pharmaceutical manufacturing process
    Quality attributes of pharmaceutical manufacturing process
    Regulatory guidelines
    Master formula
    Operating procedure
    Documents and records
    Environmental controls
    Cleaning
    Quarantine and in-process storing
    In-process quality control
    Identification and tagging
    Contamination and cross-contamination
- Control of quality variation in the pharmaceutical manufacturing process
    Operational excellence
    Process evaluation
    Continuous processing
    Production procedure control
- Control of sterile and non-sterile manufacturing process
    Master batch and completed batch records
    Production operations

KEY POINTS

- As the marketing and sale of pharmaceutical products are under regulatory control and pharmaceuticals are legally bound to strictly control the quality, purity, and stability of formulations. Quality standards of the pharmaceutical products are designed after a long process of research and development with the investment of a lot of resources. Product quality variation is any deviation from pre-defined standards or non-conformance with the specification. As quality depends on factors like facility, material, equipment, process, tests, and personnel, these are also the most common sources of quality variation.

- Quality variation is an issue of concern for the pharmaceuticals in the long run and can be eliminated with a detailed understanding of various sources. Most effective ways to reduce quality variation is to identify, characterize and prevent sources by the implementation of robust process design and management practices that are possibly insensitive to uncontrollable variation.

- Quality attributes of pharmaceutical raw and packaging materials, manufacturing process, equipment,and personnel are identified. Preventive measures are implemented as system improvements to control quality variation. Quality by design concept emphasizes on building quality by a thorough understanding of product and process along with the risks involved.
- Traditionally process control was achieved through tight control on key process parameters at predetermined set points or ranges, i.e. raw material properties, temperature, humidity or pH, that effects the process outputs. Advanced process control uses mathematical algorithms of predictive, adaptive and optimization techniques to control multi-input, multi-output processes.
- The USFDA encourages adoption of process analytical technology; A system developed based on an understanding of how the Critical Process Parameters (CPP) affects the variability in the critical quality attributes (CQA). PAT aims at the assurance of product quality in 'real-time' while batch manufacturing process despite variations in materials and processing.

QUALITY VARIATIONS IN PHARMACEUTICAL PRODUCT

The quality of a pharmaceutical product is standard in itself, which is designed after a long process of research and development. Quality not only concerns with active substance but also depends on many other factors such as excipients, equipment, facility, and procedures. The pharmaceutical industry invests many resources in developing and designing formulations and different dosage forms. The marketing and sale of pharmaceutical products are under strict regulatory control, and the pharmaceuticals are legally bound to follow the strict guidelines set by the regulatory bodies. The quality, purity, stability, and safety of formulations are tested for compliance within the limits of predetermined specifications while manufacturing the dosage form. The maintenance and compliance of quality standards is the responsibility of each, and every person in a pharmaceutical industry setup and is ensured by the QA department which strictly supervises all function. The function of QA is to inspect various phases of production to ensure the highest quality by monitoring records, process, material, tests, facilities, and personnel.

Variation is seen as the enemy that must be eliminated whenever it appears. Variation inevitably reappears and worsens unless fully understood with details of root causes. Variations instead are to be looked upon as an opportunity exposing error sources to become more productive. Proper identification, characterization, and quantification of variation can improve the bottom line that eventually reduces operating costs and improved customer satisfaction. Understanding of variation should be a core competency of statisticians, Six sigma, quality engineers, quality managers, and all other improvement concerned professionals.

Statistical quality control has three key elements, i.e. process, variation, and data. The process produces the variation acting as the sources of the variation and the data generated are used to deal with it. Professional approach towards minimization of variation should be guided by the aspects that cause variation occurrence:

- Variation can be quantified
- Variation can be predicted
- Sources of variation are additive if not controlled properly
- A small number of sources contribute most of the variations
- Process data reflects variation produced by the process as well as a measurement system.
- Process input variation effects to cause variation in process output

- Variation affects the quality management system.

Quality variation is a deviation from defined standard and non-conformance with the specification. Quality control efforts in pharmaceutical are mostly focused on control of quality variation sources. Quality variation can occur due to a mistake in any step starting from the receipt of raw material to the distribution of the final product. The risk of variation increases when the source is a raw material or the method and become very complicated. Causes of variations are sometimes *Deliberate* but in most of the cases *Accidental*.

SOURCE OF QUALITY VARIATION

The sources of variation, most notably are the difference in material lots, machines, operating lines and human behavior. The guiding rule for the identification of various source, that is, all potential sources of variation are guilty until the data proves them innocent. Machines often act a typically potent source of variations in the pharmaceutical industry. Variation in operating lines, both in manufacturing and services results from variations in human behavior. Human resource differs from day to day, group to group and organization to organization. The general sources causing product quality variation in pharmaceuticals are categorized as raw material, packaging material, equipment, process, personnel, environment and miscellaneous:

Raw and Packaging Material

- Inherent variability in components
- Variations between different suppliers for the same substances.
- Alteration in supplier qualification
- Batch to batch variations by same suppliers.
- Variations within a batch.

- Inadequate monitoring of quality attributes
- Improper characterization of excipient quality
- Poor understanding of component variability on processability
- Alteration in suppliers product qualification
- Multivariate interactions
- Inadequate understanding of packaging material characteristics
  - Unintended changes in packaging components affecting the operation downstream
  - Inadequate communication of changes in packaging components and lack of understanding of its unintended but adverse impact on drug product quality
  - Improper dissemination of supplier change communication
  - Components of undefined physical properties
  - Characteristics robust during design but does not hold up later
  - Inadequate characterization of functional properties of excipients with API compatibility

Equipment

- Variation in equipment performance
- Poor functional adjustments
- Aging and improper care
- Lack of adequate preventive maintenance
- Lack of adequate calibration
- Disregard for limitations imposed by OQ/PQ
- Poorly defined operational requirements
- Improper measurement and data presentation
- Misinterpretation
  - Wrong application of statistics
  - Too much data (can change knowledge base)

- Inadequate sampling scheme
- Human error (intra or inter-operator variability)
- Inappropriate interface with process and equipment
- Incorrect process attribute
- Inadequate analytical qualification

Process

- Inadequate or wrong procedure description
- Negligence in following standard procedures
- Improper/inadequate adjustment of the manufacturing process to accommodate material variability
- The process not developed to be robust
- Complexity and multistep product formulation procedure
- Formulation process not suitable for available manufacturing equipment
- Poor or operators unfriendly design
- More emphasis on manual operations rather than automation
- Lack of risk management
- The inadequate Change Management system
  - Improper circulation of information between the workers
  - Workers not well versed with the change management system
  - Lack of best practice models for change management and risk assessment
  - Lack of implementation of detection systems to identify potential problems downstream
  - Unable to recruit a workforce with the right skill sets to determine change implications
- Inadequate monitoring of change management
  - Trending of "special" attributes as the indicator of the positive/negative

impact of the changing enforcement on a validated process
  - Variations introduced by unknown factors

Personnel

- Improper working conditions
- Inadequate training
- Lack of interest and emotional upheavals
- Dishonesty, fatigue, and carelessness
- Poor procedural understanding
- Unable to follow or understand procedures
- The work force is not well qualified to adopt with procedural changes when steps are critical vs. trivial (shift change procedures)
- Inadequate resources/poor work environment/rigid schedule
- Poor monitoring of training effectiveness
- Lack of skill leading to poor execution (lack of procedural control)
- Attrition (acquisitions, mergers, etc.)
- Operators error and performance non-conformance
  - Performing ad hoc changes
  - Poor follow up of SOPs
  - Poor documentation practices
  - Poor supervisory controls
  - Insufficient training for using current methodologies

Environment

- Inadequate or poor understanding of environmental control aspects
- The sensitivity of specialized dosage forms to humidity, temperature, etc.
- Effects of seasonal variation not adequately monitored
- Needs for specialized equipment (FBD) for proper environmental control
- Effect of poorly controlled environment on sensitive processes like coating
- Insufficient resources for implementation and monitoring of environmental controls

- Inadequate and insufficient validation of environment control factors

Laboratory

- QC laboratory controls
  - Ambiguity in method instructions/SOP leaving room for multiple interpretations
  - Multiple sources of procurement for critical reagents used for testing
  - Inadequate training of analyst and chemists
  - Poor monitoring of the effectiveness of training
  - Poor maintenance and inadequate calibration of instruments
- Research and development laboratory
  - Inadequate instruments and resources
  - Time and cost crunch/pressures during development timeline follow up
  - Failure to define critical points during Process Development
  - Lack of management support (Financial limitations)
  - Inadequate knowledge and understanding of formulation factors
  - Lack of multidisciplinary expert team approach at R&D for integration of steps from scale-up to commercialization
  - Inadequate knowledge transfer from R&D to pilot scale

Miscellaneous

- Unable to do immediate cause vs. root cause solutions analysis for complaint and recalls
- Right quality output vs. large quantity output policy adoption by management
- Ambiguous quality culture followed by management and its propagation between the staffs

- Change in regulatory requirement can also introduce or give the perception of variability

The most effective way to reduce variation is to anticipate, identify and prevent it in advance by implementation of robust process design, products quality control and management practices in that areas as much as possible insensitive to uncontrollable variation. This concept of adoption of measures that are insensitivity to variation is called robustness which is the crucial aspect of statistical quality control. A robust process or product is designed to be insensitive to a range of variations under all conditions of manufacture, distribution, use, and disposal. Robust process is expected to show resistance towards uncontrollable variations in process inputs, external factors, and transformations in the course of the process. A robust management system can be created when all the working procedures involved in a project system are developed in such a way that is insensitive to changes in personnel and working conditions.

QUALITY VARIATION IN RAW AND PACKAGING MATERIAL

High-quality starting materials are an essential prerequisite for any scientific processing method to be reliable and reproducible. For therapeutic and diagnostic pharmaceuticals this is of paramount importance. Though standard laboratory chemicals are usually perfectly satisfactory, it is necessary for a QC laboratory to invest substantial effort in setting in-house testing procedures and preparation of standard reagents. According to cGMP, all raw materials that come into contact with medicinal products need to be controlled and tested for purity and identity.

Quality Attributes of Raw and Packaging Materials

Quality of any drug formulation or medicinal product depends on the quality of raw material, that is why testing of raw materials for its quality is most important. Quality variations can be controlled, minimized or eliminated by eradicating mistakes following good material control procedures. Material control starts immediately after receipt of materials like API, excipients, packaging and printed items from suppliers. There should be well established and validated system for the receipt, storage, testing and release of all these materials. All the procedures are required to be completely recorded and reviewed time to time for compliance (Fig. 5.1).

All the incoming materials are kept in store arranged alphabetically or differentiated depending upon physical nature. Samples are withdrawn for laboratory testing from the container, and a 'Sampled' label is fixed on the material container. In the case of active constituents, percentage purity, expiry date, lot number, exact packing conditions are checked. In the case of printing and packaging material especially the color of label, weight mentioned in the label and cartons and grammage is checked. When the material found up to the mark, it is labelled as 'Passed' and is placed at the proper location. On the other hand, if it is found substandard, then labeled as 'Rejected' and kept in a designated area for rejected items for further disposal or sent back to the supplier.

Receipt

1. The receipt of each consignment delivery of individual raw material should be recorded separately.
2. Visual inspection should be carried out for the exact label, container damage and contamination, if any.
3. Damaged material should be kept in a separate area and sent back to the supplier or destroyed.
4. The control reference number is assigned to each raw material throughout its presence in the premises.
5. Records are maintained that contain all relevant information regarding a particular raw material starting from receipt to final use.
6. Different batches of a particular raw material are to be considered as separate batches.
7. Following details are incorporated in records.
   a. Name of the material
   b. The quantity of material received and number of containers

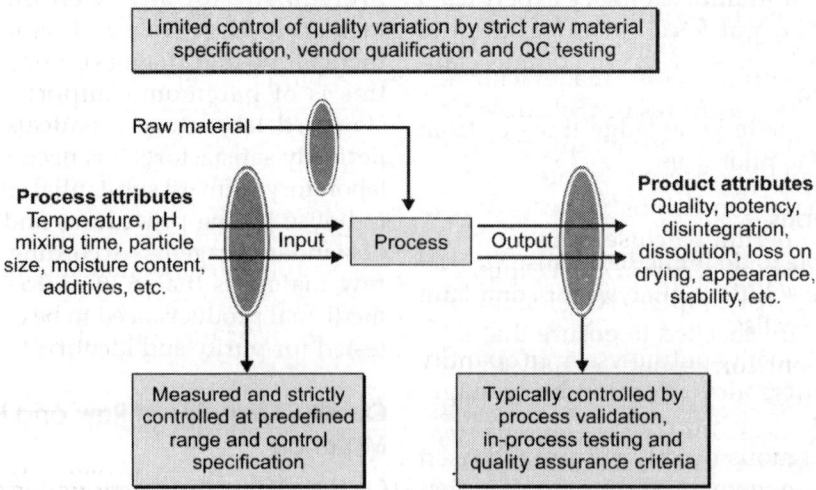

Fig. 5.1: A paradigm of source control responsible for quality variation in pharmaceuticals

c. Date of receipt
d. Name and address of the supplier and manufacturer.
e. The supplier reference number/batch number as assigned by the manufacturer.
f. Results of tests/analysis carried out.
g. Release status of material (approval or rejection of consignment/batch).

8. Every raw material should be held in quarantine until released for use by QC manager. Usually, in pharmaceuticals, yellow color label is attached to designate quarantine materials. Such labels should be different from supplier labels and applied by QC people only.

9. Once the status of the material changes, status label should be immediately changed accordingly and pasted near the original/previous labels (e.g. under test, approved, rejected, etc).

10. Labels should never be pasted overlapped. Along with manufacturers original label, all other labels should be visible simultaneously.

11. Pallets are advised to be utilized to keep the raw materials in the storage area.

Good storage control practice

1. The licensee is required to keep an inventory of all raw materials used at all the stage of drug product manufacturing and maintain records as per Schedule U.

2. All incoming materials are quarantined immediately after receipt, stored under appropriate conditions in an orderly fashion to permit batch segregation and stock rotation by a 'first in/first expiry'—'first out' principle. All incoming materials are checked to ensure that the consignment corresponds exactly to the order placed.

3. All incoming materials are to be purchased from approved vendors under valid purchase vouchers. It is recommended to purchase raw materials preferably directly from the producers.

4. Authorized staff appointed by the licensee in this behalf, mostly personnel from the QC Department, examine each consignment on receipt and check each container for the integrity of package and seal. Any container damaged are identified, recorded and segregated.

5. When a single delivery consignment of material is made up of different batches, each batch shall be considered as separately for sampling, testing, and release.

6. Raw materials stored in the central storage area shall be appropriately labeled in different colors as per status for easy identification. Labels are marked with the following information:
   a. Designated name of the product and the internal reference code, and analytical reference number when applicable.
   b. Manufacturer's name, address, and batch number.
   c. The status of the contents (e.g. quarantine, under test, released, approved, rejected) must be accessible in the label.
   d. The manufacturing date, expiry date the re-test date.

7. Adequate separate areas should be provided for materials 'under test' 'approved' and 'rejected' with arrangements of equipment to undertake a clear, orderly placement of stored materials and products, wherever necessary under controlled temperature and humidity.

8. Containers from which samples have already been withdrawn shall be identified.

9. Only raw materials formally released by the QC department and are within their shelf-life should be used. It should be ensured that the shelf life of formulated

product must not exceed that of active raw materials used.

10. Ensured proper placement of all the containers of raw materials on raised platforms/racks but not preferably directly on the floor.

The objective of testing raw material is:

1. Identity confirmation of the material.
2. Retaliation of the product physico-chemical characteristics to ensure the desired qualities in the produced dosage form.
3. Assurance of desired biochemical properties of the final product.

Testing

1. Raw materials are not to be sent to the production department until it is sampled, analyzed and found to be satisfactory as per specification and released by QC department.
2. Standard operating procedure for sampling is prepared and authorized by the QA manager.
3. SOPs are reviewed periodically, and the current one is adopted.
4. Identification test on the content of every container must be carried out.
5. Every raw material must be checked for
   a. Identity
   b. Purity
   c. Contamination with dirt, microbes and insect infestation
6. Approved active raw materials are stored with an assigned re-test duration if not used immediately and over the recommended re-test period are only used after QC approval.
7. The approved active raw material sample is retained for re-examination during the shelf life of the material.

Sampling

The sample is taken from a lot for testing purpose. Sampling is the process of collecting a portion of material from a larger quantity:

1. The sampling plan is decided on the basis of the nature of the material, the number of batches in a consignment, history of supplies from each source and manufacturer's reliability on the material.
2. Every batch must be sampled, and if possible, every container of the very batch is sampled.
3. The quantity of sampled material should be sufficient to analyze and to keep for reference purpose. Usually, it should be twice the requirement.
4. The sample should be collected in two separate containers, so that later examination if required, can be carried out on an unopened container.
5. Properly suitable sampling equipment should be used for the materials looking in the chemical nature of the substance.
6. Adequately trained samplers conduct sampling operations. The sampler should strictly follow the standard sampling procedure approved by QC personnel.
7. Sampler needs to ensure proper adoption of precautions that are to be taken while performing sampling.

Release

1. Batch or lot of any raw material which meets the approved specifications as ensured by testing is approved and released for use. QA department attaches authorized passed labels.
2. After the release of material when not used immediately, storage conditions should be adequate to ensure that deteriorate of material will not take place during storage.
3. When quarantine or under test status label has been used it should be replaced by or canceled with the passed labels.
4. Adoption of "First In First Out" system is a recommended method for good

inventory control. For this stability conditions and expiry period of raw materials are considered.

5. If the material is not used up to expiry period, it is to be retested and if found up to the quality parameter then only can be used. Wording on such labels should be "Valid up to" or "Re-tested on" with appropriate date inserted.

6. As a basic principle and common rule, any material should not have a retest date of more than 12 months.

7. Material not found up to the specified requirements are rejected and should have the rejected label. In such cases quarantine or under test status label are canceled with rejected label and material removed to the rejected area.

8. The usual color scheme adopted for different types of materials maintained in the store is:
   – Passed material: Green color
   – Rejected material: Red color
   – Quarantine: Yellow color
   – Under test: Pink color

CONTROL OF QUALITY VARIATION IN RAW MATERIAL

The chemical, physical, and biopharmaceutical characteristics of the active drug and other components is characterized in order to design a suitable manufacturing process that ensures to provide finished product with consistent quality attributes. Although the science of analyzing chemical attributes such as identity and purity is well developed, specific physical attributes such as solid form, particle size, and particle shape are more challenging to analyze and control. Effective quality implementation is based on the detailed, science-based understanding of the chemical and mechanical properties of all elements that are to be incorporated in a proposed drug product.

Source control: Many of the raw materials used in pharmaceutical processes today are either natural products or are derived from natural products. As such, their variation needs to be closely monitored in order to maintain the highest quality. Traditionally, this is carried out using wet chemistry methods such as solubility, melting point, pH, TLC, etc. Nowadays, these labor intensive methods have been complemented or superseded by rapid and automated instrumental techniques such as spectroscopy and/or particle size distribution analysis. These multivariate quality defying signals require proper treatment using *multivariate analysis* to provide real-time quality monitoring, forward control and a starting point for the *design of experiments*.

Pharmaceutical formulation manufacturing processes require a variety of chemical or biological materials. The quality control system of materials and formulations for pharmaceutical use include, i.e. confirmation of chemical purity, polymorphism, and water content, etc. Some important physical characteristics are functionality-related properties that can vary between different grades of the same chemical entity. Such characteristics include dissolution rate, physical state (dispersed/aggregates), thermal stability (thermal transition), and particle size. In particular with biologically active macromolecules such as proteins, polysaccharides or synthesized polymers, this is very true. The specific physical and functionality-related properties are tested by different methods such as ultraviolet (UV)/visible spectroscopy, nuclear magnetic resonance (NMR), laser diffraction, calorimetry, and dynamic rheology. All have their limitations and therefore, search for new, fast and effective methods for wide-range characterization of material (raw materials, intermediates, excipients, and active ingredients) is a prime issue in drug R and D, production and quality control. The consistency of product quality can only be assured with regular and constant maintenance of physicochemical properties of the API and other raw materials. The principal strategy in ensuring product quality is tight control over raw material specification. The critical factors that are to be considered:

- Study different solid forms attainable by raw material and their relevance to the manufacturing process and final use of the product
- Select the optimum solid form of raw material suitable for a particular product
- Investigate and optimize the physical properties such as particle size, particle shape, stability, drying, filterability, solubility, dissolution rate, etc. of the solid raw material
- Develop a manufacturing process or procure sourcing materials from a reliable source that consistently provides the API having the desired physical characteristics
- Develop analytical methods to verify the presence and quantify the concentration of the selected form of the API in a drug product formulation
- Finalize the aids in setting API specifications
- Determine excipient compatibility
- Optimize the aids for formulation design
- Develop the aids in setting drug product specifications
- Develop optimum product manufacturing strategies consistent with the solid properties of the API.

Monitoring of raw material specifications with conventional spectroscopic methods in conjunction with multivariate sophisticated analytical methods can more efficiently monitor raw materials and ascertain their impact on product quality.

High-Resolution Ultrasonic Spectroscopy: High-resolution ultrasonic spectroscopy (HR-US) is a non-destructive technique with enormous potential for the analysis of materials and formulations used in the pharmaceutical industry. This technique is based on precision measurements of acoustical wave parameters at high frequencies propagating through materials. Unlike current analytical methods, optical transparency is not required because ultrasonic waves can propagate through opaque samples. These instruments require small sample volumes, down to 0.03 ml and give an excellent resolution. HR-US is used for analyzing composition, aggregation, gelation, micelle formation, crystallization, dissolution, sedimentation, enzyme activity, conformational transitions in polymers, ligand binding, antigen–antibody interactions and many other processes that play a crucial role for functional properties of the material used in drug production. This instrument is capable of dealing with a wide range of samples and dynamic processes. HR-US generates product quality information in real process time allowing fast analysis of formulation consistency, batch-to-batch variation, stability assessment and so forth.

Scanning Electron Microscopy: Scanning electron microscopy (SEM) helps manufacturers to identify and analyze the presence of foreign particles in the formulation by automated analysis of acquiring images, morphology, and elemental composition information. This way, the QC can quickly identify the presence of foreign particles that would compromise final product's quality. As the SEM can identify particles as small as 0.1 microns, it is an ideal tool for micro-contamination quality control.

Multivariate calibration: Traditional analytical technique can measure one single variable and to avoid error due to interference samples needed to be purified which is a time to consume and expensive endeavor. Multivariate calibration is a chemometric method designed for quantitative analysis based on the powerful mathematical tool. Chemical concentrations can be determined rapidly and reliable by combining information from several measurement variables eliminating systematic errors. Multivariate calibration is a technique that reduces the need for sample preparation and replaces the wet chemistry measurements with spectroscopic (or other multidimensional) sensor arrays because various systematic noise types can be eliminated mathematically. Unexpected problems in unknown samples can be detected automatically thus reliable quantitative measurement is possible even with unpurified mixed samples. Multivariate calibration technique uses a set of calibration samples data with known composition feed in the mathematical model of a microcomputer to remove systematic errors due to interference in the measured data. The mathematical results are used to get a rapid determination of the chemical composition of similar unknown samples regardless of the level of interference. Multivariate calibration combines data from several channels, in order to overcome selectivity problems, gain new insight and allow automatic outlier detection which is the basis for the present success of high-speed near-infrared (NIR) diffuse spectroscopy of intact samples. The main advantages of multivariate calibration techniques are non-destructive analytical measurements that allow for accurate quantitative analysis in the presence of high interference by other analytes.

Process analytical technology (PAT) is the system for design, analysis, and control pharmaceutical manufacturing process by estimating critical process parameters that affect critical quality attributes. In a typical PAT application, a multivariate calibration model provides a real-time analysis capability during pharmaceutical production stages, e.g. granulation, drying, synthesis. Simple spectroscopic data are translated back to concentration, solvent content, etc. for end-point detection, monitoring, and control.

Various process parameters are acquired by using multiple analysis techniques like IR, UV-VIS, Raman, HPLC and Mass spectroscopy. Out of all the analytical technologies utilized in PAT, application of spectroscopy is most extensive concerning money value, whereas near infrared (NIR) by far is the most common technique. Electrochemistry is also commonly applied due to lower cost and relative technical simplicity. Analytical techniques like particle size analysis, HPLC, mass spectrometry are now having a significant application with the fast growing technique of thermal effusivity. The market scope of software for instrument control, process modeling, data collection, and analysis lags significantly behind the instrument technologies regarding development and is primarily the realm of software consultants who develop highly customized solutions for individual manufacturers. PAT is a landmark in the control, supervision, and monitoring of process systems with best-established practices in modern pharmaceutical manufacturing. PAT uses high-level quality specifications typically obtained by multiparametric *in situ* on-line techniques such as process spectroscopies. PAT strategy developed for a dynamic process strongly depends upon the starting conditions of the raw materials.

SOURCE AND CONTROL OF QUALITY VARIATION IN THE CONTAINER CLOSURE

A *container closure system* is the summation of packaging components that together contain and protect a dosage form which is also called the *packaging system*. It mostly includes primary packaging and secondary packaging components, where the latter is intended to provide additional protection to the drug product. The *primary packaging component* is in or may be in direct contact with the dosage form. The *secondary packaging component* is not meant to and will not be in direct contact with the dosage form.

CGMP, CPSC and USP Requirements for Containers and Closures

Drug product containers and closures shall be nonreactive, nonadditive and nonabsorptive so that they does not alter the safety, identity, strength, quality or purity of the drug beyond the official or established requirements. Container closure systems are meant to provide adequate protection against foreseeable external factors while storing and use of the product that can cause deterioration or contamination of the drug product. Drug product containers and closures must be adequately clean as indicated by the nature of the drug sterilized and processed to remove pyrogenic substances to assure suitability for intended use. Standards of specifications, methods of testing, cleaning and sterilizing, and process to remove pyrogenic substances are maintained in written and followed for product containers and closures.

Packing material includes:

1. The primary packaging material is one which comes in contact with the product (e.g. bottle, vial, ampoule, tin, tube, foil wrapping, etc,) and also the cap, wad, bung, etc. used with the container.
2. The secondary package (e.g. carton, box, catch-cover, tin, etc) including any stuffing such as shredded paper, polyurethane pads, cotton, wool or other materials used for space filling.
3. The label on the primary and/or secondary packaging along with other descriptive materials such as leaflets inserted in them.

Quality control of container closure systems is equally vital as they provide safety and protect products against harmful effects of the environment. However, while intended to provide a stable environment to the dosage form, container closures may also interact with a product, affecting performance and potentially enhancing toxicity. Therefore, rigorous safety evaluations are required not only in the context of the product but also for product containment. The choice and rationale behind the selection of the container closure system for the commercial product are considered based on the intended use of the drug product and the suitability of the container closure system at the time of storage and transportation. During product development and package finalization, a possibility of interaction occurs between product and container or label should be considered.

Selection of primary packaging materials are based on the consideration of choice of materials, protection from moisture and light, compatibility of the materials of construction with the dosage form (including adsorption to container and leaching), and safety of materials of construction. A proper justification for secondary packaging materials selection is considered when relevant. Whenever a dosing device is used (e.g. dropper pipette, pen injection device, dry powder inhaler), it is essential to demonstrate delivery of an accurate and reproducible dose of the product under testing conditions and as far as possible also in case of simulated use of the product.

The United States Pharmacopoeial Convention has established requirements for drug product containers described in *The United States Pharmacopeia/National Formulary (USP/NF)* drug product monographs. The requirements generally relate to the design characteristics of the container (e.g. tight, well-closed or light-resistant) for solid dosage form like capsules and tablets. Whereas materials of construction (e.g. "Preserve in single-dose or multiple-dose containers, preferably of Type I glass, protected from light") is crucial for injectable products. These requirements are defined in the "General Notices and Requirements" (Preservation, Packaging, Storage, and Labeling) section of the *USP*. The requirements for materials of construction are defined in the "General Chapters" 4 of the USP.

QUALITY ATTRIBUTES OF PACKAGING COMPONENTS

Description

Description of the container closure system material of construction and quality attributes for individual Packaging Component generally includes the following:

- Specified name of component, product code, and physical description
- Manufacturer name and address
- Materials of construction
- Description of any additional treatments or preparations

Suitability

Protection: By each component and/or the container closure system, as appropriate

- Light exposure
- Reactive gases (e.g. oxygen)
- Moisture permeation
- Solvent loss or leakage
- Microbial contamination (sterility/container integrity, increased bioburden, and microbial limits)
- Filth
- Seal integrity or leak testing of tubes (ophthalmic, topical drug products) and unit dose containers (liquid-based oral drug products)

Safety: Material of construction, as appropriate

- Chemical composition of the material
- Extractables potential as appropriate for the material like plastics, elastomers, adhesives, etc.
- Toxicological evaluation, as appropriate
- Appropriate pharmacopoeial testing
- Appropriate reference to the food additive used as per regulations
- Other studies as appropriate

Compatibility: Component and/or the packaging system, as appropriate

- Interaction with other component and/or dosage form
- If required, post-approval stability studies
- Coating integrity testing for coated metal tubes
- Evaluation of swelling effects for elastomeric components
- Physicochemical tests for plastic components (including tube coatings)
- Particulate matter and eye irritants for ophthalmic

Performance: For the assembled packaging system

- As appropriate, functionality and/or drug delivery

Quality control

For Each Packaging Component Received by the Applicant:

- In house tests and acceptance criteria
- Dimensional (drawing) matching
- Evaluation of performance criteria
- Monitor consistency in composition, as appropriate
- Manufacturer's acceptance criteria for release, as appropriate
- A brief description of the manufacturing process

Stability

Test for non-reactivity, non-leaching, non-absorbent properties in an environment of high temperature and humidity.

CONTROL OF QUALITY VARIATION IN THE PHARMACEUTICAL CONTAINER CLOSURE

Specifications

In consultation with production and marketing team, QC manager lay down specifications in writing for any packaging materials.

1. Designated name of materials.
2. Description of the nature, dimensions, and material of construction of the component with the relevant standards and applicable control limits
3. Testing for compliance with the specifications
4. Any other details such as drawing, etc.
5. Sampling instructions
6. Storage conditions
7. The frequency of re-examination of the stored material.
8. Date of issue of specification
9. Approval of the QC manager.
10. Printed packaging material must have identification code numbers or marks on the printed copy of the text.

The possible defects are to be identified as major or minor defects.

Specification for Different Types of Packaging Material

Bottle
- Capacity
- Material (glass, plastic, aluminum)
- Weight of bottle
- Thread of bottle
- Cap material (rubber, plastic coated)
- Thickness

Silica bag
- Weight
- Capacity

Carton
- Dimensions (notches, locking system)
- Quality of Board (grammage)
- Printings
- Color (reflection color measurement by tintometer; some local industries use color album)

Label
- Dimensions
- Printing
- Weight
- Striations (lines on paper)

Sampling

Statistical plan basis sampling for physical tests are preferred with pre-determined and specified Acceptable Quality Levels (AQL) after consultation and agreement with the QA personnel. A representative sample is taken from each lot.

Testing

Each batch of packaging material are given a reference number which permits access to records that provide full details including the results of testing of the respective batch and tested for:
- Physical characteristics such as dimensions, color variation, gauge of material, appearance, etc. are tested,
- Chemical and biological tests on aqueous extracts as detailed in the pharmacopeia must be carried out for glass vials, ampoules, bottles are plastic containers.
- Printed packaging material is checked for text matter.

The test report contains:
- Name of packing material and date of testing or inspection mentioned.
- The reference number noted for identifying the batch.
- Results of testing or inspection are documented including the classification of defects, if any.
- The name of the person (s) carried out the testing/inspection.
- QC signed decision of release or rejection of the material.

Shipment

- The container closure system mostly used for storage or shipment of bulk solid drug substance are drummed with double LDPE liners usually heat sealed or closed with a twist tie.
- The container closure system typically used for storage or shipment of a bulk liquid drug substance is plastic, stainless steel, glass-lined metal container or

epoxy-lined metal container with a rugged, tamper-resistant closure.

- Appropriate desiccant is placed when required between the bags.
- Qualification of the container closure system includes characterization for solvent and gas permeation, light transmittance, closure integrity, ruggedness in shipment, protection against microbial contamination through the closure, and compatibility and safety of the packaging components as appropriate.
- In all cases, container closure system used for bulk drug products storage before packaging or for shipment to repackagers and contract packagers should be constructed of materials that are compatible and safe to protect the dosage form adequately.
- Similarly container closure system for the transportation of bulk drug products to contract packagers should be adequate to protect the dosage form, and the materials to be compatible with the product and safe for the intended use.
- A container closure system intended specifically for transportation of large volume solid or liquid dosage form of drug products to a repackager, C&F or wholesaler is considered a market package. The package should also meet the same requirements for protection, compatibility, and safety as other packaging material and should also be included in the stability studies for approval application and in the long-term stability protocol.

QUALITY VARIATION IN PHARMACEUTICAL EQUIPMENT

The Good Laboratory Practice regulations impose that all pieces of equipment utilized for generation, measurement or assessment of data shall be adequately tested, calibrated, and/or standardized. All the equipment

qualification must be defined and documented. Documentation must contain provisions for the qualification, operation, and maintenance of all equipment used to collect data for regulatory submissions related to the drug product manufacturing and QC control. This accomplished by using a Standard Operating Procedure (SOP) that describes the overall program and schedule. Master SOPs are used to describe the compliance requirements for a variety of equipment, and any specific equipment SOP can be created as separate documents similar to test methods as required. All equipment placed in side pharmaceutical manufacturing or quality control sections must be tagged or labeled with maintained relevant records in the form of log book documenting all critical activities such as qualification, testing, location, custodian, failures, maintenance and so forth. Labeling serves the purpose of equipment identification helps in easy traceability of the unqualified or non-performing equipment. It prevents use of such equipment while it is not in its optimal operating condition.

Quality Attributes of the Pharmaceutical Equipment System

Instrument: Instrument is defined as a device (chemical, electrical, hydraulic, magnetic, mechanical, optical, pneumatic) used to test, observe, measure, monitor, alter, generate, record, calibrate, manage, or control physical properties, movements or other characteristics. Devices taking a physical measurement and displays a value or have no control or analytical function, e.g. stop watches, timers, and thermometers are called instrument.

Equipment: Equipment is a device or collection of components that perform a process to produce a result. Collectively the analytical measurement instruments, in conjunction with firmware is assembled to perform some particular mechanical process.

Computerized equipment is controlled by the computer system that also collects data measurement by the equipment. Equipment qualification is the action of proving evidence that the equipment works correctly and leads to accurate and reliable results. It includes design qualification (DQ), installation qualification (IQ), calibration, operational qualification (OQ) and performance qualification (PQ).

Equipment Qualification

Design qualification (DQ): It defines the functional, operational and design specifications of the instrument. It specifies the quality attributes based on which selection of the manufacturer or supplier is made for the purchase of a particular instrument.

Installation qualification (IQ): It establishes the specification that the instrument is delivered as designed and specified, that it is installed correctly in the selected environment, and that the environment is suitable for the operation and use specified. Documented verification ensures that all critical aspects of hardware had been installation and adhered to appropriate codes. IQ establishes confidence that equipment process and ancillary systems are capable of consistently operating within established limits and tolerances.

Operation qualification (OQ): It is the process of demonstration that equipment will function according to its operational specifications in the selected environment. Documented verification assures that the equipment system or subsystems operate as specified in the specifications throughout the representative or anticipated operating ranges.

Performance qualification (PQ): It is the process of demonstrating that an instrument consistently performs according to specifications as defined and appropriate for its routine use. Documented verification ensures that the integrated system performs as intended in its defined operating environment.

Process performance qualification: It concerns with establishing confidence that a process used for the manufacturing of a particular product with a specified line of equipment is efficient and reproducible.

Product performance qualification: It relates to establishing confidence through appropriate testing that the finished product produced by a specified process using a particular equipment line meets all release requirements for functionality and safety.

Calibration and Validation

Calibration: Under specified conditions establishment of a relationship between values indicated by a measuring instrument or measuring system, or materials measured with the corresponding values of the measure following a particular set of operations. Calibration refers to the process of checking or adjusting instruments as per the requirement of regulatory agencies.

Validation: It is the process of establishing documented evidence providing a high degree of assurance that a specific process consistently produces a product meeting its predetermined specifications and quality attributes.

Requalification and revalidation: Requalification is a repetition of the entire qualification process or a particular selected portion of it. Revalidation is similarly repetition of the entire validation effort or a selected portion of it.

Standardization: The assignment of a compositional value of one standard equipment based on another standard.

Verification: The process of establishing conformance by examination and procuring evidence that specified predecided requirements have been met.

Change control: It is a formal monitoring system of the qualified representatives of appropriate disciplines (usually QA) to review the proposed or actual changes that might affect a validated status to determine the need for corrective action. Change control system is required to assure that the system retains its validated state. Change control system is required to be reviewed by qualified representatives following formalized program to assess potential effects of proposed and actual changes in products, processes, equipment or software on the validation status.

Computerized system: It is a system that has a computer as a major and integral part, and dependents on the computer software to function. Computer hardware components with a set of software programs assembled to perform alone or in conjunction with any electronic device or equipment which are collectively designed to perform a specific function or group of functions.

CONTROL OF QUALITY VARIATION IN THE PHARMACEUTICAL EQUIPMENT SYSTEM

The Analytical Research and Development Steering Committee of the Pharmaceutical Research and Manufacturers, USA, has originally developed the concept of Acceptable Analytical Practices (AAPs). This was focused to share information with ICH and other regulatory authorities worldwide about the implementation status of the CMC and Quality Guidances in the pharmaceutical industries. Previously regulations regarding qualification of laboratory and production equipment were being vague and subject to divergent interpretation. The GMP requirements on **pharmaceutical equipment system** state that "calibration of instruments, apparatus, gauges, and recording devices at suitable intervals in accordance with an established written program containing specific directions, schedules, limits for

accuracy and precision, and provisions for remedial action in the event accuracy and/or precision limits are not met". Instruments, apparatus, gauges, and recording devices became the primary source of quality variation when established specifications are not fulfilled.

Equipment Placement and Maintenance

Activities involved in equipment prepurchase are formally not required to be documented and commonly referred to as design qualification, which leads to the selection of equipment. Once the equipment arrives with the installation phase, the first part of the qualification cycle begins requiring formal documentation that is called the Installation Qualification. In addition to specific installation activities, a pivotal part of IQ is to enter the equipment details in the inventory maintained as part of the program by labeling and creating the equipment log. Vendors are required to perform the installation in the presence of operators that ensures shared documentation of IQ activities. The equipment qualification life cycle further includes components commonly referred to as operational qualification and performance qualification. Depending on the specific use of each equipment appropriate tests and frequency of testing are to be incorporated into the qualification program. Performance Qualification involves the testing of equipment using the specific method or assay to ensure that the equipment is producing valid data. The objective of OQ testing is to ensure that the equipment is capable of meeting performance criteria within the ranges established for all of the testings and assures data validity. PQ also encompasses method validation testing, system suitability testing along with analysis and trending of control samples. PQ supplements the OQ by performing checks of the specific method used, that are like:

Equipment planning: Equipment planning reviews the equipment placement location, design, construction, installation and maintenance based on the operations to be conducted.

Equipment layout: Equipment layout is planned to minimize the risk of errors facilitating effective cleaning and maintenance, and thus avoiding contamination or any other undesired effect on product quality.

Equipment change control: Equipment change control system based on different test methods verify that change control has ensured the qualified state of the equipment.

Qualification and validation: It is the practice of verifying that the qualifications and validations of facilities, equipment, and utilities are conducted in accordance to diverse requirements as mentioned in factory and site acceptance testing, installation, operational, and performance qualification (IQ/OQ/PQ) before process validation.

Equipment maintenance procedure: Equipment maintenance procedure verifies that process is in use for routine and non-routine maintenance testing of heating, ventilation, air conditioning (HVAC) systems, air, and water filters, and other GMP equipment and utilities, etc.

Equipment metrology change control: This verifies that appropriate calibration and equipment change control procedures are in place, and ensures that metrology program exists for the calibration of instruments that are in manufacturing facilities, utilities, and equipment.

Preventive maintenance is performed mainly for economic advantages because it is the most cost-effective method of maintaining equipment that requires frequent service. Components, in general, are subject to wear and tear requiring routine replacement as part of best preventive maintenance program. The preventive maintenance intervals should be defined, documented, and be an integral part of the qualification life cycle. Intervals are defined or adjusted from the actual equipment qualification or maintenance history. Equipment maintenance is done by repairing or replacing any damaged or non-working part and performing qualification test again. OQ testing that is limited to the operational functions can affect the specific maintenance procedure. This usually involves repeating the OQ tests evaluating the component that has been repaired or replaced.

Equipment Washing and Cleaning Facilities

Equipment washing facilities are verified for adequacy and appropriateness. Review of cleaning procedures following cleaning validation is required to be performed that includes:

Equipment cleaning and maintenance: Review of procedures and schedules for equipment cleaning, maintenance, and wherever specified necessary sanitization to ensure that they meet requirements.

Equipment cleaning validation and verification: Specific need based evaluation and methodology development for product-contact cleaning validation and verification of both.

Sanitization procedures: Review of the sanitization procedures developed for facilities and pieces of equipment, including details of cleaning schedules, cleaning methods, cleaning equipment used, cleaning materials used, etc. Verification of the sanitizers, disinfectants, sporicides and sterilants that are used as per marketing authorization requirements and periodic validation studies are performed.

Pest control: Pest control verifies uses of authorized rodenticides, insecticides, fungicides, fumigating agents and appropriate traps for pest elimination, etc. and periodic review of the same.

Sterilization processes: Verify that appropriate and effective sterilization processes are in place.

Automated or Computerized Systems

The automated and computerized system can also generate quality variation in data generated and archived that are required to be reviewed by:

System validation: This includes review of the procedure for validation of all systems, i.e. building maintenance, utilities, equipment, etc. to verify that critical parameters for their operation maintenance are controlled and monitored.

Open and closed computerized systems: It is the process implemented to distinguish between open and closed computerized systems.

Configuration control: Verify that version control and the latest configurations are maintained and monitored.

Security requirements: Evaluation of the computerized systems ensure that they meet requirements of regulatory guidance for key elements such as access control, data protection, change control, data archiving, maintenance, transcription, audit trail, periodic system monitoring, etc, are the important component of security control.

General Requirements of Equipment

1. The types of equipment used for storage, processing, checking and packaging should be of suitable design, size, construction and appropriately located.
2. Equipment should be constructed of a proper size that can be properly accommodated in the facility. The size should be sufficient to process a complete batch at once adoptively as per the planned capacity of a manufacturing facility.
3. The surfaces of the equipment should be non-reactive, non-absorptive and non-additive.
4. The equipment should be constructed and fitted in a way providing easy assess for washing/cleaning, operation, unloading and part replacement.
5. To check cross contamination and mix-ups different formulations should be manufactured in a separate section, i.e. the tablet and liquid section should be totally separate. Segregation should also be ensured when a particular section is having multiple facilities, i.e. if the manufacturing facility has more than one tableting machines, they should be placed in complete separation as in separate cabinets.
6. As per the cleaning and sanitation requirements, all the pieces of equipment are supplied with cold, hot and purified water along with steam and dry air. The proper outflow of water and drainage facility is needed to be maintained.

QUALITY VARIATION IN THE PHARMACEUTICAL MANUFACTURING PROCESS

Excellence in overall manufacturing performance can only be achieved by enhancing process capability. Keeping track with the latest scientific advances in pharmaceutical manufacturing technology and real-time adaptation enhances the core value of the organization. Efficient use of the current pharmaceutical science and engineering principles throughout the Product Life Cycle guarantees improvement in the efficiencies of both manufacturing capacity and adherence to regulatory guidelines. Product quality is more desired than reaching maximum manufacturing efficiency and profitability. It is a safe approach to be acquainted with a technological edge to ensure the highest level of product quality, but it does not always provide with the immediate benefits of being using the established concepts. The pharmaceutical manufacturing process is always in a cross-road balancing between maintaining desired product quality and achieving maximum production capacity. The guidance documents of FDA, WHO, USFDA or EMEA provide the framework to aid pharmaceutical manufacturers to assess the planned or existing documents describing the methods followed to manufacture, test, and administratively control distribution of medicinal products.

Quality Attributes of the Pharmaceutical Manufacturing Process

Regulatory guidelines

GMP covers all aspects of the manufacturing process, viz. defining manufacturing procedure, validation of critical manufacturing steps, suitability of premises, storage and transport, need of qualified and trained personnel, adequate laboratory facilities, approved written procedures and instructions, records to assure following all steps of defined procedures, full traceability of products through batch processing records and distribution records, and systems for recall and investigation of complaints. WHO defines GMP as "part of quality assurance which ensures that products are consistently produced and controlled to the quality standards appropriate to their intended use and as required by the marketing authorization." Quality must be built into a product and not just tested in a finished product is the guiding principle of GMP. Eventually, GMP assures that products not only meet the final specifications but also it has been manufactured following the same approved and validated procedures under the same conditions every time. This can only be ensured by a multidirectional control, controlling the quality of the facility and its systems, starting materials, production at all stages, the identity of materials by adequate labeling and

segregation, materials and product by adequate storage and testing. All of these controls must follow prescribed, formally approved procedures written as protocols, SOPs or master formulae describing all the tasks to be carried out in the entire manufacturing and control process of the drug manufacturing and quality control process.

CDSCO provides general information and guidelines regarding drug regulatory requirements in India. The Drugs and Cosmetics Act, 1940, regulates the import, manufacture, distribution, and sale of drugs in India. The Ministry of Health, along with Drugs Controller General of India (DCGI) and Indian Council for Medical Research (ICMR) has come out with draft guidelines for research in human subjects to control clinical trials in India. The Good Clinical Practices (GCP) guidelines are mainly based on the Declaration of Helsinki, WHO guidelines and ICH requirements clinical practices. WHO guidelines provide policy on technical cooperation, traditional medicines regulation, intellectual property rights, financing, and supply management, quality and safety, selection and rational use of medicines in an international drug regulatory aspect. US Food and Drug Administration controls the quality of drugs manufactured by license holders in the USA as well all over the world approved by USFDA for the marketing of products in the USA. European Medicines Agency (EMEA), a decentralized body of the European Union, prescribes guidelines for inspections and general reporting and all aspects of human and veterinary medicines in the European Union. Medicines and Healthcare products Regulatory Agency (MHRA) is responsible for ensuring efficacy and safety of medicines and medical devices in the UK provided with news, warnings, information, and publications related to UK government guidelines.

Glossing over regulatory control issues related production and distribution of pharmaceutical products are critical as various regulatory guidelines make it clear that manufacturers, distributors, and sellers must comply with the regulations or otherwise may face legal sanctions if found violating regulations. Regular inspection of the manufacturing facilities is being undertaken by regulatory authorities to check for GMP compliance in the manufacturing process. Adverse inspections reports trigger recommendations for corrective action, and if not implemented within the said period, the FDA can take regulatory action like suspension of a manufacturer, distribution, wholesale or retail license. Compulsory variation in the license can also be evoked to exclude certain activities and legal sanctions against the responsible person. In case of most serious offenses license can also be canceled permanently.

Master formula

Master formula document or set of documents are developed for a particular product specify starting and packaging materials with their quantities together with a description of the procedures and precautions required to be followed to produce a specific quantity. It also contains processing instructions including in-process controls. Master formulae and batch processing records are prepared as written instructions for the production and control process. Master formulae is an approved master document that describes the full process of manufacturing for a batch of a specific product and in different scales of production batches or lots. Individual companies may give internal names like manufacturing instructions, monographs, etc., to these documents. Separate Master Production Formula and Master Packaging Formula are generally prepared for WHO, EU, PICs, and Health Canada, whereas USFDA regulations do not distinguish between production and packaging master formulae. The master formula includes the name of the product with product reference code, testing specification, dosage form description, product strength, batch size, list of all starting materials to be used, expected final yield with the acceptable limits, principal equipment to be used, detailed stepwise processing instructions and special precautions to be observed. Approved and signed master formulae are kept under the control of QA and copies are not allowed to be stored in the production areas checking uncontrolled use. While revision (following the change control and document control process), the new version is assigned a revision (or edition) number, approval signature and effective dates are added, and the previous version is archived.

Operating procedure

Pharmaceutical manufacturing operations must be carried out under the supervision of technical staff approved by the Licensing Authority. Pharmaceutical manufacturing is a multi-step process and these steps are called "Unit Operation". All critical process steps related to weighing, measuring, addition of raw material during various stages of operation and mixing must be performed by trained personnel under the direct personal supervision of approved technical staff. Each unit operation produces an intermediate with pre-determined quality specifications that ultimately ensures the quality of the finished product. All vessels and containers used in manufacturing and storage of semi-finished products during various manufacturing stages are conspicuously labeled with the product name, batch number, batch size, and stage of manufacturing signed and dated by the authorized technical staff. Product manufacturing operations are performed sequentially to process a "lot" with the objective of reducing the between (inter) lot variability and the within (intra) lot variability. For example, one of the unit operations in the process of manufacturing tablets is the tablet compression using compression machine. Designated equipment is used to apply a compression force to the powder mixture containing the active pharmaceutical ingredient with other ingredients. The compression process produces a solid entity known as a table. These tablets have a number of critical quality attributes that gave the product its identity, i.e. dimension, hardness, friability, disintegration, and dissolution are some of the critical quality attributes to ensure the suitability of the tablet for the intended use.

Tablet hardness (tensile strength) is one of the critical quality features affecting tablet coating, disintegration, dissolution, handling, packaging, and transportation. Therefore, monitoring this attribute is critical during the lot compression process. The product is sampled by collecting representative tablets from specifically targeted locations during the compression operations at predefined intervals. The test results are used to monitor the manufacturing process output related variations that are more likely to cause finished product variability. Process control charts are used to accomplish routine quality monitoring of a production process. Depending on the number of processes attributes to be monitored, mostly two types of control charts are used. The first is referred as a univariate control chart, with a graphical presentation (chart) of only one quality characteristic. The second is referred to as a multivariate control chart with a graphical presentation of statistic that represents more than one quality characteristic.

Documents and records

Documentation is the key to compliance with GMP requirements while operating in a pharmaceutical company. Documentation systems are devised with the primary objective of establishing, monitoring and recording of all quality related aspects of the production. In order to control quality variations in the pharmaceutical manufacturing

process, several types of documents are needed, viz. standard operating procedures (SOP), specifications, master formulae, labels, and forms. Descriptive documents provide detailed instructions and description for performing a procedure or a study like SOP, protocols (for validation, stability, safety studies) or master formulae (manufacturing instructions). Specifications describe the requisite characteristics composition of a product or material or test. These documents provide specific details defining the quality of incoming materials, production environment, production, control process, and the final product attributes. Forms are used for recording data obtained during performance of a task, test or event. Forms are data sheets, reports, batch processing records, equipment log books, etc. These documents are crucial for archival of evidence that the raw materials, facility environment, production process, and the final product consistently meet the established quality requirements.

Batch Record: Review of batch records and data for conformance with written procedures, operating parameters and product specifications prior arriving at the final release decision for an aseptically processed product is done for process and system performance analysis in a given cycle of manufacture. All in-process and laboratory control results are recorded in the batch record documentation section for a particular product. Environmental and personnel monitoring data review ascertaining for acceptability of support systems output (e.g. HEPA/HVAC, WFI, steam generator, etc) and proper functioning of equipment (batch alarms report, integrity of various filters, etc) are considered essential elements of batch release decision.

Record Review: All production control, packaging and labeling records are reviewed and approved by the quality control unit to determine compliance with all established and approved written procedures before a batch is released or distributed. Any unexplained discrepancy in theoretical yield (exceeding the maximum or minimum percentages established in master production and control records), batch failure or any case of production component failure for specifications adherence are thoroughly investigated. The investigation shall also extend to other batches of the same drug product and other drug products that may have been associated with the specific failure or discrepancy. Investigation report is prepared, signed and kept for future reference that also include the conclusions and follow-up actions recommended.

Interventions and Change Control Records: Interventions and/or stoppages of any kind are recorded in the batch record, in particular, line stoppages and any unplanned interventions should be sufficiently documented with the associated time and duration of the event. Written procedures describing the need for line clearances in the event of particular interventions, such as machine adjustments and repairs are established and documented in more detail than minor events. A full line clearance process is to be undertaken when any intervention results in substantial activity near exposed product or container closures lasting beyond a reasonable exposure time. Any disruption in the power supply is a manufacturing deviation, however momentary but could affect product quality and must be included in batch records.

The WHO guidelines for Good Manufacturing Practices and all other national and international GMP guidelines and regulations emphasize the requirement for complete documentation. A well-structured documentation system, including SOPs for the regular document review and revision, provides a framework for recording the evidence supporting quality of the product.

All documentation must be organized into files and maintained for specified periods after the expiry date of the product. The documentation system must include quality assurance procedures to ensure that instructions are followed, labels and numbering systems are appropriately used and recorded, and that data record forms and batch processing records are assembled and reviewed. Strict control and periodic evaluations of documentation system itself is a critical management tool for ongoing assessment of the changes and revisions necessary to be undertaken to remain in compliance and to obsolete unnecessary or redundant procedures for overall improvement in processes.

Environmental controls

Manufacturers need to develop process and environmental control activities in the processing operation. These activities need to be strictly implemented on a daily basis. Pharmaceutical products sterility and overall freedom from contamination depend on both the quality status of the components incorporated and the environmental conditions under which the process is performed. Optimum environmental condition standards are developed depending upon the extent of anticipated product exposure to the immediate environment during processing. Control of environmental conditions for operations using sterile components requires strict supervision.

Critical sites: The degree of exposure to the product during processing depends on the length of exposure time, size and nature of the critical site exposed. A critical site is an opening in the processing equipment providing a direct pathway between a non-sterile/sterile product and the environment or any surface coming in direct contact with the product and the environment. The risk of picking up contamination from the environment increases with time and area of such site exposure. This should be given due consideration in processing plan in order to keep such exposure time to a minimum. The nature of a critical site (rough/permeable) also affects the risk of contamination. Elimination of airborne particles from the immediate manufacturing environment or prevention from coming in direct contact is given high priority. Airborne contaminants are much more likely to reach critical sites than contaminants that adhere to the floor or other surfaces below the work level. Relatively large or high density particles more quickly settle from the airspace and easily removable from the vicinity of critical sites.

Cleaning

Equipment cleaning instructions and records for manual cleaning methods are documented in detailed stepwise format. For automated cleaning systems, it is defined in sequential operation stages. Each significant cleaning cycle for equipment should be recorded completely either manually (initial, date and time) or using a validated computerized system. Such instruction records should include the parameters, name of cleaning and sanitizing agents, concentration, amount used, contact time, quality of water or other solvents used, etc. Consideration for removal requirements of microbiological organisms and cleaning agents (when used), including any non-active drug product such as granulating or film-coating solutions must be directed. Documented and approved risk assessment study should be performed to determine the microbial acceptability limits required for cleaning validation of non-sterile product contact equipment. Risk assessment tools are useful in documenting the rationale supporting the cleaning program, for example; the probability of residual cleaning agent to be a contaminant based on its solubility in cleaning media, amount present and toxicity impact as per minimum therapeutic dose are assessed.

Documentation used to describe and justify the cleaning validation approach are subject to site change control procedures following which they are reviewed and approved by the quality control and production authority. SOP describes the types of the cleaning process for specific facilities and cleaning agents used for different process equipment and their validation. Complete instruction on cleaning validation, calculation of acceptance limits for rinse and swab samples, calculation of acceptance limits for swabs, analytical method validation for cleaning, cleaning validation test protocols and change control for revalidation are to be documented.

Quarantine and in-process storing

Along with environmental controls, the temperature is one of the most crucial variables needed to be precisely controlled. In particular, drug products should be stored in clean, dry place having adequate circulation and maintained within acceptable temperature limits. General storage areas are maintained well lit to reduce chances of human error. Latest guidelines describe aseptic storage facility for vaccines, antisera and parenteral products. These must be handled aseptically as well as stored at specific temperatures and in a controlled environment. The warehouse refrigeration equipment needs to be securely locked to prevent any malicious contamination or theft. Biological standards should be followed for such material handling and storage in order to assure safety and the quality. The correct climate controlled containers for storing vaccines are vital. Good practices, policies, procedures, and climate controlled containers are needed to ensure that vaccines are stored at the correct temperature.

All quarantine and in process drugs should be stored according to conditions specified, controls for humidity, light, etc. should be in place. Preventative conservation storage ensures dust free temperature controlled secure storage for items ranging from quarantine collectibles to in-process samples. Stability storage includes walk-in size storage containers such as freezers and refrigerated areas with temperature as well as humidity control. Long-term storage of items such as susceptible and thermolabile pharmaceutical supplies or quarantined materials should be done in stability controlled conditions. Ambient temperature storage generally has moderate temperature control in the range of 15°C down to negative 2°C. Pharmaceutical items like solvents, dry materials, nasal sprays, tablets, and capsules should be stored at the refrigeration grade temperature of 2–8°C. Low-temperature storage from negative 2°C down to around negative 15°C along with humidity control is considered ideal for vaccines, serums, toxins, and parenteral pharmaceuticals.

Refrigerators and freezers used to store drugs must be well maintained, equipped with alarms and free from excessive frost buildup. Orderly storage with adequate space allocation within the refrigerator chamber allows proper air distribution. Storage practices and container loading configurations should not lead to obstruction of air distribution. Critical refrigeration equipment needed to be equipped with a backup power source to tackle the event of power failure and premises must have alternate storage facility available for both walk-in and stand alone refrigerators/freezers in warehouses.

In-process quality control

In-process methods are vital components of quality control in a pharmaceutical manufacturing plant. These methods ensure that the production process steps conducted by trained operators within the entire validated process will produce a quality formulation within the defined specification. Process performance variability ultimately depends on the choice of manufacturing technology. Well-designed processes reduce the chances of human mistakes contributing to high robustness.

Critical quality attributes are process parameters, capabilities, technologies, and infrastructure controlling product and process. Product manufacturing process development studies the inputs and outputs of the process to determine the critical process parameters attributes, tolerances for those parameters and the best measures to control them.

Sources of variability: Typical sources of variability are equipment capabilities, calibration limits, testing method, raw materials, sampling techniques, and environmental factors.

Critical quality attributes: Identified and measured attributes that are deemed critical to ensure the quality requirements, viz. purity, efficacy, and safety of an intermediate or final product are called critical quality attributes (CQA).

Critical process parameters: Critical process parameters (CPP) has a direct and significant influence on a critical quality attributes when varied beyond a limited range. All the production processes are required to report the overall yield from bulk to the semi-finished or finished product. It is essential to distinguish between parameters that affect critical quality attributes and that affecting efficiency, yield, worker safety or other business objectives. Understanding the impact of raw materials, manufacturing equipment, the degree of automation or prescriptive procedure on final product quality is necessary to assure adequate control.

Proven acceptable range: The body of experimental data generated at the time of product development is initially selected to define the tolerance parameter which becomes the proven acceptable range (PAR). Operating range is set for given parameters based on the normal operating range (NOR) considering the PAR.

In a robust process, CPPs are being identified and characterized so the process can be controlled within defined limits. A process operating consistently in a narrow NOR demonstrates low process variability and excellent control. The functional ability of operating in a NOR depends on the process equipment, defined process controls, and process capability.

Setting Tolerance Limits: Acceptable attributes are established between upper and lower tolerances around a midpoint within the PAR of a parameter. The defined limits selected to accommodate the expected variability of parameters are needed to be practical while conforming to the quality attribute acceptance criteria.

Identification and tagging

Identification number: Identification systems or codes are devised to track information and documents with numbers. These are SOP numbers, equipment numbers, form numbers, receiving codes, batch/lot numbers, etc. Numbering systems are designed to trace procedures, processes, and materials throughout the data recording.

Labels: Labelling systems are practiced to identify the status of the equipment or facility and restricted areas. These permit the identification and tracking of materials, progress of a production process and assurance of the proper functioning of equipment. Labels should be printed in bright colors in a legible manner carrying all the prescribed details about the product. Different color-coded labels shall be used to indicate the status of a product (for example, under test, approved, passed, rejected) to avoid the chance of a mix-up. Printed packaging materials and product leaflets relating to different products shall be stored separately. The label indicates, in general, the concentration, lot number, potency, date on which containers were first opened and storage conditions, where appropriate. The labels mostly required in the pharmaceutical manufacturing facility includes raw material

tags, quarantine labels, release labels, reject labels, labels to identify specific storage areas, biohazard or radioactive labels, restricted access labels, equipment "cleaned" or "waiting for cleaning" labels, process intermediate label, final product labels, etc. Records for receipt of all labeling and packaging materials are maintained individually for each shipment indicating receipt date, control reference numbers and accept or reject decisions. Unused and/or damaged labels and packaging materials are recorded and destroyed.

Batch/Lot Number: The term "batch" more appropriately refers to intermediate or finally formulated bulks contained in one or a few large containers, while "lot" usually refers to the final product in the final marketable container. The term batch or lot generally refers to all production intermediates, finally formulated bulks and final packed products. As explained in the WHO definition, a final "lot" is the product filled during the same continuous process at the same time having unique numbers to identify. On occasion, when a large final bulk is processed in parts, the lot numbers for these bulk parts have a common identifier with a suffix ("–1" or "a")

Contamination and cross-contamination

A pharmaceutical manufacturer must consistently reproduce the desired quality of products over the period without deviation. The cGMP regulation astringently complies strict control over contamination and Cross-contamination of pharmaceutical products. All raw materials and products needed to be protected from contamination and cross-contamination through full manufacturing stages. Contaminants may result from inappropriate premises design (e.g. design, layout, finishing), poor cleaning procedures, unskilled personnel, and improper functioning HVAC system. External airborne contaminants can be controlled through effective ventilation and further removed by effective filtration of the supplied air. The manufacturing process core area is regarded as the most stringently controlled clean zone which should be protected by surrounding clean areas with an area of lower classification or by ancillary area. The process core area is protected with double corridor premises designed with a shell-like layout. Internal contaminants are removed by dilution and flushing of the room or by displacement airflow. Critical parameters are airborne particulates and the degree of filtration concerning the level of product protection required.

Contamination: Undesired introduction of impurities of a chemical or microbiological nature or foreign matter, into or onto starting or intermediate material during production, sampling, packaging, repacking, storage and transportation of pharmaceutical formulation is called contamination. The most typical sources of contamination are a faulty design of building and premises, personnel, HVAC system, manufacturing operations, clothing, utilities, and services. The design of premises should be such that it provides separate entry for personnel and material, and there should not be any crossing over between at any level of production. Entry of unauthorized persons is blocked in production, packing and quality control areas. Persons do not work in these areas are not allowed to use them as a passageway.

Cross-contamination: The manufacturing of pharmaceutical products involves a series of processing steps and the use of various equipment. Equipment and ancillary systems may be used for manufacturing single dedicated product or multiple products. The inadequate cleaning process may lead to the residue to get carried forward as a contaminant in the next batch to be manufactured with the same equipment. Cross-contamination is contamination of a starting material, intermediate product, finished product with another starting material or a product or its residue. Control of cross-contamination plays a critical role in maintaining the quality of product and is one of the utmost concerns for pharmaceutical manufacturers. Contamination of starting material or a product by another material or product must be avoided. This risk of accidental cross-contamination may arise from situations like the uncontrolled release of dust, gases, particles, vapors, sprays or organisms from materials and products in process, residues on equipment, intruding insects, and from operators clothing or exposed skin, etc. The significance of contamination risk varies with the type of contaminants and the product being contaminated. Biological preparations such as containing living organisms, certain hormones, cytotoxic substances, and other bioactive highly sensitizing materials are the most hazardous contaminants. Products like injections, topically applied to open wounds, given in large doses and/or over a long time, are likely to have the most significant issues with contamination.

The prime source of cross-contamination is improper change over and line clearance practice. Cleaning validation is crucial to identify and correct the potential unsuspected problems compromising the safety, efficacy, and quality of subsequent batches of drug product produced using the same equipment assembly. Validated cleaning procedures and analytical verification techniques are used to prevent such occurrence. Careful evaluation of current cleaning procedures in use is essential to assure that it is effective and reproducible and allow active compound of the previous process to get dissolved in a suitable solvent before changing over to another formulation. Cleaning process development studies must evaluate the solubility of the drug substances in a variety of solvents including water, acids, bases, and alcohols. Qualification of the cleaning materials should be done to make sure that the cleaning materials used for equipment cleaning are suitable and of consistent quality. Operators performing sampling of cleaned equipment should be trained and qualified. Designing of a cleaning procedure essentially needs consideration to be given to the equipment to be cleaned. The areas "difficult-to-clean" are located during initial operational qualification (OQ) of the equipment. Often a water-soluble UV active placebo is used to "dirty" the equipment and following that equipment is cleaned and inspected to check for any area that is still showing evidence of the placebo. Overheads, vent lines, vacuum lines, and valves are notoriously difficult to clean, and particular attention needs must be given to these sites while cleaning and sampling.

Cleaning validation requires a pre-approved protocol, which details who will be responsible for what, procedures to be followed, the number of cleaning cycles to be run, the time frame for validation and the acceptance criteria. Considering what levels of residue can be tolerated in the equipment after cleaning, any exceptional condition, procedure or sampling should be discussed. Toxicity data are useful in calculating permissible residue limits. The protocol also indicates a summary report to be written once the validation procedures are completed. Forms are maintained to document all cleaning activities, i.e. the personnel responsible, materials to be used, cleaning procedure, sampling procedure, analytical results specification, conformance to the permissible limits, securing of the cleaned equipment, maintenance and identification so to get it ready for the next operation. After completion of cleaning and analysis, the record is reviewed by the Quality Assurance.

CONTROL OF QUALITY VARIATION IN THE PHARMACEUTICAL MANUFACTURING PROCESS

The perspective of process variation control relies on the context of problem solving and process improvement as well as the pedigree of the data generated. Most importantly, proper identification of causes behind process variables increase the likelihood of problems to be solved successfully. The most preferred way for important process variable identification is to track the key input and output variables at each process step and to prioritize the input variables using cause and effect matrix. Principle sources of variation are often identified by making a chart of key process output variables and looking for out of control signals indicating notable variation. Analysis of the data can detect critical sources of variation and uncontrolled noise as in process input material, operating personnel and specification of equipment.

Operational Excellence

Operational excellence is achieved by the use of an Integrated System Approach towards product quality regulation, based on sound science and engineering principles for assessing and mitigating risks of poor quality product due to inadequate process quality. Approach to manufacturing regulations titled as risk-based cGMP solicits to free the industry from unnecessary perspective rules and to direct the quality control efforts where the most substantial risk persists. The following points are to be considered for achieving operational excellence:

1. Systematically revealing exact root causes of unwanted variations in manufacturing processes, e.g. errors in weights (apothecial), while raw material was dispensed process loss, etc. and to improve quality by getting a thorough understanding of the variation creating sources in the process and then reducing variations to a minimum level.
2. Implementation of process analytical technology (PAT) for continuous monitoring of the manufacturing process.
3. Elimination of waste for sustainable performance improvements.

4. Use of Agile Manufacturing concept helps to prevent and maintain the sub-optimizing and non-value-added steps.

Four crucial levels of operational excellence can be implemented to improve plant capabilities. By adopting and following four levels, a company can achieve the goal **effectiveness** and **efficiency** in the process.

1. Performance of internal and external quality audits helps in achieving the main objective of **regulatory requirements** compliance.
2. Developing capabilities to get a scientific understanding of the **process and root causes of deviations** to move towards predictive performance rather than reactive compliance.
3. Understanding the value of good quality from the viewpoint of customer satisfaction, inventory management, waste reduction and **problems related to processes**.
4. Identify all significant deviation root causes and simultaneously **managing to prevent deviations re-occurrence** throughout its operations.

Process Evaluation

Pharmaceutical process evaluation utilizes a multi-scenario approach to generate data for critical evaluation of the batch process sequence. To reduce the size of the multi-scenario problem, identification of the most significant parameters such as lack of concentration, improper training, incompetence, etc., are essential. The following points are considered during process evaluation:

1. Identification of high risk related to unacceptable performance that is devoted to the failure of crucial expectation thresholds leading to noncompliance of proposed operations and existing equipment.
2. Prediction of causative components and process uncertainty that are responsible for adverse process variations and correction of which can achieve the final objective of a best expected end product.
3. Track progressive reduction in uncertainty while promoting process alternatives by incorporating new data from scale-up experiments.

Continuous Processing

It is the next logical step in achieving pharmaceutical manufacturing excellence. A process has a chain of activity with multiple interlinked sub-activities that generate data that can be used for efficient production control. It is one of the best mechanisms to ensure consistent product composition. It offers the potential to reduce cost, maximize facility utility, energy efficient working and also minimize batch-to-batch variations.

Production Procedure Control

The manufacturing processes should strictly be operated according to the established rules from the reception of material up to the delivery of the final product.

1. Both QC and production departments are responsible for the production procedure control.
2. Complete list of all required ingredients along with quantity is delivered to the production department according to the batch master formula. It contains all the information of that batch, i.e. procedures, equipment, testing to be performed and precautions to be taken, etc.
3. According to the master formula, all the materials for the batch are weighed and delivered to production department from the store. All ingredients are rechecked and ensured for pretesting and released tag from the laboratory.
4. In the production process stage, some tests are done for procedure control, which is called in-process quality control (IPQC) test by the QC department.

CONTROL OF STERILE AND NON-STERILE MANUFACTURING PROCESS

Master Batch and Completed Batch Records

Elements check requirements: Batch records are reviewed for elements like proper material issuance, yields on different unit operations, critical manufacturing step verification, processing instructions, hold times, etc. to ensure a tight hold on in-process control elements.

Record processing requirements: Analysis of batch records to confirm that it meets all requirements for execution, review and disposition decisions should be done at regular intervals.

Production Operations

Regulatory requirements: Designing of production operation is based on the description of differential requirements for manufacturing processes according to their application as human or veterinary drugs or biologics. The specific guidelines by the regulatory authority mandate the production and quality control of medicinal products defining the specific requirements for specific types of formulations.

Utility requirements: Appropriate production environments, facilities, and utilities are required for particular product types. Identification of specific requirements for nonsterile manufacturing, solid and semisolid dosage forms, liquids, creams, ointments, combination products, etc. ensures consistency in product quality. Production operations require special provisions for gowning, sanitization, hygiene, and other product-protective steps. Identification of all these requiments and their sensible application ensure quality compliance.

Requirements for Critical Process Parameters (CPPs)

Unit operating procedures: Review of qualification and validation results and analysis for conformance are eventually reflected in operating procedures. Assess of unit processes or their validation for deviations requires investigation and analysis. Monitoring is required for Critical Process Parameters (CPPs) for such unit processes as filtration, depyrogenation, lyophilization, drying processes, emulsification, granulation and compression, aseptic filling, filtration sterilization, terminal sterilization, etc.

Environmental monitoring: Different environmental monitoring requirements are to be in place for different product manufacturing area, based on classifications. Application of various monitoring tools for measuring viable and nonviable particulates, pressure differentials, temperature, humidity, etc. are included in the operational procedure.

Validation studies: Explanation and evaluation of the validation studies, specifically the methodologies and acceptance criteria are required before implementing critical unit processes. Evaluation of validation studies is required for aseptic processes including process simulations. Appropriate criteria and frequency for re-evaluation and revalidation of unit processes should be established and evaluate periodically for the outcome.

Control of Contamination and Cross-Contamination

Identification of potential sources for contamination and cross-contamination is the first step in the control of these events. Application of various techniques for mitigating the risk of these events, including cleaning, facility and equipment design, qualified disinfectants, operator training, validation, monitoring is essential.

Reprocessed and Reworked Materials

Appropriate documentation, approval, and disposal methods should be developed and maintained for reprocess and rework. Following specific requirements for segregation and secure storage of these materials are crucial.

CONTROL OF FILLING, PACKAGING AND LABELING OPERATIONS

Filling Operations Controls

Environmental monitoring: Various monitoring techniques (active air sampling, settle plates, nonviable particle counting, contact plates for surfaces and people, etc.) are applied to determine what appropriate environmental conditions are to be maintained in various operations.

Materials control: Material control systems are created ensure the identity, strength, and purity of specified materials and to prevent them from being altered. Regular review of these procedures is also needed to be done.

Filling operation control: All staged materials should be reviewed to confirm that they are approved for use. Proper status labeling should be applied throughout the process. Analysis of the controls is needed for various types of production equipment and processes to ensure that appropriate controls are in place to verify filling criteria. Control measures should be applied to prevent microbial and other contamination at all stages of filling.

In-process and Finished Goods Inspections

Inspection staff: Proper manual and automated inspection processes are to be developed and written down in the form of SOP. Manual inspection staffs are appropriately trained to ensure that their inspections meet reproducibility requirements. Automated inspection processes should be validated for performance compliance. The inspectors should be provided with frequent breaks from inspection. Periodic eye examinations of visual inspectors (parenteral and liquid formulations) are conducted and documented.

Finished goods inspections: In-process product testing and final finished packaged materials (i.e. seal test, torque test, bottle rejection systems, etc.) for inspection criteria are developed and validated to follow in regular practice.

Failure detection systems: Qualified, calibrated and challenged detection systems are required for failure detection. Defect characterizations and identification for each product is required to ensure that a defect can be detected by inspection or test.

Packaging Operations Controls

Packaging component should be stored in such environment that it prevents the occurrence of events responsible for altering the identity, strength, and purity of the packaged content. Specified criteria for checking the identity and quality of packaging material are developed and performed as qualified.

Equipment qualification and maintenance: Before starting packaging operation it is to be ensured that packaging line setup instructions are appropriate for all components. Equipment used in packaging operations should be qualified and maintained to ensure proper working status. Line clearance is performed as per SOP and documented. Appropriate procedures are followed for applying cut labels, splices, etc., and hand-applied labeling procedures are 100% inspected before release.

Tamper-evident packaging: Tamper-evident and child-proof packaging requirements are to be ensured for required products.

Filling and packaging records: Proper understanding of defined terms related to filling and packaging records maintenance, evidence of line clearance, printed material reconciliation, yields, etc. are to be ensured in record maintenance.

Labeling Operations Controls

The process of label printing over packaging should be performed as per documented procedure. Conformance of printing is done separately or in the course of packaging under strict vigilance.

Artwork development controls: Proper understanding of defined packaging terms related to artwork/graphics, offline printing, roll label splicing, gang printing should be cultured in operators with regular training and follow-up. Ensure limited access to artwork and label control for the creation and use of artwork. Secure storage and when required in particular destruction process should be in place.

Quality of print: All printed information (engraved, embossed, etc.) on packaging materials must be clear and resistant to fading, smudging or erasure.

Label reconciliation: Strictly confirm label reconciliation after each labeling operation. Unused labels and labeling materials must be placed and destroyed according to the documented method and record maintained.

QUALITY VARIATION IN PHARMACEUTICAL PERSONNEL

The strength and asset for any organization are the qualified, well trained, dedicated, hardworking, knowledgeable, skilled personnel with positive attitude. It is not the product that competes and succeeds in the market; it is the people who put their ideas to make it a success. In a pharmaceutical industry professional working at every level is responsible for meeting standards of quality. Quality work begins with the conscious efforts of the staffs to execute the specifications of the product in practicality.

Quality Attributes of Pharmaceutical Personnel

Qualifications

Each person engaged in the processing, manufacturing, packing, supervising or holding of drug product should have an adequate educational qualification, training, and experience, or a combination thereof. While selecting the individuals, these points should be given preference. This enables the persons to perform the assigned functions in such a manner as to assure drug product safety, identity, strength, quality, and purity that it purports or is represented to possess. All working staff in pharmaceuticals should know English writing, reading and good in numeracy (mathematics).

1. The organization chart represents the work position arrangement for management, production, quality control, quality assurance including and other supporting personnel.

2. Qualification, experience, and responsibilities of key personnel are to be defined and documented.

3. Manufacturing operations are conducted under the direct supervision of an adequate number of competent technical staff with prescribed qualifications. Technical staff must have adequate practical experience in the relevant dosage form and/or handling active pharmaceutical products.

4. The head of the QC Laboratory works independent of the manufacturing unit. Material and product testing are conducted under the direct supervision of competent technical staff as permanent employees of the licensee.

5. Personnel working in QA and QC operations shall be suitably qualified and experienced.

6. Production and QC department supervisors should be B. Pharm. or B.Sc. with specified experience (according to the Drugs and Cosmetics Act)

7. While selecting the individual in pharmaceuticals, candidates previous records must be identified, reference should be collected and criminal nature should be investigated as Pharmaceutical

companies manufacture many controlled substances like narcotics and psycho-tropics, steroids, etc.

Responsibilities

1. Personnel engaged in the manufacturing, processing, packing, or holding of a drug product are required to wear clean clothing appropriate for performance of duties. Protective apparel such as head, face, hand, and arm coverings, shall be worn as necessary to protect drug products from contamination.
2. Written duties of technical and QC personnel are laid and followed strictly.
3. Personnel shall practice proper sanitation and health habits.
4. Only authorized personnel are entitled to enter the areas of the buildings and facilities designated as limited-access areas.
5. All personnel are instructed to report to the supervisory personnel about any health conditions that may have an adverse effect on drug products.

Recruitment process

Recruitment process should always ensure recruitment of confident best possible candidates with appropriate educational qualification, experience, and other required skill to meet the specific requirements. Recruitment process starts by obtaining a total understanding of the requirements of the candidate required for specific departments. The selection process should not just be based on basic requirements, organizations culture and business strategy should also be taken into account for selection of the ideal candidates. Maintaining a database of aspiring candidates with the help of modern recruitment software can also support to call up candidates according to the exact criteria that the company is looking for. CVs of the prospective candidates should be reviewed, shortlisted

and matched against skill profile. There should be a well reformed contractual agreement between employee and employer describing the terms and conditions along with responsibilities from both the sides.

Training

Training shall be provided for the particular operations that the employee is assigned to perform as per the cGMP:

1. cGMP training are conducted by qualified individuals with sufficient frequency to assure that employees remain familiar with cGMP requirements applicable.
2. The licenses shall ensure that all personnel in the production area and QC laboratories receive regular in-service training appropriate to the duties and responsibility assigned to them as per written instructions.
3. All persons are trained in personal hygiene practices before and during employment. High level of personal hygiene is to be observed by all staff engaged in manufacturing processes. Instructions for appropriate hygienic practices are needed to be displayed in change-rooms and other strategic locations.

Adequate number

An organization should have sufficient and adequate number of qualified personnel to perform and supervise the manufacturing, processing, packing or holding of drug products. The number of personnel employed shall be adequate and in direct proportion to the workload. Manufacturing operation shall be conducted under the active direction and personal supervision of competent technical staff who is a full-time employee as per the Rule 71 of Drug and Cosmetic Act 1940. The Licensing Authority permits manufacturing of formulations under the personal supervision of the competent technical staff who is approved by the Licensing Authority when having adequate experience in the manufacture of such formulation.

Health, clothing, and sanitation

Before employment, all personnel shall undergo medical examination including eye examination, and shall be free from tuberculosis, shin and other communicable or contagious diseases. They should also be medically examined periodically, at least once a year and records maintained thereof. The licensee is required to assure the availability of qualified physician services for assessing the health status of personnel involved in different activities.

1. The personnel handling beta-lactam antibiotics are needed to be tested for penicillin sensitivity before duty assignment and those handling sex hormones, cytotoxic substances, and other potent drugs shall be periodically examined for adverse effects. The personnel should be moved out of these sections (except in dedicated facilities), by rotation, as a health safeguard.

2. Persons diagnosed to have any apparent illness or open lesions are excluded from direct contact with components, drug product containers, closures, in-process materials, and drug products as this may adversely affect the safety or quality of drug products. This is to be followed until the condition is reversed as determined by competent medical personnel not to jeopardize the safety or quality of drug products.

3. Direct contact with raw materials, intermediate or finished, unpacked products with unprotected hands of personnel are avoided.

4. Before entering into the manufacturing area, all personnel shall wear clean body coverings appropriate as per duties.

Separate change rooms are to be provided for male and female staffs with adequate facilities for personal cleanliness. The change rooms generally have wash basin with running water, soaps, disinfectants, clean towels and/or hand dryers. The change room also has cabinets for storage of personal belongings of the staffs.

5. Smoking, eating, drinking, chewing, keeping plants and personal medicines are not permitted in production, laboratory, storage and other areas where they can adversely influence the product quality.

CONTROL OF QUALITY VARIATION IN PHARMACEUTICAL PERSONNEL

Quality defect and variation attributable to personnel are mostly related to unskilled workers, physical fatigue from extended manual working hours, misplacement of a worker at the workstation, lack of training, the absence of engineering knowledge of basic pieces of equipment and poor compliance of written instruction are the few factors directly related to product quality. Quality control in concern to the human resource is as important as of material and premises management. These following measures can help in minimizing generation of quality variation due to inadequate personnel management:

1. A well-updated organizational chart can guide the employees to know their rights and responsibilities. Organizational chart not only divides the functions of the different departments but also shows the relationships between the staff members of individual departments. This chart helps to improve employee performance, understand and enhance the coordination in the organization.

2. Desired qualifications, experience and responsibilities of all the key personnel should be well defined and documented.

3. Properly review system should be in place for the identification of external training needs, and the responsible person should work to execute training conduction as per preplanning. Brief details of the training programme are mentioned which should include course study material and evaluation process.

4. Provision and method for basic and in-service in-house training should be developed and practiced. Training must include practical exposure and expertise in newly introduced equipments and instruments. Methods to evaluate the efficacy of in-house training should be developed, i.e. MCQ questionnaires or written test. All the records of the training programme should be maintained.

5. Personnel welfare is a critical issue related to productive work output of the workers in all industry setting. Overwork generated physical fatigue of the workers can cause severe manual mistakes in the manufacturing process and testing, in turn, resulting in a quality defect. Misplacement of a worker at a workstation regarding working experience in a particular formulation or equipment will generate variation in quality aspects due to improper process step following and equipment handling.

6. Strictly following the health requirements of personnel engaged in the pharmaceuticals are very important to reduce the chances of contamination. Responsibility to monitor the health status of employees is to be assigned to a suitably qualified person as approved by the management. A pre-employment medical examination is to be done mandatorily and records maintained along with routine health examination. Properly validated and documented method for the workers is to be followed for reporting sickness or contact with sick people before working in a critical area. A formal method of reporting back after illness should be in place with the approval of the person responsible for monitoring the health status of employees in the manufacturing premises. The person designated to work in clean areas is required to go through additional monitoring.

7. Employees should be provided with suitable washing, changing and rest areas. One of the vital quality compliance issues is to ensure proper following the approved gowning procedure by the workers. The suitability of clothing to work in production, QC and packing are determined based on their non-shedding lint-free material. Explicit instruction should be provided regarding wearing and change guidelines of protective clothing. Proper laundry facility should be in place in-house or external for washing to prepare them for reuse.

8. The most important aspect of quality variation due to personnel arise from poor and improper compliance of the written instruction related to different process and methods. Interpretation of written instructions varies person to person creating deviation and changes, only strict vigilance and training can reduce such possibilities. Sometimes instructions are not followed correctly due to sheer negligence or some malicious intentions, that should be dealt with strict disciplinary action.

Quality Personnel System

Supportive, problem-solving and communicative organizational culture inculcated by the senior management can effectively develop quality personnel system. Managers are expected to encourage inter-personnel communication by creating an amicable environment that values employee suggestions and also acts on suggestions for improvement. Management is also expected to develop cross cutting groups to share ideas to improve procedures and processes. It is recommended that personnel assigned to an operation should be qualified to do that concerning with the nature and potential risk to quality presented by the operational activities. Managers define appropriate qualifications for each position to help ensure individuals are assigned with appropriate responsibilities. Personnel must be trained and educated to understand the impact of their activities on the product quality and customer safety. The parameters of the quality systems should be based on the cGMP regulations, which identify specific qualifications, i.e. education, training, and experience or any combination thereof. In a quality system, continued training is critical to ensure that the employees remain proficient in their operational functions and is updated with their understanding of cGMP regulations. Typical quality systems training addresses the policies, processes, procedures and written instructions related to operational activities. Designing of a training program for a particular industry always depends on the products/services, quality system, and the desired work culture (e.g. team building, communication, challenges, behavior). Training is expected to focus on both the employee's specific job functions and the related cGMP regulatory requirements. Management is expected to establish training programs that include the following:

- Evaluation of training needs
- Provision of training to satisfy these needs
- Evaluation of the effectiveness of training
- Documentation of training and /or re-training

When operating in a robust quality system environment, it is vital that supervisory managers ensure that skills gained from training be incorporated into the day-to-day performance.

QUALITY VARIATION IN THE PHARMACEUTICAL MANUFACTURING ENVIRONMENT

Environment of manufacturing premises are composed of both viable and non-viable particulates, mostly dust, molds, microorganisms, etc. Environmental parameters inside manufacturing, storage, and other relevant areas is maintained complying to the pre-established set of specifications under FDA regulations and guidelines. Significant lapses from the standards in any of these areas can render the product unsuitable as per quality specifications giving rise to recall of the product. The actual contaminated product comes under a Class I recall. This is a situation with reasonable probability that the use of or exposure to the violative product can cause serious adverse health consequences or death. Whereas in Class II recall the use of or exposure to a violative product may cause temporary or medically reversible adverse health consequences. With Class II recall the probability of serious adverse health consequences is remote. The issue depends on the degree of risk the product would pose for the user, and in cases of actual product contamination, the risk is obvious. Manufacturer's responsibility is to control, maintain and monitor environmental conditions inside the premises as per recommendations. When a pre-established set of specifications for environmental parameters under which a product is mandated to be manufactured is not met, a judgment call must be made concerning the suitability of the product for use. Individuals knowledgeable in the issues should make this call to assess potential product contamination, the likely outcome of such contamination, and the risk posed by the identified scenario. Risk assessment should focus on the identification and control of critical factors that affect process and product quality. Presence of environmental contaminants does not result in a uniform pattern of contamination, as this is affected by both equipment functional speed and process design. Usually, the demonstrated presence of viable particulates in a particular environment does not equate to the level of product contamination.

QUALITY ATTRIBUTES OF THE PHARMACEUTICAL MANUFACTURING ENVIRONMENT

In the pharmaceutical industry, the ambient environment must be controlled and monitored to provide the highest level of cleanliness for the production of drug substances and formulations. The environmental conditions for the non-sterile pharmaceutical operations are not much well defined as that of aseptic or sterile manufacturing. The environmental conditions guided for sterile pharmaceutical production operations are rigorously defined and are primarily intended for aseptic filling operations. Contamination originating in the surrounding environment is extremely unlikely to result in contamination of the unsterile materials contained within the facility. The risk of surrounding environment related contamination is very high with sterile material, biologics, steroids, etc.

Design and Construction of an Area

Pharmaceutical product manufacturing premises are designed to be of suitable size, construction, and location to facilitate cleaning and maintenance that permit production of drugs under hygienic conditions. The building shall conform to the conditions laid down in the Factories Act, 1948 (63 of 1948). Proper building design having a plan for separate personnel, material, and equipment flow is essential for maintaining cleanliness and pressure gradients. Monitoring of storage and production environments has become an important issue in the pharmaceutical industry.

Storage: Manufacturers, authorized distributors of drugs and their representatives need to store and handle all drug samples in such conditions that can maintain their stability, integrity, and effectiveness, and ensure that the drug samples are free of contamination, deterioration, and adulteration. Storage areas are designed to accommodate for sufficient and orderly warehousing of various categories of starting and packaging materials, and sometimes if required for intermediates, bulk, and finished products. Products in different stages like quarantine, released, rejected, returned or recalled should be stored in designated areas with proper segregation. Warehousing areas shall be clean, dry and maintained with acceptable temperature limits, where special storage conditions are required (e.g. temperature, humidity), there shall be provided, monitored and recorded. Storage areas must have proper housekeeping and rodent, pests and vermin control procedures and records are to be maintained. Separate sampling area is required for active raw materials and excipients in such a way as to prevent contamination, cross-contamination, and mix-up. Highly hazardous, poisonous and explosive materials like narcotics, psychotropic drugs and substances presenting potential risks of abuse, fire or explosion are stored in safe and secure areas. Adequate fire protection measures must be installed in the warehouse as per conformity of the concerned civic authority rules.

The Medicines and Healthcare Products Regulatory Agency (MHRA) reports that temperature rises above the desired parameters are the most frequently occurring critical deficiency in pharmaceutical warehouses. Normal temperature conditions within the operational space do not affect product quality adversely, but extremes of temperature does it rapidly. Temperature excursions are dangerous because non-compliance with the manufacturer's storage recommendations may destroy affected products promoting health risk to patients which can ultimately lead to expensive product recalls.

Production: Pharmaceutical manufacturing areas are classified as different "clean areas." All pharmaceutical starting materials, intermediates, in-process materials, finished products, product contact utensils and equipment are exposed to the clean area environment. Achievement of a particular clean area classification depends on number of criteria, viz. design of building, outside air quality and filtration facility, air change rate, room pressure, pressure differentials, location of air terminals, airflow direction, temperature, humidity, material flow, personnel flow, equipment movement, type of process being carried out, etc. The production area is designed to allow the production preferably in uniflow and with a logical sequence of operations. Working and the in-process area should be adequate to permit orderly and logical positioning of equipment, materials and smooth movement of personnel to avoid cross-contamination and to minimize the risk of omission or wrong application of any manufacturing and control measures. For the production of sensitive pharmaceutical products like penicillin and biological preparations with live microorganisms separate, dedicated and self-contained facilities are provided to avoid risk of cross-contamination.

The pipeline, electrical fittings, ventilation openings, and other similar service lines are designed, fixed and constructed to avoid the creation of recesses. Services lines should be marked/indicated with color codes as per the nature of the supply and direction of the flow. Risk of insects and pests entry inside the manufacturing area is to be eliminated by suitable design of facilities and services equipped with maximum protection. Entry of unauthorized person should be restricted in production, packing and quality control areas. Interior surfaces of all walls, floor, and ceiling are required to be smooth, free from cracks and open joints, and must not shed any particulate matter of paint. The internal surface of manufacturing area should permit easy and effective cleaning. Ventilation and light points are designed to avoid creation of recesses which are difficult to clean.

Quality control: Every manufacturing establishment shall establish its quality control laboratory equipped with standard instruments along with the qualified and experienced staff. QC is concerned with sampling, specifications, testing, and documentation to ensure that necessary and relevant release procedures tests are performed. Finished pharmaceutical products are released for use, sale or supply only after specified quality tests been performed and satisfactorily certified by the authorized person(s) following the requirements of the standards laid down.

QC laboratories shall be independent of the production areas and are designed appropriately for the operations intended to be carried out. QC laboratory is preferably divided into chemical, instrumentation, microbiological and biological testing areas. The microbiology section should have airlocks and laminar air flow workstations.

Separate areas shall be provided for physicochemical, biological, microbiological and radio-isotope analysis. Separate instrument room with an adequate area is provided for sensitive and sophisticated instruments employed for analysis. Sufficient and suitable storage space is made available for test samples, retained samples, reference standards, reagents, and records. The laboratory shall be provided with a regular supply of water of appropriate quality for cleaning and testing purpose. Standard operating procedures are made available for sampling, inspecting and testing of raw materials, intermediate bulk finished products, packing materials and for monitoring of environmental conditions. QC department is also responsible for conduction of stability studies of the finished products to ensure and assign shell life at the prescribed conditions of storage. All instruments are calibrated and testing procedures validated before adopting for routine testing. Periodical calibration of instrument and validation measures are carried out following approved schedule and method. Specification for raw materials, intermediates, final products, and packing materials are developed, approved and maintained by the QC department. Pharmacopeias, reference standards, working standards, references, spectra, technical books, and other reference materials as required must be available in the QC laboratory.

Temperature and Humidity Control

Environmental conditions are of primary importance as they directly impact the quality of the products manufactured. Space pressurization and volumetric air flow rate are controlled to prevent contamination by dirt and pathogens, as well as cross-contamination from the production rooms of other drugs in the facility. Temperature affects drug products directly or indirectly by fostering growth of microbial contaminants. Room temperature (T) is not considered critical as long as it provides comfortable conditions for the staffs. Temperature along with relative humidity are controlled, monitored and recorded as recommended, in order to ensure compliance with materials and products requirements. Maximum and minimum room temperatures ranges and relative humidity should be appropriately designated. Temperature conditions are adjusted to suit the protective clothing worn by the operators. The operating band or tolerance between the acceptable minimum and maximum temperatures should not be too close or too far. Generally, manufacturing areas are designed to set temperatures from 67 and 77°F with a control point of 72°F. Lower temperature level may be required where people are very heavily gowned and would be uncomfortable at "normal" room conditions. Each environ-

mental parameter is controlled and evaluated in light of its potential to impact product quality.

Humidity affects the efficacy and stability of drugs. Humidity control aims at removing excess moisture from the air or adding moisture to the air as relevant. Dehumidification (moisture removal), may be achieved using either refrigerated dehumidifiers or chemical dehumidifiers. Appropriate cooling media for dehumidification is used such as low-temperature chilled water/glycol mixture or refrigerant. Humidification is done utilizing steam injection into the air stream. Humidifiers are mostly avoided as far as possible because it may become a source of contamination by microbiological growth. Evaporative systems, atomizers or water mist sprays like humidification appliances are not used due to the possible microbial contamination risk. Humidification systems should be equipped with well water draining measures preventing accumulation of condensate in air handling systems. Final air filters are not allowed to install immediately downstream of humidifiers. Air filters should have insulation of cold surfaces in order to prevent condensation within the clean area or on air-handling components, where high humidity is required. Chemical dryers can be used to achieve conditions lower than 45% RH at a temperature of 22°C. Chemical dryers or dehumidifiers equipped with silica gel or lithium chloride desiccants should have a non-shedding type desiccant wheels that do not support microbial growth. Appropriate air filters are to be used downstream to prevent desiccant particulates from entering the production premises.

Temperature Profiling of Storage

Temperature profiling studies are performed demonstrating suitability for areas in controlled room temperature designated explicitly for storing pharmacopoeial article.

Temperature and humidity profiles are developed archiving the data received from temperature and humidity recording instruments installed in sufficient numbers. Temperature recording is required for establishing mean kinetic temperature in compliance with the warehouse's written procedures. A reporting mechanism should be in place ensuring that the management is immediately informed in the event of predefined high or low temperatures or humidity limits are exceeded. Records are reviewed periodically as decided by the management, following established guidelines. The persons involved in the recording of temperature should be suitably trained. Regular quality accountability and tracking systems are maintained for temperature regulation.

Temperature profiles are prepared by using a suitable number of thermometers or other temperature recording instruments. Temperature recording devices are placed throughout the warehouse in divided sections to record the maximum and minimum temperatures during 24 hours. The recorded data for a total of three consecutive 24-hour periods, some of which may give rise to extreme temperatures are considered during the process of temperature profiling. Size of storage space, the location of heaters, sun-facing walls, low ceilings or roofs and geographic location of the warehouse effects the temperature variation possibilities inside the storage area.

Temperature profiling for warehouses already in use must be done at known times of external temperature extremes, when air temperatures were higher than 25% or lower than 15% for more than 3 hours. Profiling should be conducted in both pick summer and winter. Mean kinetic temperature is obtained for the separate critical areas within the warehouse. The temperature profile report provides recommendations for optimal use of each area and also identify areas found unsuitable for storage.

Temperature and Humidity Controlled Storage

Equipment used for storing pharmacopoeial articles at low temperature should be qualified according to written procedures. Recording devices are installed within the equipment that is enabled to record both air and product temperatures at regular intervals. Required number and location of monitoring devices are determined based on the temperature profiling result. Temperature records must be examined at least once in every 24 hours or as recommended in the equipment protocol as per the cool or cold conditions and moisture-condensing conditions. Humidity-monitoring devices are used for pharmacopoeial article that is humidity-sensitive or labeled to avoid moisture.

Temperature-monitoring and humidity-monitoring alarm devices are installed wherever necessary for alerting personnel in the event of compromised controls. Protocols are developed to address procedures for responding to failed temperature, and humidity ranges both for regular working hours and outside of regular working hours. Temperature and humidity profiles are reviewed at predefined time interval as per established protocol. The calibration of all temperature and humidity monitoring devices including alarms and other associated equipment should be done on an annual or semi-annual basis. Regular maintenance protocols for refrigeration equipment should be in place. There should be written agreements for all maintenance and evaluation procedures that should also include an emergency handling protocol.

Temperature and humidity excursions and the duration of excursion are considered critical when it triggers audio/visual alarms. Production operators and other staffs working on the premises must take concern of the alarms promptly in order to take corrective and/or mitigating actions.

HVAC system

The building management system captures the temperature and humidity data. Temperature, relative humidity, and ventilation must be appropriate and should not adversely affect the quality of pharmaceutical products during their manufacture and storage and also allow accurate functioning of equipment. Heating, ventilation, and air-conditioning (HVAC) system play a vital role in supporting the production of quality pharmaceutical products. HVAC system design influences the architectural layouts about items such as airlock positions, doorways, and lobbies. The architectural components affect room pressure differential cascades and cross-contamination control. Essential design consideration for the HVAC system is the prevention of contamination and cross-contamination. HVAC system plays a critical role in controlling the three primary aspects of pharmaceutical production, e.g. product protection, personal protection, and environmental protection.

Particulate and Microbial Contamination

Non-sterile pharmaceutical manufacturers need to develop microbial environmental Control program to identify, investigate, and trend the contamination events encountered during manufacturing. Raw materials, excipients, and drug substances are the primary source of microbiological contamination. Specifications should be established to guarantee that material meets the desired microbiological attributes. Written procedures are established and followed to minimize objectionable microbiological contamination in APIs and intermediates that are of biologic origin, sensitive to microbiological deterioration should have established microbiological specification. Environmental monitoring is regularly performed for drug fill/finish in clean-rooms, formulation tank rooms, laminar flow hoods, biological safety hoods, isolators, glove boxes, molding machines, kit assembly lines, intravenous (IV) compounding critical areas and sterile packaging to control the viable (living microorganisms) and non-viable particles. Monitoring of viable particulates refers to testing for the detection and enumeration of bacteria, yeast, and mold. It also includes monitoring of personnel, air and area surface for microbial contamination. Viable counts provide metrics on the contamination potential of a product as well as demonstrate the veracity that a clean room is functioning as designed and being adequately maintained. Non-viable environmental monitoring refers to particle counts measured by a laser counter. Monitoring of working surface and air quality exhibit the asepsis of the product manufacturing operation.

Personnel: Personnel is the biggest source of contamination in production areas. Personnel harbors millions of bacteria carrying them in the body part to the manufacturing facility. Strict following of gowning practice is the most effective way to protect the manufacturing environment from ourselves. The effectiveness of the gowning practice is assessed by monitoring the personnel on a regular basis for viable counts. Personnel monitoring employs contact plates tests to assess microbial contamination of personnel working in the clean room and other sections.

Air Flow: Air flow and temperature throughout the operational space is maintained at ±1°C within the desired level. The level of manufacturing area protection and air cleanliness required for different areas are evaluated based on the product being manufactured, process and susceptibility to degradation. Attainment of clean area classification is ensured by air filtration efficiency and air change rates. Manufacturers determine the optimum air change rates required taking into account the various critical parameters at the design stage. Primarily air change rate is set to a level required to achieve the particular clean area classification. Directional air flow within production or packing areas additionally assists in preventing possible contamination. Airflows directions are planned considering the operator's locations to minimize operators chances of contaminating the product and also to protect the operator from product fine dust inhalation. HVAC air distribution components are designed and installed in defined locations to prevent spreading of contaminants generated within the room. Exhausting air from rooms at a low level is recommended wherever possible. Unidirectional airflow protects the product by supplying clean air over the product and minimizing the ingress of contaminants from surrounding areas. Where appropriate the unidirectional airflow should also protect the operator from contamination by the product.

Air filtration: Air quality in different sections of the manufacturing facility is controlled and monitored on a regular basis daily, weekly or quarterly, based on area specification and guidelines requirements for particle counts, viable counts, temperature, and humidity. High-Efficiency Particulate Air (HEPA) filters are used to control the viable and non-viable particulate counts in air. HEPA filters have the capability to filter out particulates down to 0.2–0.45 µm in size. HEPA filters run continuously at a calibrated flow rate to maintain the required air quality within the room. Humidity is usually kept at a low level within the room to prevent proliferation of microbes such as bacteria and mold which tend to prefer damp conditions in order to replicate. Air quality is controlled and monitored following regular sampling by using air samplers (active air sampling). Air samplers draw a predetermined volume of air over a sterile media plate, which is later incubated to reveal the number of viable organisms per cubic feet or liter. Currently, in pharma industries, agar impaction is the method of choice. A specially designed, calibrated equipment holds the media plate

under a perforated lid and draws in a known amount of air. After incubation one can accurately measure the number of viable bacteria within the air. The other method can be settling Petri dishes containing sterile growth media exposed to the environment for a specific period. It is usually between 30–60 minutes but can be exposed up to four hours before compromising the integrity of the media itself. Viable microorganisms settle onto the media surface and grow when the plates are incubated. However, passive air sampling tends to be phased out because it does not reflect microbial contamination with an accurately measured volume of air.

Air pressure differential: Infiltration of unfiltered air into the pharmaceutical manufacturing plant must not be allowed as it may act as a source of contamination. The inside environment of manufacturing facilities are maintained at a positive pressure relative to the outside, in order to limit the ingress of air contaminants. In order to prevent the escape of harmful active compounds (such as penicillin and hormones) into the outside environment, these facilities are maintained at negative pressures relative to ambient. Location of the negative pressure facility is carefully considered concerning the areas surrounding it, and particular attention is given in ensuring that the building structure is well sealed. Negative pressure zones should be as far as possible, encapsulated by surrounding areas with clean air supplies, so that only clean air can infiltrate into the controlled zone.

Area: Surfaces (floors, walls, equipment, etc.) are cleaned and monitored on a regular basis for viable counts by using specially designed contact plates containing Trypticase Soy Agar (TSA) and Sabouraud Dextrose Agar (SDA) growth media. TSA growth medium is designed for bacteria, and the SDA is a growth medium designed for mold and yeast. TSA plates are typically incubated at 30–35°C which is mainly the optimal growing temperature for most environmental bacteria, and SDA plates are incubated at 20–25°C which is the optimal growing temperature for most mold and yeast species. This technique is widely used to detect the number of viable microorganisms present on a particular surface.

Cross-contamination: Cross-contamination can be avoided by taking appropriate technical or organizational measures. While manufacturing dry materials and products, special precautions should be taken to prevent the generation and dissemination of dust. Provision is made for proper air control (e.g. supply and extraction of air of suitable quality). Production of a particular product should be carried out in dedicated and self-contained areas (especially for products such as penicillins, live vaccines, live bacterial preparations, and biologicals). Appropriately designed airlocks, pressure differentials, proper air supply, and extraction systems can effectively control cross contamination. The risk of contamination is high with recirculation or re-entry of untreated or insufficiently treated air. Adoption of common protective measures like wearing protective clothing before products or materials handling, using cleaning and decontamination procedures of known effectiveness, using a "closed system" in production, testing for residues, using cleanliness status labels on equipment are necessarily needed for control of contamination and cross-contamination. While conducting campaign manufacturing (separation in time of production) series of batches of the same product is produced in a predefined time period followed by appropriate cleaning as per validated cleaning procedure is done by pharmaceuticals to minimize the risk of contamination.

Containment can typically be achieved by adopting displacement concept (low-pressure differential, along with a high airflow rate), or pressure differential concept (high pressure differential, low airflow), or physical barrier concept. In a multi-product manufacturing site when different products are manufactured at the same time in different areas/cubicles, measures are taken to ensure that dust cannot move from one cubicle to another. Correctly directional air movement and pressure cascade system assist in preventing cross-contamination. Airflow is directed from the clean corridor to the cubicles maintaining pressure cascade resulting in dust containment. The corridor is maintained at a higher pressure than the cubicles, and the cubicles are at higher pressure in respect to the atmospheric pressure. The choice of pressure cascade regime and airflow direction are considered about the product and processing method in use. Highly potent products are manufactured under a negative pressure cascade regime relative to atmospheric pressure. Assessment of pressure cascade for each facility is done individually according to the nature of the product handled and the level of protection required. For effective functioning of the pressure cascade building, structural design is especially important. Airtight designing of ceilings and walls, close-fitting doors and sealed light fittings is must for achieving pressure cascade goals. Measures to prevent cross-contamination and their effectiveness are checked periodically according to standard operating procedures. Susceptible products processing and production areas should undergo periodic environmental monitoring for microbiological and particulate matter monitoring wherever applicable.

Cleaning and Sanitation of the Sterile Area

The responsibility of cleaning and sanitation of the direct and contiguous compounding areas are assigned to trained operators and are done following written procedures. All compounding surfaces are cleaned applying residue-free sanitizing agent leaving on the surface for a time period sufficient to exert its antimicrobial effect. Other work surfaces in the buffer or clean area like counter tops, supply carts, storage shelving are emptied of all supplies, cleaned using approved agents and sanitized at least weekly. Floors in the buffer or clean area are cleaned by mopping once daily using approved agents as described in the written procedures when no aseptic operations are in progress. For all cleaning processes only approved cleaning and sanitizing agents are used with careful consideration of compatibilities and effectiveness. Cleaning and sanitizing must not leave over with any toxic residues. Cleaning schedule and methods of cleaning agent application should be in accordance with written procedures. All cleaning tools, such as wipers, sponges, and mops should be non-shedding and dedicated to being used in the buffer or clean area only. Before reusing cleaning tools, their cleanliness is to be ensured by thorough rinsing and sanitization. These devices are properly clean again after every use and stored in clean environment between uses. Trash is collected in suitable plastic bags and removed with minimal agitation. Supplies and equipment removed from shipping cartons are wiped with a sanitizing agent, such as sterile 70% isopropyl alcohol, which is checked periodically for contamination. External shipping materials or cartons are not allowed to be taken into the buffer or clean area. Cleaning and sanitizing of the quarantine area is performed at least weekly by trained staff and supervised by custodial personnel, by written procedures. Storage shelves are emptied of all supplies, cleaned and sanitized at planned intervals, preferably monthly.

Cleaning and Sanitation of the Non-Sterile Area

Non-sterile manufacturing premises are maintained in an orderly manner and cleaned to make free from accumulated waste, dust, debris and other similar materials. The manufacturing areas are not permitted to store any materials except for the material under process. A routine sanitation program shall be drawn up, observed and properly recorded indicating; specific areas to be cleaned and cleaning intervals, cleaning procedure, equipment and materials to be used for cleaning, and personnel assigned and responsible for the cleaning operation. The working and in-process storage space are designed accordingly to permit orderly and logical positioning of equipment and materials. This is important to minimize the risk of mix-up between different pharmaceutical products or components and also to avoid the risk of cross-contamination. It also helps in minimizing the risk of omission or wrong application of any of the manufacturing or control steps. Outside air entering the clean room is filtered to exclude dust. Inside air is continuously recirculated through HEPA and/or ultra-low penetration air (ULPA) filters to remove the internally generated contaminants and also to maintain moisture level to prevent microbial growth. Airlocks and air showers are provided at the entrance and all the staff working inside are required to wear protective clothing such as hoods, face masks, gloves, boots, and cover all as required. Equipment inside the clean room is designed and placed in a way that generates minimal air contamination. Clean room furniture is also designed to produce minimum particles and to be easy to clean. Though non-sterile clean rooms are not free microbial contaminations but must not have the uncontrolled presence of microbes and airborne particles. Particle levels are tested using a particle counter. Mostly clean rooms are kept at a positive pressure to prevent unfiltered air coming in. Low-level contamination clean rooms require special shoes having completely smooth soles with the track of dust or dirt. Entering a clean room usually requires wearing a clean room suit requiring an anteroom, known as a "gray room," in which the special suits must be put on, before the personnel walk in.

Environmental Monitoring of the Sterile Area

Environmental monitoring is the process of assessing the clean rooms and other controlled environments in the pharmaceutical facility to evaluate the effect of controls on the manufacturing environment. A clean room is part of sterile area environmental control system with defined particulate and microbial contamination. Clean rooms are constructed and used in such a way as to reduce the introduction, generation, and retention of contaminants within the sterile area. The clean room serves as an adjunct to the sterility assurance program of the aseptic area for the microbial quality control of drugs. Evaluation of sterile area environmental air quality is performed by measuring total number of particulate matter and viable microorganisms in the controlled compounding area. Environmental monitoring data of sterile area helps in determining the effectiveness of the cleaning procedures and validation of established cleaning and sanitization procedures. This also ensures the effective removal of the drug product and detergent residue after completion of a proper cleaning procedure. Assessment and verification of the sterile compounding environment of the sterility adequacy are essential, especially for preparing high-risk formulations. Verification of each laminar airflow workstations (LAFW) and barrier isolator for proper functioning and compliance with air quality requirement is performed at least every six months by a qualified operator(s) using state-of-the-art electronic air sampler, re-verification have to be performed when the LAFW or barrier isolator is relocated. Similarly, the air quality of the buffer, clean and quarantine area is also evaluated periodically. These records are maintained and reviewed by the supervising personnel or other designated employee.

Written environmental monitoring schedule and plan are established and followed. All compounding personnel is trained in and made well versed about the importance of the environmental monitoring process. Airborne microorganisms count in the controlled air environments (LAFW, barrier isolators, buffer or clean area and anteroom area) is performed using suitable electric air samplers or by exposing sterile nutrient agar plates for a suitable period by adequately trained individuals. Air sampling is performed at locations most prone to contamination during compounding activities like the zones of air backwash turbulence within LAFWs and compounding area. Such evaluations are performed as a regular interval in the ongoing process, i.e. at least monthly for sterile compounding areas used for manufacturing of low- and medium-risk preparations and at least weekly for areas used for high-risk preparations. Working instructions and verification requirements for electric air samplers that actively collect volumes of air for evaluation must be followed properly. While passive exposure of sterile nutrient agar settling plates, the covers are removed, and media is exposed usually for one hour or longer as required to collect viable microorganisms as they settle down.

At the end of the designated exposure period, the plates are recovered and incubated at 30 to 35°C temperature for 48 hours conducive to multiplication of microorganisms on the nutrient agar. The number of discrete microorganism colonies developed is counted and reported as colony forming units (CFU). The level of microbial contamination in the air of the tested environment is expressed as CFU/cubic meter or millimeters. Limits for microbial and particulate count should be consistent with regulatory and compendia guidelines. Alert limits should be set from monitoring histories at an interval between 95% percentile. The reaction should be to consecutive for out-of-limit and not for individual results. Validation and periodic qualification are must for working personnel, environment, HVAC systems, media fills and utilities.

An increasing trend in CFU counts over the time is sufficient to alarm for a prompt re-evaluation of the adequacy of cleaning functions, operational procedures, and air filtration efficiency within the sterile compounding area. Action may be warranted when an increasing trend to 50% above the baseline for areas used for high- and medium-risk preparations or to 100% above baseline for areas used for low-risk preparations is found. Written corrective action plans are maintained for investigation of the status of the environmental control systems undertaken in response to excursions outside the action limits and out-off-trend results. Development of checklists for systems review and corrective action is part of good practice. Identification of the microorganisms from isolates and determination of their possible origin and occurrence of atypical activity in the processing area helps in the systematic review. Review of product and component sterilization and the aseptic filling process should be undertaken if required. Investigations are also directed for assessment of media fill record, equipment and facilities maintenance, sanitization record, training status of the personnel and level of supervision. All corrective actions must be completed and documented in a timely fashion for additional environmental controls like more intense sampling, a revision to aseptic practices, review of cleaning and sanitization practices, sensitivity determination of the isolate to disinfectant, enhanced supervision, retraining of clean room personnel and additional product testing.

Environmental Monitoring of the Non-Sterile Area

Monitoring of non-sterile environment is performed for nonviable airborne particles, viable airborne particles, presence of a viable contaminant on surfaces, introduction of a viable contaminant from personnel, temperature and relative humidity. Nonviable and viable contaminants should be controlled in an area where non-sterile products, in-process materials, and product-contact equipment surfaces, containers and closures are exposed to the environment to reduce product bioburden. These non-sterile areas are maintained as Class 1,00,000 or Class 10,000 environment. Dust control measurements are necessary for adjacent or ancillary areas. Study in static conditions, as part of HVAC qualification is done periodically to ensure that area meets acceptable conditions after cleaning and before use. Clean room environment is typically suitable for pharmaceutical manufacturing of products having a low-level liability for environmental pollutants such as dust, airborne microbes, aerosol particles, and/or chemical vapors. Clean room has a controlled level of contamination defined by the number of particles per cubic meter at specified particle size. An ISO 1 clean room does not allow any particle above the size range 0.5 μm and larger in diameter, and can contain only maximum 12 particles the size range 0.3 μm and smaller per cubic meter. The ambient outside air in a typical urban environment contains 35,000,000 particles in the size range 0.5 μm and larger in diameter per cubic meter that corresponds to the ISO 9 clean room as a perspective.

Products not required to be manufactured under aseptic conditions are essentially required to be free from pathogens like *Salmonella, Escherichia coli, Pyocyanea*, etc. Microbial monitoring is done for viable airborne contaminants, surface contaminants (in walls, equipment surfaces, drainage, and floors) and personnel contaminants. Methods used for monitoring viable contaminant should be capable of detecting molds and yeasts. Frequencies of monitoring may vary depending upon the risk of exposure. Routine monitoring during operations for airborne contaminants and immediately after operation and cleaning should be performed for surfaces and personnel. Monitoring frequencies and procedures are influenced by stage of manufacturing, i.e. open or closed manufacturing step and utilization capability for single or multiple product manufacturing. Microbial monitoring devices used are slit-to-agar (STA), sieve impactor, centrifugal sampler (taking the known volume of air), sterilizable microbiological atrium (SMA), settle plates, and surface monitoring by contact plates (for regular surfaces) and swabs (for irregular surfaces). Establishment of normal flora with the identification of bacterial isolates to the species level and fungi at least to the genus level is performed in case of out of specification performances.

Air conditioning system is maintained between 10–20 air changes per hour. Temperature is maintained between 15–30°C for non-sensitive products and 20–25°C for sensitive products. Considering human comfort aspect RH is maintained between 40 ± 10% for sensitive products and between 50 ± 10% for non-sensitive products as RH above 65% promotes microbial growth. For HVAC validation and maintenance, considerations are given to air velocity, airflow patterns, and turbulence.

Smoke studies are done to determine flow patterns during static and dynamic conditions. HEPA filter integrity testing, filter efficiency testing and air pressure differentials are also monitored. As per WHO guidelines dust and vapor control measures are monitored at the point of extraction, close to the generation point fixed high-velocity extraction point or articulated arm with movable hood. Sufficient transfer velocity, e.g. 15–20 m/sec as per density is maintained. Airflow design should be such that product had minimal chances of getting contaminated by the operator. Generally, unidirectional airflow is maintained to remove dust and vapors. For turbulent airflow, air is introduced from ceiling diffusers and extracted at a low level.

For manufacturing of potent products such as penicillin, hormones, enzymes, etc enclosed facilities are required where harmful/potent substances are exhausted. The final filters should be a HEPA filter. For particularly identified hazardous component it may be necessary to install two banks of HEPA filters in series, to provide additional protection in case the first filter fails. Environmental monitoring requirement for non-sterile areas is less as compared to aseptic operations. Monitoring is only restricted to temperature, relative humidity, and microbial contamination. Adequate monitoring is required for products containing penicillin, or cephalosporin drug categories. Differential pressures control limits should be realistic. Along with the settle plate method, there should be provision for fumigation and de-fumigation along with regular monitoring of compressed air.

CONTROL OF QUALITY VARIATION IN A PHARMACEUTICAL MANUFACTURING ENVIRONMENT

Quality by Design (QbD) concept was first outlined by well-known quality expert **Joseph M. Juran** in notable publication, *Juran on Quality by Design.* Juran believed that quality could be planned and that most quality crises and problems relate to the quality planning measures in the first place. As per his concept quality should be built into a product with a thorough understanding of the **product** and **process**. The practice of this concept requires an overall understanding of manufacturing process along with knowledge of the risks involved and sound technical command on best possible measures to mitigate those risks. This is a successor to the "quality by inspection" (or "quality after design") approach that the FDA has taken until the late 1990s/early 2000s. The QbD is a systemic approach to pharmaceutical development that emphasizes product and process understanding and process control based on modern science and quality risk management principals. The QbD approach ensures the presence of predefined product quality in formulations inculcated through its design, development and manufacturing processes. QbD helps to gain enhanced knowledge of product performance over a range of material attributes, manufacturing process options and process parameters considering the appropriate use of quality risk management principles. Some of the QbD elements include:

- Defining the target product quality profile
- Designing product and manufacturing processes
- Identifying critical quality attributes, process parameters and sources of variability
- Controlling manufacturing processes to produce consistent quality over time

QbD principles have been adopted by the USFDA as a vehicle for the transformation of a drug discovered through development phases to commercial manufacturing. QbD in the pharmaceuticals provides a push towards process understanding that results in assuring product quality in the manufacturing level rather than Quality by Inspection (QbI) which takes place after production. This assures the pharmaceuticals that with the development of intricate knowledge of the design process can enable to analyze the quality components during manufacturing as opposed to relying on final product testing to assess the quality of the product. Working with the European Medicines Agency, EU and FDA Japan have been instrumental in furthering QbD objectives through the Technical Requirements for Registration of Pharmaceuticals for Human Use of ICH. ICH guidelines Q8 (pharmaceutical development), Q9 (quality risk management), and Q10 (pharmaceutical

quality system) are aimed at assisting manufacturers in implementation QbD principles into their operations. The QbD devised practical input helps to ensure use of quality risk management fundamentals in making necessary lifecycle adaptations to achieve process control and maintain product quality, implementation of rapid corrective and preventative action (CAPA) to assure sustainable cGMP compliance:

- **Manufacturing process improvements:** QbD provides an assortment of diagnostic tools to identify manufacturing parameters that influence product quality and variation of product quality.
- **Manufacturing production control:** Using the multivariate data analysis and machine learning tools QbD enables assembly of reliable prediction models, which can be used by plant operators for production control.
- **Real-time process monitoring:** Pharmaceutical manufacturing entails a complex sequence of unit operations usually carried out in batches. Unit operations are typically monitored by process analytical technology as a time series. The trajectory of these batches from initiation to completion can be summarized into a multivariate process signature, a fingerprint. Multivariate analysis of these fingerprints and comparison to historical fingerprints of successful and failed batches can provide a mean to ascertain the status of a current batch in real time.
- **Approaches for environment management:** The current regulatory guidelines highlighted innovative ideas regarding process development and manufacturing process control. These concepts are thought provoking regarding practicalities of implementation. It has also focused renewed attention on these significant areas of the process sciences that have been somewhat neglected in the pharmaceutical industry.

Design Space Development

Design space is the multidimensional combination of process parameters and interaction between input variables (e.g. material attributes) that are essential for product quality assurance. Design space is an individualistic approach that is proposed by the applicant and is subject to regulatory assessment and approval. Controlling the interacting parts in a manufacturing space depends on an understanding of variables that affect product quality attributes. Methods to monitor and process control strategy that falls within the boundaries of knowledge, i.e. in established design space are:

Starting materials: Particle size distribution, specific surface area or other functionality related characteristics, the ratio of ingredients to each other, etc.

Process operations: Water content of mass/granule over time, blending profile over time, etc.

Machine parameters: Weight discharged by blender, feedback control of compression force, etc.

An approved manufacturing process operated strictly within the control space producing materials meeting the required identity, potency, quality specifications. The maturity of product life cycle, the scale-up, economic and/or other factors can demand changes in the control scheme of the process, moving it from old control space to a new control space. The new control space is usually developed out of necessity to cope with process shortcomings sometimes long after the original process development being done. Working within design space (multidimensional region) not generally considered as a change. Movement out of design space is a change, and regulatory postapproval is needed for such change process. It is needed to be reviewed and approved by the regulatory authorities before the process could be operated commercially in the new control space. The process development and manufacturing teams must develop and document the scientific basis for approval of the design space in the chemistry manufacturing and controls (CMC) section of the regulatory submission.

Appropriately designed experiment test and defined the outer limits of the intended design space. This information is used to understand the effects on the critical quality Attributes (CQAs) and characterize any new Critical Process parameters (CPPs) that might arise in a new control space.

Design for Manufacturing

Development and approval of a control space and/or a design space depend on full utilization of prior knowledge and experience of the process development of the manufacturing teams. Previous process behavior data when subjected to the constraints of full-scale commercial operations act as a vital source of guidance while designing subsequent process to operate successfully within those constraints. The term "design for manufacturing" is used by FDA to describe the utilization of this process information to achieve an acceptable quality standard consistently. Assessment and analysis of actual data generated by prior manufacturing processes operating under similar conditions help in archiving information useful for the current process under development.

Process improvement and Process Analytical Technology (PAT)

The usefulness of PAT or other process improvement initiative in QbD depends on all data (discrete, replicate, continuous and paper-based) on process trending, reporting, descriptive analysis, univariate and multivariate cause-and-effect analysis, and parameter relationship modeling generated in the same integrated environment. The process scientists need to work with continuous, discrete and replicate data together for quantitative analysis. Process improvement following PAT technique needs a framework for managing both the manufacturing process and enabling collaborative analysis of the resulting data to improve the predictability and quality of operations. The key is to provide on-demand access to not only the summary production data but also to the individual underlying data elements in a context that is natural to users. The critical success factor for process improvement is easy, on-demand access to all the data and data types in the infrastructure systems, including supervisory control and data acquisition (SCADA), laboratory information management systems (LIMS), enterprise resource planning (ERP), manufacturing execution systems (MES), and electronic batch record (EBR) systems and of other manufacturing control and data acquisition systems. On-demand access allows a multi-disciplinary team of users to extract information in context and use it to understand cause-and-effect relationships. The data access method must directly enable users to identify and understand cause-and-effect relationships between CPPs and CQAs without spending excessive amounts of time on manual programming tasks or manually collecting and reconciling data. Collaboration between participants of the process development, manufacturing and quality teams is most useful when technology platform is used to access data and share ideas between the diverse group of users; production engineers, statisticians, and quality professionals.

Advantages

Using QbD fundamentals a pharmaceutical manufacturing unit is assurance of understanding and controlling formulation and manufacturing variables. Product testing confirms product quality, but the implementation of QbD enable the transformation of the chemistry, manufacturing, and controls (CMC) into a science-based pharmaceutical quality assessment. When fully implemented, QbD assures that all the critical sources of process variability have been identified, measured and understood so that the manufacturing process itself can control them. The resulting business benefits of the manufacturer implementing QbD to the manufacturing process are plentiful and significant:

- Superior quality.
- Higher level of product quality assurance throughout product lifecycle and supply chain.
- Reduced batch failure rates, less final product testing efforts, and lower batch release costs.
- Lower operating costs due to fewer failures and deviation investigations.
- Reduced need for final product testing, this will end up with lower costing to the manufacturer and the consumer.
- Since there is also increased predictability of product quality in the manufacturing process, there can also be faster approval for new products and reduced time to reach the market.
- Increased predictability of manufacturing output and quality.
- Reduced raw material, WIP and finished product inventory costs.
- Documentation of QbD during the pre-IND meeting and at the end of phase II meeting before regulatory submissions allow early review and analysis of the CMC section of an NDA.
- Faster regulatory approval of new product applications and process changes.
- Fewer and shorter regulatory inspections of manufacturing sites.
- Faster technology transfer between development and manufacturing.
- Addressing issues of concern and further QbD implementation results in the classification of the drug substance and

drug process manufacturing process as low-risk.

- Expected to have less comprehensive or eliminated preapproval inspection.

These benefits can translate into significant reductions in working capital requirements, resource costs and time to value. In a pharmaceutical manufacturing unit operations are typically carried out in batches, and the trajectory of these batches from initiation to completion can be summarized into a multivariate signature, or fingerprint, using specified software. Historical fingerprint provides quality assurance of new batches and indicates the state of the process. These batch models may be executed in real-time using on-line software, with diagnostic tools for identifying the root cause of problems as they occur.

Disadvantages

It is expected that adopting QbD together with ICH Q10 'Pharmaceutical Quality Systems,' can assure achievement of the "desired state" of pharmaceutical manufacturing control. The emphasis on QbD requires pharmaceutical manufacturers to make large investments at earlier stages of process development in a product life cycle in advance of any approved commercial operations. Development of a sound scientific basis for the "control space" accommodating the whole range of defined variability in the commercial process operations targeting to produce a product of the right quality is very difficult though achievable. The current QbD methodology requires processes and inventories that need infrastructure to support quality pharmaceutical production. This early phase investment can, in turn, make the consumers pay for it, but lately, QbD can be equated to just in time (JIT) as the industry will have total control of the manufacturing process. The value of JIT has been addressed by many researchers written in scientific publication as it eventually soothes out the total business process.

ADVANCED PHARMACEUTICAL PROCESS CONTROL

The pharmaceutical industries continue to evolve and grow to meet the requirements of a new era. ICH guidelines of Q8, Q9, and Q10 provides scientific, risk-based approaches for development, risk management, and quality systems empowering manufacturers for continuous improvement and technical innovation throughout the product life cycle. Key factors driving the evolution of the pharmaceutical industry include competition, cost containment, quality, and regulatory considerations. New technological initiatives provide capabilities with the potential to enhance productivity by improving the process capability, quality control, robustness reducing cycle times and improving consistency, while at the same time ensuring compliance. In the pharmaceutical manufacturing sector, new technologies are being introduced, and the process scientists develop sophisticated approaches to process analytical technology (PAT). New technologies in combination with strategic use of design space and advances in PAT and implementation of quality risk management, enabled QbD to achieve astringent process control for the desired quality state of manufacturing.

Traditional Process Control

Traditional process control approach works through tight control of key process parameters at predetermined set points or ranges. It focuses on the establishment of a relationship between process outputs as crucial product attributes with the process input variables like raw materials and API properties, process parameters such as temperature, humidity or pH. This control strategy, however, does not allow for mid-course correction for variations in starting materials or other process upsets, nor does it allow flexibility within or between production design space concepts. The set points for critical process parameter are commonly determined during development stage typically performing experiments, and the process is validated using a three batch validation approach. Reduction of common cause variations in such traditionally controlled process requires significant effort. Control strategies that are based on fixed process parameters can result in higher variability of product attributes due to less flexibility.

Advanced Process Control

Advanced process control (APC) describes mathematically advanced control algorithms that use predictive, adaptive and optimization techniques to control multi-input, multi-output processes. APC is a well-practiced commonly used technology in many industrial sectors for improving quality, consistency, and process efficiency, though it is relatively a new concept in the pharmaceutical industry. APC as a control strategy manipulates process parameters (process inputs, Xs) within the required constraints utilizing PAT, process models, and other techniques in order to actively control the drug product attributes (process outputs, Ys) like an active pharmaceutical ingredient and raw material variations at a set point or within a tight range. APC overcome traditional control strategy limitations and improve capabilities by real-time monitoring of process outputs and prediction of process endpoints to determine any potential deviation from desired range and calculate the changes needed in process inputs to minimize the potential deviation in process outputs. APC offers a new and promising paradigm in the field of pharmaceutical processes efficiency enhancement providing tangible quality and business benefits. APC enable to achieve higher process capability while maintaining the process attributes close to specification. The APC advanced strategy offers a wide range of benefit with improved product quality, lower common cause variations, greater product consistency, higher yield, and close adherence to cycle time.

Process Analytical Technology

The USFDA is encouraging the pharmaceutical industries to achieve an optimum level of "real-time" product quality while a batch is being manufactured (RTQA) enabled with consistent process understanding and controlling process variability. Ideally, a standardized process must assure the appropriate level of quality in real-time despite variations in materials and processing. In the traditional approach, such variations would have resulted in unacceptable and rejected product batches following QC laboratory testing of the finished product. In the current practice APC functions based on the fact that appropriate quality outcome must be designed into the process itself rather than relying on final product testing. The developers to produce the desired state of the product, need to have a complete understanding of all the pieces involved in the process, both of the raw materials and the intermediates as well as the interactions between the two. In other words, they must understand how the critical process parameters (CPP) affects the variability in the critical quality attributes (CQA) so that these can be measured and controlled in the manufacturing process. Process analytical technology (PAT) is a system for designing, analyzing and controlling manufacturing processes developed based on the identification of the variables that affect product quality with an understanding of the scientific and engineering principals involved in manufacturing technology. According to the USFDA draft guidance, the optimally desired control state in pharmaceutical manufacturing is:

- Ensuring product quality through effective design and efficient performance of manufacturing processes

- Defining product and process specifications based on mechanistic understanding of process factors that affect product formulation performance
- Continuous and real-time quality assurance
- Procedures are tailored to accommodate the current scientific knowledge relevant to regulatory policies
- Application of risk-based regulatory approaches recognizing both the level of scientific understanding and the process control capabilities related to product quality and performance

Specifically, the guidance document discusses PAT tools, the need for process understanding, risk-based management, integrated systems thinking and real-time product release. With PAT the reduced time and operational cost of taking a product from one end of manufacturing to the other end of the marketplace have captured the interest of the industry. PAT requires planned generation and effective utilization of all of this data in order to be able to minimize the risks associated with manufacturing process variations. The paramount goal of PAT is to provide a standardized process capable of generating products of predetermined quality consistently. Identifying the source of quality variation followed by effective control of parameters, in turn, improve quality and efficiency as off:

- Cycle time reduction using on-, in-, or at-line measurements and controls
- Prevention of product rejection and resource wastage
- Increased use of automation
- Real-time product release
- Continuous processing results in improved energy and material utilization with increased capacity

Process controls when applied will produce a consistent quality product with no or minimal in-process testing. PAT represents the single most significant change in drug development in the last 30 years. Other industries have been driven toward PAT due to customer or market pressure. Only by complete understanding and characterization of critical variables, it is possible to develop and implement solutions which will anticipate product performance and realize both the compliance benefit of PAT as outlined in the agency guidance and financial benefit of having a faster, cheaper delivery to market. Newly emergent PAT-based approaches are pushing the boundaries of process design and redefining the process control strategies. Coherent with the improvement of reliability and performance of PAT systems, it has the potential to serve as an integral part of pharmaceutical processes. In this context, PAT is increasingly paying its part to replace off-line final product tests with at-line, or on-line PAT-based release tests providing the basis for process control strategy and enabling continuous quality verification (CQV) and real-time release (RTR). Continuous manufacturing concept works on the combination of multiple unit operations in a manufacturing process following a single integrated system. In continuous process design sources of variation are defined and controlled based on QbD principles, and the end product variations are minimized by controlling the process within the design space. Driven by cycle time reduction and capacity enhancement, as well as reduced off-line analytical testing and minimized change over time, it results in capital and operating cost reductions. Integration of on-line PAT tools acts as a foundation for the development of more advanced process control strategies resulting in CQV that in turn leads to RTR.

CONTINUAL IMPROVEMENT OF THE PHARMACEUTICAL QUALITY SYSTEM

In pharmaceutical quality system, continuous efforts are to be directed towards improvement of the quality system.

Corrective Action and Preventive Action (CAPA) System

Every pharmaceutical manufacturing facility must have a system for implementing CAPA activities. The CAPA requirements generally results from the following review and verification process, i.e. investigation of complaints, product rejections, non-conformances, recalls, deviations, audits, regulatory inspections and findings, trends from process performance and product quality monitoring. A structured approach for investigation of the process is used with the objective of determining the root cause and the level of effort that are commensurate with the level of risk. Investigation of CAPA is carried out by the following:

Investigation is needed to identify trigger events and to evaluate the implications of the event and also to determine the underlying cause for the event.

It defines the needed immediate action, corrective action and preventive action to be undertaken. It also explains their importance regarding management responsibility and methods of implementation.

This describes the relationship of trending used in the interpretation of CAPA data. Use of investigation feedbacks and CAPA results to modify appropriate quality system elements to create an error-free system. CAPA methodologies result in product and process improvements and enhanced product and process understanding.

Change Management System

Product quality monitoring and CAPA drive changes are the steering wheel of continual improvement that shows their outputs in process performance. In order to evaluate the root cause and implement the approved changes correctly, pharma manufacturing units should have an effective change management system. The formality of change management processes before the initial regulatory submission generally differs from the after submission requirements where changes to the regulatory filing are required to be modulated as per regional requirements. The change management system ensures implementation of continuous improvement in a timely and effective manner along with assurance that there are no unintended consequences of the change. The change management system includes the following, as appropriate for defining the product life cycle stages:

- Quality risk management approach is utilized to evaluate the proposed changes and the level of effort and formality of the evaluation commensurate with the level of risk.
- Proposed changes are evaluated relative to the marketing authorization requirements, design space implemented and/or current product and process understanding. The assessment must also be directed to determine whether changes to the regulatory filing is required under regional requirements. Working within the defined design space is not considered a change (from a regulatory filing perspective) as stated in ICH Q8, however, from pharmaceutical quality system standpoint all changes should be evaluated by an approved change management system.
- To ensure that the changes are technically justified, the proposed changes are to be evaluated by expert teams having appropriate expertise and knowledge of relevant pharmaceutical development, manufacturing, quality, regulatory affairs, and medicinal product registration areas. Prospective evaluation criteria for a proposed change should be set forward based on approved changes as per CAPA analysis.
- Following implementation, evaluation of the changes should be undertaken to confirm that change objectives were achieved and there was no deleterious impact of change on product quality.

1. **Pre-change analysis:** It assesses the impact of proposed changes on the products, processes, facilities, utilities, etc. It analyses the CAPA data to ensure risk minimization and ongoing regulatory compliance.

2. **Post-change analysis**
   - Deviation, change management processes, CAPA, complaint, and recall;
   - Feedback on outsourced activities;
   - Implementation of self-assessment processes like risk assessments, trending, and audits;
   - External assessments including regulatory inspection findings and customer audits.

   This analyses data and other inputs to determine the results of a change, and evaluate if there are chances that the change can create any new risk factors.

3. **Review of the quality management system:** Quality assurance section in coordination with quality control needs to develop a formal periodic review process for the pharmaceutical quality system. The review primarily includes assessment of quality system objective achievement based on the following performance indicators commonly used to monitor the effectiveness of processes within the pharmaceutical quality system:

4. **Monitoring of internal and external factors impacting the pharmaceutical quality system:** External and internal business and financial factors impacting the quality system are:
   - Emerging regulation changes, new guidance release and other financial related quality issues effecting the quality system;
   - Adoption of innovations for enhanced performance of quality system;
   - Changes in the business environment and objectives;
   - Changes in product ownership.

5. **Outcomes of management review and monitoring:** The higher management reviews the outcome of improvements of the pharmaceutical quality system implementation and monitor internal and external factors related to processes.

Statistical Process Control (SPC)

To determine if variability occurring in a process is stable over time is useful to detect and identify the source of abnormal events. Multivariate analysis reduces the number of variables by combining correlated variables, which is used in combination with SPC. Variations can be off, common cause variation due to random fluctuation of response caused by unknown factors or special cause variation due to non-random variation caused by a specific factor. Statistical methods are applied to identify and control the particular cause of variation in a process, like the identification of issues before they become problems and track process performance for potential improvements:

- Allocation or reallocation of resources
- Personnel training on new guidance and regulatory policies;
- Revision of quality policy and quality objectives;
- Documentation and timely communication of the management review results and actions, including escalation of appropriate issues to senior management.

Audits and Self-Inspections

1. **Audits processes and results:** It defines the need to carry out different types of audits (systems, product, and process) and to analyze audit results for assessing conformance to requirements.

2. **Audit follow-up:** Uses various methods to evaluate and verify the adequacy of corrective actions taken.

3. **Ineffective corrective actions:** When the implemented corrective actions are not

sufficient to determine the appropriate strategies to use.

Documents and records management

1. **GMP document system:** Review and checking of the GMP documentation system, including corporate standards, master plans, procedures, manufacturing, and test instructions, etc., to analyze the compliance with regulatory requirements.
2. **GMP compliance of records:** Analyze and review various records (logbooks, tags, training evidence, etc.) to confirm compliance with requirements.
3. **Record retention:** Identify any gap between actual practice and regulatory requirements for GMP compliance in record retention.

Product Quality Complaints vs. Adverse Event Reports

1. **Quality complaints:** Describe and distinguish between product complaints and adverse events, and evaluate complaint-handling processes.
2. **Adverse events and pharmacovigilance:** This understands the severity and after effects of adverse events and identifies the regulatory reports for these events and analyze the pharmacovigilance data.
3. **Problem response:** Evaluates the level of action that needs to be taken in response to the types of events, including corrections, product removal, etc.

Product Trend Requirements

Describe and distinguish between components of the Annual Product Review (APR) and the Product Quality Review (PQR) about data trends and other required review methods and to understand the requirement.

CONTROL OF LABORATORY SYSTEMS

Compendia

Required vs. informational compendia: Describe and distinguish between required

and informational (general) compendial chapters.

Marketing requirements vs. compendia: Understand and distinguish among the US Pharmacopoeia (USP), European Pharmacopoeia (PhEur or EP) and Japanese Pharmacopoeia (JP) regarding requirements for marketing authorization.

Compendial methods review: Evaluate and review compendial methods to ensure that they are verified as suitable for use in the testing lab.

Compendial requirements review: Review and analysis of test methods, qualifications, and validations actually in practice against the required compendial or informational general chapters when specific tests are not prescribed in the product compendial monograph.

Biological, microbiological, chemical, and physical test methods: Identify, interpret and apply results for compendia identification tests, quantitative analysis, qualitative analysis, and other tests or studies for biological, microbiological, and chemical and physical parameters testing purposes.

Laboratory Investigations of Aberrant Results

Test data: Analyze, describe and distinguish among biological, microbiological, and chemical test data, and develop procedures for investigating each type.

Aberrant results: Identify, analyze, evaluate and interpret data on processes or products that are out-of-specification or out-of-trend, and determine the outcome of the laboratory test results and the criteria for further investigation.

Instrument Control and Record-Keeping

Instrument control: Examine and apply operating procedures for instrument identification, classification and calibration, to meet requirements.

Instrument calibration: Determine instruments calibration results are within the specified range of operation and are accurate and precise.

Specifications

Types of specifications: Analyze and determine that approved specifications exist for raw materials, intermediates, packaging components, finished products, etc.

Test data and specifications: Analyze and compare test data with specifications to determine that raw materials, intermediates, packaging, or products meet requirements.

Specifications revision: Review, evaluate and update specifications when methods are revised, or compendia are changed.

Laboratory Record-Keeping and Data Requirements

Record review: Analysis and review laboratory records to detect errors or falsification and to prevent loss of data.

Record-keeping requirements: Identify and review record-keeping requirements for data acquisition systems.

Certificates of analysis (COA): Periodic review of COA of the API and raw materials to ensure accuracy and an appropriate record retaining.

Laboratory handling controls

Sample identification: Determine that the samples are identified and handled in accordance with the requirements, including name, sample identification, chains of custody, etc.

Reagents, solutions, and standards identification: Determine that reagents, solutions, and standards are identified and labeled in accordance with requirements as of opened-on, expiry, (validated) use-by, or recertify-by dates.

Storage requirements: Describe and use procedures to store samples, reagents, solutions, and standards in appropriate environmental conditions (e.g. temperature, humidity, light exposure, the absence of oxygen, etc.) to maintain the material's characteristics for testing.

Stability Programs

Release tests vs. stability-indicating tests: Define and distinguish between these two types of tests.

Stability test data: Evaluate and review stability data and identify trends that support or challenge an expiry date.

Stability-point failure: Evaluate and identify the stability-point failure of a product or material and evaluate the implications for regulatory compliance.

Reserve samples and retains: Describe the various current regulatory requirements for retains and reserve samples.

INFRASTRUCTURE: FACILITIES AND UTILITIES

Facilities

Buildings: Determine requirements for appropriate size and construction of buildings and areas allocation for controlled system operations. Ensure that construction and proper facility location and operations minimizing the risk of errors and cross contamination.

Manufacture and storage environment: Identify requirements for appropriate lighting, ventilation, and drainage and proper functioning to avoid an adverse effect on product quality (either directly or indirectly) during manufacturing and storage.

Facilities change control: Assessment of various methods to verify that change control practices are in use to maintain the qualified state of the facilities.

Utilities

Water supply systems: Identify and interpret regulatory requirements proper design of water supply systems, with specific requirements of various unit operations (e.g. dechlorination, reverse osmosis, deionization, distillation, etc.). All the delivery lines, backflow or back-siphonage prevention and drainage systems, should be appropriate for the type of water (potable, purified, water for injection, etc.) needed in various processing operations.

Compressed air and gas systems: Identify and apply regulatory requirements related to compressed air and gas systems, including storage, flow regulation, filtration, venting, and purging, etc.

Utility design for production: Identify and select utility designs related to production steps (e.g. washing, sterilizing, depyrogenation, etc.) for use with specific materials and processes.

Utility design specifications: Review operations of utilities to ensure that they meet design specifications.

Utilities change control: Identify and apply various methods to verify that change control practices are in use to maintain the qualified state of affected utilities.

Computers and Software used to Control Laboratory Equipment

Current regulations require validation of computers and software that are used to control laboratory equipment or process data. Systems that acquire, process, or store data also have additional requirements defined by 21 *CFR*. Although computer and software qualification is considered a subset of validation, it requires additional documentation in case of change control procedures. Guidance for validation of computers and software for general computer-related systems and data acquisition systems are described in Parenteral Drug Association technical reports. These guidance documents provide procedures for the documentation, qualification, and change control aspects of validation.

When multiple laboratory computers are maintained with the same configuration of hardware and software, complete validation on a single representative unit can be performed. All other identical configurations would require only the IQ portion of the qualification. All such computers must be maintained in the same system of change control, which requires the appropriate revalidation when any change in configuration is made.

BIBLIOGRAPHY

1. Agalloco J. Closed Systems and Environmental Control: Application of Risk Based Design. American Pharmaceutical Review; 1-4. http://www.medinstill.com/pdf/Agalloco_Closed.pdf.

2. Bedson P. The Development and Application of Guidance on Equipment Qualification of Analytical Instruments. Accreditation and Quality Assurance 1(6); 1996: 265–274.

3. Box GEP, Hunter JS, Hunter WG. Statistics for Experimenters: Design, Innovation, and Discovery. 2nd Ed. Wiley-Inter Science, London; 2005.

4. Booth CM. Designing An Environmental Monitoring Program For Non-Sterile Manufacturing: A Risk-Based Approach. Pharmaceutical Online; 2017. https://www.pharmaceuticalonline.com/doc/designing-an-environmental-monitoring-program-for-non-sterile-manufacturing-a-risk-based-approach-0001.

5. European Commission, Brussels. XXX Com, 650 Annex I, 4th Volume, Proposal for a Regulation of the European Parliament and the Council; 2011.

6. European Medicines Agency 7 Westferry Circus, Canary Wharf, London, E14 4HB, UK http://www.emea.europa.eu. European Medicines Agency 2008.

7. Farrington JK. Environmental Monitoring in Pharmaceutical Manufacturing—A Product Risk. American Pharmaceutical Review; 2008. http://americanpharmaceuticalreview.com/ViewArticle.aspx?ContentID=254 .

8. Friedli HM, Kickuth M, Stieneker F, Bastoen B, Chick SE, Friedli T, et al. Operational Excellence in the Pharmaceutical Industry. Der Pharmazeutische Betrieb; 2006. http://www.item.unisg.ch/org/item/tectemw.nsf/SysWebResources/Publikation+OPEX+ Leseprobe/$FILE.

9. Glodek M, Liebowitz S, McCarthy R, McNally G, Oksanen C, Schultz T, et al. Process robustness – A PQRI white paper. Pharmaceutical Engineering 26(6); 2006: http:// www.ispe.org/pe_online_exclusive.

10. Guidance for Industry: Container Closure Systems for Packaging Human Drugs and Biologics. Chemistry, Manufacturing, and Controls Documentation. U.S. Department of Health and Human Services. Food and Drug Administration Center for Drug Evaluation and Research (CDER). Center for Biologics Evaluation and Research (CBER); 1999.

11. Guidelines on GMP for HVAC systems for non-sterile dosage forms. Appendix to main guidelines" (Working document QAS/02.048/ Figs/Rev.2), WHO; 2005.

12. ICH Q10: Pharmaceutical Quality System.4th Version, 2008: http://www.ich.org/fileadmin/ Public_Web_Site/ICH_Products/Guidelines/ Quality/Q10/Step4/Q10_Guideline.pdf

13. ICH. Quality Guidelines. https://www.ich.org/ products/guidelines/quality/article/quality-guidelines.html.

14. Innovation and Continuous Improvement in Pharmaceutical Manufacturing (Pharmaceutical CGMPs for the 21st Century) The PAT Team and Manufacturing Science Working Group Report: A Summary of Learning, Contributions and Proposed Next Steps for moving towards the "Desired State" of Pharmaceutical Manufacturing in the 21st Century. http://www.2004-4080b1_01_manufSciWP.pdf .

15. International Cleanroom Standards. ISO 14644; Parts 1 to 6: 2015. https://www.iso.org/ standard/53394.html

16. ISPE Baseline Pharmaceutical Engineering Guides for New and Renovated Facilities. 1st Edition, 3rd Vol. Sterile Manufacturing Facilities; 1999.

17. Juran JM. Juran on Quality by Design: The New Steps for Planning Quality into Goods and Services. Free Press, New York; 1992.

18. Kudryashov E, Smyth C, O'Driscoll B, Buckin V. Analysing Raw Materials and Formulations Using High-Resolution Ultrasonic Spectroscopy. Pharmaceutical Technology Europe; 2005. http:// www.pharmatech.com .

19. Laboratory Controls, General Requirements. Code of Federal Regulations, Part 211.160, Title 21, Rev; 2000.

20. MacLeod P. Temperature control in pharmaceutical warehouses. 2015. https:// www.shdlogistics.com/news/temperature-control-in-pharmaceutical-warehouses

21. Maintenance and Calibration of Equipment. Code of Federal Regulations, Part 58.63, Title 21, Rev: 2000.

22. Moshgbar M. Advanced process control can improve pharmaceutical manufacturing. Pharmaceutical Formulation and Quality; 2009. http://www.pharmaquality.com.

23. Nadpara NP, Thumar RV, Kalola VN, Patel PB. Quality by design (QBD): A complete review. International Journal of Pharmaceutical Sciences Review and Research 17(2); 2012: 20–28.

24. National Conference of Standards Laboratories. Establishment and Adjustment of Calibration Intervals, NCSL RP-1; 1996.

25. National Conference of Standards Laboratories. General Requirements for the Competence of Testing and Calibration Laboratories, ANSI/ISO/ IEC 17025; 2000.

26. PDA, Validation, and Qualification of Computerized Laboratory Data Acquisition Systems, Technical Report No. 31. PDA Journal of Pharmaceutical Science and Technology 53(4); 1999: 1–12.

27. PDA, Validation of Computer-Related Systems, Technical Report No. 18. PDA Journal of Pharmaceutical Science and Technology 49(1); 1995: S1–S17.

28. Pharmaceutical Inspectorate Convention/ Pharmaceutical Inspection Co-operation Scheme Guide to Good Manufacturing Practice for Medicinal Products. Rev. 3; 2002: 1–97.

29. Pharmaceutical Quality for the 21st Century: A Risk-Based Approach. Department of Health and Human Services. U.S Food and Drug Administration September; 2004.

30. Quality Assurance of Pharmaceuticals. A compendium of guidelines and related materials. 1st Vol, World Health Organization, Geneva; 1997.

31. Quality Assurance of Pharmaceuticals. A compendium of guidelines and related materials. 2nd Vol, Updated Edition. Good manufacturing practices and inspection. World Health Organization, Geneva; 2004.

32. Robert RR, Michael JM, Hal P. Developing a viable environmental monitoring program for non-sterile pharmaceutical operations. Pharmaceutical Technology 27(3); 2003: 92.

33. Sangshetti JN, Deshpande M, Zaheer Z, Shinde DB, Arote R. Quality by design approach: Regulatory need. Arabian Journal of Chemistry. 10(2); 2017: S3412–S3425.

34. Sigvardson KW, Manalo JA, Roller RW, Saless F, Wasserman D. Laboratory Equipment Qualification. Pharmaceutical Technology; 2001: 102–108.

35. Snee RD. Creating Robust Work Processes. Quality Progress 26(2); 1993: 37–41.

36. Takahashi H, Hiroshi Sakai PE, Gold DH. Case Study: Beta-Lactam Decontamination and Cleaning Validation of a Pharmaceutical Manufacturing Facility. Pharmaceutical Engineering 28(6); 2008.

37. The Rules Governing Medicinal Products in the European Community, Volume IV. Good Manufacturing Practice for Medicinal Products.

38. Tierney P, Burke R, O'Donnell B, McAteer J. Environmental Monitoring - Maintaining a Clean Room. 28; 2010. http://www.pharmpro.com/articles/2010/06/clean-rooms-Environmental-Monitoring-Maintaining-a-Clean-Room.

39. United States Pharmacopeia. 32nd Edition, 3rd Vol, National Formulary 27; 2010.

40. United States Pharmacopeia. Microbiological Evaluation of Clean rooms and other controlled environments. 32nd Edition, National Formulary 27; 2010.

Documentation

Laboratory record
Distribution records
Complaint files
- Document hierarchy
  Level 1: Manual
  Level 2: Policy

Level 3: Procedures
Level 4: Working instructions
Level 5: Records/specification/validation
- Document checklist
- Forms and Tables

KEY POINTS

- Good manufacturing practice compliance necessitates maintenance of documentation system covering all aspects of pharmaceutical production activities for traceability of all development, manufacturing and testing activities. Documentation includes all procedures, instructions, specifications, and records with complete and accurate information entered at the time of actual work performed.
- Manufacturer formulates standard operating procedure (SOP) to describe the format and design of all documents to be maintained in a particular site. Documentation format should include all information necessary to define its purpose, traceability, legibility, validity, and authorization.
- Documentation system is intended to fulfil the statutory regulatory requirement like permanent traceability of records, as a training aid, auditing, investigation and tracking of batch history, control of deviation and changes that can affect the quality, safety or efficacy of products.
- Documentation database is used to facilitate the creation, control, maintenance, tracking of all master file documents. Document control system implemented by the QA department ensures complete control over all the documents by identifying with a unique title and document number.
- Pharmaceutical as per cGMP maintain quality management system (QMS) documentation in a hierarchical manner starting manual and policies followed downward to more specific quality related documents like procedures, work instructions, and records.

SCOPE OF DOCUMENTATION

Documentation is the fundamental and integral part of good manufacturing practices. Good documentation system covers all the aspects of pharmaceutical production. Specifications, manufacturing formulae, procedures, and records must be free from errors and available in writing. A vital aspect of a GMP facility is well-written procedures. Procedures should be clear, concise, unambiguous, and easy for employees to follow. Documentation defines a system of information and control so that misinterpretation or error in oral communication is minimized. Documentation results in consistent quality and prevents errors. Documentation enables investigation of problems, errors, defects, complaints, etc., thereby determining the best corrective and preventative actions to be taken. Documentation should be available for all aspects of the manufacturing activities performed. Documentation consequently strengthens the quality and consistency of all activities associated with the manufacturing of pharmaceutical preparations including active drug substances, as it is legally mandatory. Documentation is the key to GMP compliance and ensures traceability of all regulatory, manufacturing and testing activities. Auditors assess overall quality of operations performed within a company while manufacturing a finished pharmaceutical product by routing the documentation.

Good documentation encompasses practically all the aspects of pharmaceutical production.

1. Buildings and premises: Design, validations, cleaning, and maintenance.
2. Personnel: Responsibility, training, hygiene, clothing.

3. Equipment: Installation, calibration, validation, maintenance, and cleaning.
4. Materials: Warehousing, specifications, testing, acceptance/rejection, and disposal.
5. Processing: Individual steps of the manufacturing process and controls thereof.
6. Finished goods: Specifications, testing, storage, distribution, rejection/disposal.
7. Complaints: Investigations, actions (including recall, if necessary).

GENERAL REQUIREMENTS

- Documents should be clear, concise and unambiguous
- Documentation overall includes procedures, instructions, specifications, and records.

Specifications

Specifications describe in detail the quality attributes and other requirements with which materials used during manufacturing or product obtained after manufacture have to adhere.

Specifications serve as foundation for quality evaluation of all the materials that are concerned with the production of a pharmaceutical formulation.

Manufacturing Formulae, Processing, and Packaging Instructions

Manufacturing formulae describe all the starting materials to be used for manufacturing of a particular formulation along with the processing instructions for manufacturing and packaging operations.

Procedures

Procedures give directions for performing a particular operation, e.g. cleaning, clothing, environmental control, sampling, testing, and equipment operation.

Records

Records provide a history for each batch of product, including its manufacturing, quality testing, distribution and all other relevant information pertinent to the quality of the final product. Records are also maintained for every function performed in a manufacturing facility, i.e. cleaning, training, facility maintenance, etc.

- Complete and accurate information is to be entered at the time actual work was performed. Entry of signature or initials is must (according to the procedure). When one or more persons complete a task, everyone must sign in the designated place.
- All the entries must be legible and indelible or non-erasable. Use of ballpoint ink in the approved color is recommended (other inks may smudge and cause the entry to be illegible).
- Limit the use of abbreviations and acronyms.
- Recording of information on scrap pieces of paper is not permitted. All recorded information relevant to the batch history of a product must only be made on controlled documents, logbooks or workbooks.
- Documents are custom designed, prepared, reviewed and distributed with proper supervision and authentication. Documents should comply with the relevant section of the manufacturing and marketing authorization dossiers.
- Documents are approved, signed and dated by appropriate and authorized persons.
- Documents should not be handwritten except the parts that require the entry of specific data at the time of actual performance of activities. Entries to be made in clear, legible and indelible handwriting. While preparation of a document proforma sufficient space should be provided for such entries.

- Be consistent with date and time. Always use the current version. Never use deleted or obsolete document.
- Documents including logbooks and work books that require data or any other information to be entered manually must be designed in a way that allows:
  - Sufficient space for the entry
  - Adequate spacing between entries, and
  - A clear indication of what is to be entered.
- Any corrections made to a document must be initialed or signed and dated by the person making the changes. The correction if required must be done in such a way that permits reading of the original information also. Only a single line through the middle of the original, incorrect entry should be made. If an entry error is made, no explanation for the correction is required. If the error was made for any other reason, a detailed reason for the error and correction must be recorded.

  The following are few a examples of notations that may be used to describe error corrections.
  - Transposition
  - Illegible entry
  - Scale zero error
  - Non-calibrated instrument
  - Calculation error
  - Wrong instrument
- The use of correction fluid or "liquid paper" is not allowed for correcting errors or for any other reason. The use of erasers is also prohibited.
- Documents should be regularly reviewed and revised to keep it up-to-date. Implementation of document revision system must ensure prevention of inadvertent use of superseded documents.
- Documents are to be laid out and kept in an orderly fashion for easy checking and retrival. The reproduction of working documents from master documents must not allow any error to get introduced through the reproduction process. Reproduced documents should be clear and legible.
- Any alteration to a record is required to be signed and dated with the original entry still visible. Where appropriate, the reason for such alteration is to be recorded.
- Changes to official documents should be avoided and wherever necessary must be signed by an authorized person.
- Data can be recorded by electronic data processing systems, photographic or other reliable means. Detailed procedures relating to the data processing system in use are to be made available to authorized persons, and the accuracy of the records are checked time to time. Only authorized personnel should be able to assess and enter or modify data in the computer and other electronic data processing systems handling documentation. Record of any changes and deletions are maintained, and result of any critical data entry should be independently checked. Passwords or other suitable means are implemented to restrict unauthorized access to data processing system. Batch records electronically stored must be protected by back-up transfer on CD, DVD, hard disk, microchip or other suitable means. It is particularly important to ensure the ready availability of data throughout the retention period.
- A controlled document template should be created for each document type. This template can then be used by all personnel who are permitted to write or fill information in documents.
- All relevant records concerning significant activities related to manufacturing

of medicinal products are to be entered and completed at the time particular action taking place. The documents are retained for at least one year after the expiry date of the finished product.

COMMON GUIDELINES FOR THE PREPARATION OF DOCUMENTS

Standard Operating Procedure (SOP) for Documentation

For development and formatting the documents, a standard operating procedure should be followed. A standard operating procedure (SOP) is formulated to define the format of all types of in site documentation. Documents should have unambiguous content and follow a logical sequence and standard design. The following should be considered before preparing a new document:

- The method by which the documents are to be reproduced to ensure a clear and legible copy.
- The proposed use of the document to provide or to record information.
- Location of information for efficient usage.
- The size, shape, and layout to ensure that there is sufficient space to record information clearly and to be compatible with filing facilities.
- Signatures of the person prepared and authorized the document.
- Period of validity (expiry)

Information Incorporated in Documentation Format

1. The name of the company and site
2. Clear title
3. A document identification number system is needed to be established for the various types of documents that are created. Examples: GEN-001 (general SOPs), TM-001 (test methods), BR-001 (batch records), QP-001 (quality policy).
4. Space of signature of persons, i.e. prepared by, authorized by, approved by, etc.
5. Name of authorized person approving the document.
6. The date of issue
7. Record of circulation (e.g. copy number)
8. Remark column

Precautions and Practices Followed in the Documentation

1. Sufficient space should be provided for making entries (e.g. temperature, weight).
2. Instruction should be precise and not ambiguous
3. All entries should be clear and legible.
4. An error in the entry should be so corrected that the original (wrong) entry is not lost, such entry should be dated.
5. Reasons for correction should also be recorded, initiated and dated in remark column.
6. Periodic review and revision of documented system should be provided. The authorized person should also approve such revised version.
7. Updated/revised, versions shall supersede the previous edition, and the document shall indicate this.
8. Outdated/superseded document should be immediately removed from active use, and copy retained only for reference.
9. The computerized documented system should ensure correctness of data and to record changes (addition/deletion) and should restrict access only to authorized persons.
10. Documents should be kept in such a manner that permits quick, easy and reliable retrieval of data, allows review up to a predetermined time in the past and meet regulatory requirements.

TYPES OF DOCUMENT

Quality Manual

A document that describes, in paragraph form, the regulations and/or parts of the regulations that the company is required to follow. It also contains instructions written in-house to be followed for the use of equipment, systems or processes.

Quality Policies

Quality policy documents describe, in general terms, the overall guidelines for implementation of specific GMP and quality aspects (such as documentation, training, responsibilities). It is considered as the quality statement of management for implementation and application related to activities and processes carried out within the organization to achieve the common goal of the company.

Standard Operating Procedures (SOPs)

Step-by-step instructions for performing a particular operation, task or activity is compiled in the SOPs. SOPs are issued to specifically instruct the employees about responsibility, work instructions, appropriate specifications, and required records. SOPs outline procedures, which must be followed to claim compliance with GMP principles or other statutory rules and regulations. Procedures can take the form of a narrative, a flow chart, a process map, or any other suitable form, however, must be written in an appropriate, competent manner in the correct grammatical style.

Instructions and Records

Batch Records: Batch records provide step-by-step instructions for production related tasks and activities. These documents are typically utilized and data entry completed by the manufacturing department.

Method of analysis: These documents are typically developed, used and maintained by the quality control department. Test methods provide step-by-step instructions for testing of supplied, materials, products, and other production related tasks and activities such as environmental monitoring of the GMP facility. Test methods contain forms which are used for documenting the testing process and the results of the testing at the end of the procedure.

Specifications: Documents that list the requirements that the supplied materials and the finished products must comply before being released for use or sale. The quality control department compare the test results with the predefined specifications to decide if the product passes or fails the approval.

Logbooks: Logbooks are bound collection of data entry forms used to document activities. Logbooks are used for documenting the operation, maintenance and calibration of equipment. Logbooks are also used for recording of clean room activities monitoring, solution preparations, deviation and corrective action and other related assignments.

Audit Report: An audit is a systematic and independent review to verify compliance, suitability and/or data integrity. Audit report assesses the overall systems, processes, procedures, facilities, products, records and/or data for compliance with policies, standards, procedures, guidelines and regulatory submissions.

Investigation/Incident Meeting Minutes: It contains a report of the finding of investigations regarding the occurrence of incidences, causalities documented in systematic order.

Quality Template: Template used for creating a particular document.

Vendor Audit Report: Audit report prepared after vendor evaluation.

DOCUMENT PREPARATION

Document communicates information concerning a wide range of activities carried out during pharmaceutical manufacturing and control operations, providing detailed and clear instructions. Written statements, whether maintained on hard copy or generated electronically it is always intended to avoid the risk of misinterpretation inherent in oral communication. Comprehensive guidance on requirements of document preparation procedure is essential for the development of errorless documentation system in manufacturing and control of medicinal products. Regulatory monographs are useful reference sources for preparing documents.

Policy documents of a company give an overview of the company's organization which aids in the achievement of management policy goal, personnel department activities and the persons accountable for ensuring proper functioning of the administration. Specifications are documents which describe starting materials, packaging materials, intermediate, the bulk or finished products regarding their chemical, physical and when appropriate biological characteristics. Specification usually includes descriptive clauses and numerical clauses, which define standards and permitted tolerances. Procedures are formal written instructions, with detail on how an operation is to be performed. These are required for all operations, which can affect the safety, identify, strength, quality and purity standards of medicinal products. Such documents are often termed SOPs or standard operating procedures. Work instructions are batch-related documents, which lists all the starting materials to be used and the steps of production operations.

Records are completed documents like reports, instructions, protocols, logbooks, log sheets, etc., that are used to record performance information. They provide a history of each batch of the product together with data pertaining to the quality of the final product. Documentation system is intended to fulfil the following requirements.

Regulatory requirement: Statutory regulations regarding the manufacturing and sale of pharmaceutical products need a detailed documentation system to be implemented and maintained for further verification.

Permanent traceable record: Records enable information to be recorded clearly and unambiguously in documented form, enabling tracing the events that happened during pharmaceutical production operation. Documentation provides an accurate record of observed values and events.

Consistent training: Documentation serves as a useful training aid. Legibly written documents are a prerequisite of effective training procedures. They help to ensure that personnel, when required to undertake a new task, are provided with the necessary information on how the task should be completed.

Auditing: Documentation is essential for maintaining the 'audit trail' which allows subsequent investigation and tracking of batch history.

Control of deviation and changes: Accidental, unintentional deviations or planned changes in an operation must be recorded, reviewed and authorized to ensure that they do not have an adverse effect on the quality, safety or efficacy of the product.

CONTROL OF DOCUMENTATION

It is critical for any pharmaceutical manufacturing facility that all activities that are performed should be clearly defined. Written procedures should be defined for controlling the preparation, approval, issue, updating, and change of all documentation. The procedures should also ensure that only current and approved documentation are to be issued or used. All completed records should be securely achieved to ensure availability for inspection or review as and when needed. Control of documentation must be assigned as responsibilities of one particular department, preferably the QA, and the system must be implemented to ensure consistency (Fig. 6.1).

Document Preparation

The preparation of documents is best done by those involved in and are familiar with the processes and procedures. There should be a guide for the preparation of all types of documents in the form of standard operating procedures, containing details of the sources of information required to prepare a particular document. The guide should also provide guidance on style and formatting of the document. Preparation of document should be done using means that minimize the risks of reprocessing and rechecking.

Indexing and Numbering

Master documents should be indexed, and this may be done in a number of ways. Editions (versions) of the document should be differentiated; it is best to use a numbering system. A computer database is a suitable mean of storing the series of numbers, as updated and reviewed for a comfortable and rapid referral. The numbering system should embrace documentation for all company activities which have an influence on good manufacturing practice, for example, SOPs, manufacturing and packaging documents, quality control specifications and methods, sampling procedures and record sheets.

For example, SOPs could be 001 to 999; manufacturing document could be 1000 to 1999, etc. Further sub-division can also be done as per requirement within a particular section, like SOPs can be subdivided by different departments, for example, QC specifications and sampling procedures may be divided into starting materials, intermediates or packaging components, etc., with particular subseries of numbers.

Approval of the Document

Authorized persons from appropriate departments should approve all documentation, and the scope of their approval must be defined

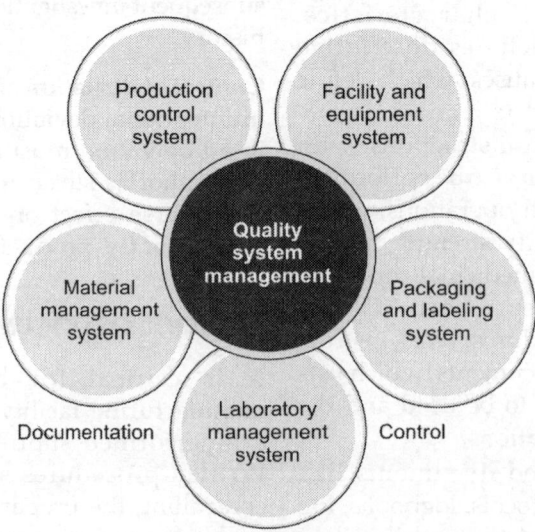

Fig. 6.1: Quality system management based on documentation control

in the procedure. The level of authority of the approver depends on the document or section in question. Whenever contract work is carried out for a third party, a responsible person in the contract-givers company should also approve the documents.

Distribution and Control of Copies

Copies of documents should be available in the relevant departments other than that no unauthorized copies should be retained. This enables systematic issuance of reviewed and updated documents and the withdrawal of superseded ones in an orderly fashion. It also prevents the use of outdated documents. There should be a proper procedure for authenticating official copies and maintaining a list of recipients and return dates. Batch-related documents, e.g. manufacturing or packaging instructions are commonly produced by photocopying a master document or by computer copy generation from a database for each batch to be produced.

Document Review

A document review mechanism is must for regular updating of all procedures. The review should be carried out by those who are directly involved in procedure implementation. Batch-related documentation should be reviewed frequently taking into account process data generated and experience gained since the last review, bearing in mind the impact of the implication of any proposed changes on the consistency of regulatory status of the product in the marketing segments. The QA, QC and/or production department should approve all changes as appropriated by the regulatory affairs department. Specification review should take into account data, experience and issues such as changes in regulatory requirements or changes in the official monograph for the product. The QA department should approve changes and if

appropriate also by the regulatory affairs department.

Organization

One department should have control over document issue and archival. While internal control rests with the appointed department, as much of the pharmaceutical documents are developed by the department, which ultimately uses it.

Storage and Archiving

Storage of documentation is achieved by using hard copies, in a magnetic disc, microfilm, microfiche, optical disc or in the digital storage device. As a precaution against loss of stored documents, duplicate copies are to be made and kept in a separate location. Caution is necessary when new technology is being utilized to ensure consistency and reliability. Copies of all editions (versions) of master documents should be stored for five years from being superseded, although product liability law, and health and safety considerations may call for more extended storage. This may be achieved by storing in hard copy, in microfilm or by electronic means. Batch related documentation should be stored for at least six years beyond the manufacturing date of the batch. Samples of raw materials and finished products both as bulk and in the pack also constitute part of the batch records and should be retained for a similar period as do associated chart record/print-outs which may be stored separately.

Document Entries

Persons making entries on documents should use clear and legible writing to confirm the entry with initials or signature and where appropriate the date. Entries should be made with ink or another permanent medium. Positive entries should be made in writing or with ticks, but ditto marks are avoided. Errors should be corrected such that the original entry is not lost and the correction is signed and dated. Where appropriate the reason for the change should be added. Correction fluids must not be used. If a page becomes illegible or otherwise unacceptable, a new page can be added, but the old page should also be retained and endorsed as the original to this effect.

Documentation Database

The documentation database is used to facilitate the creation, control, maintenance and tracking of quality, external and master file documents. These are also referred to as 'Controlled Documents'. The documentation database has three major areas of control:

1. Quality documents (in-house and external): This area of the documentation database stores data for controlling and maintaining quality related documentation. Quality documents are prepared for control methods, raw material specification, test methods, finished goods specification, test reports and stability specifications.

2. Quality audits: This area of the documentation database facilitates control of the quality audit program including scheduling and auditor assignment.

3. Master file documents: This documentation database stores data for controlling and maintaining a master file which comprised of both technical and quality documents needed for manufacturing a product (Fig. 6.2).

DOCUMENT CONTROL SYSTEM

Document control system ensures complete control over all the authorized documents. A unique title and document number should identify all documents. The document should be designed, prepared, received, approved, signed and dated by authorized persons and distributed to concerned departments. Approved documents are not allowed to correct manually with a pen or pencil for any possible reason. The QAs role in documentation system is to manage and overview the implementation. QA ensures that all documents are maintained in a controlled fashion. The subject matter experts approve all procedures used within a company, that should be of the most current version and consistent with all other documents. One way by which QA ensures this is by checking the last signature on all approved documents. All documents, i.e. current, obsolete, superseded, as well as all the history on the creation and revision of the document are kept with quality assurance.

Creation

Experienced and knowledgeable employees are given the responsibility to write or revise documents as needed. All the relevant changes are made with red ink or redline along with detailed justification of the changes while revising a document.

Routing

The document control persons of QA is responsible for routing documents for review and approval. A pre-route should be ensured including all affected parties in agreement before the document is submitted to QA. There should be a documented process detailing with how documents are to be submitted for review and approval.

Approval

The MASTER document is routed for approval signatures. Typically the approval signatures are made by the respective department and QA head. Usually, the approval signatures mostly appear on the first page of the document. Following approval signature of the master document, effective date is stamped onto each page of the document. The documents are cirlulated in advance of the effective date so that all the effective

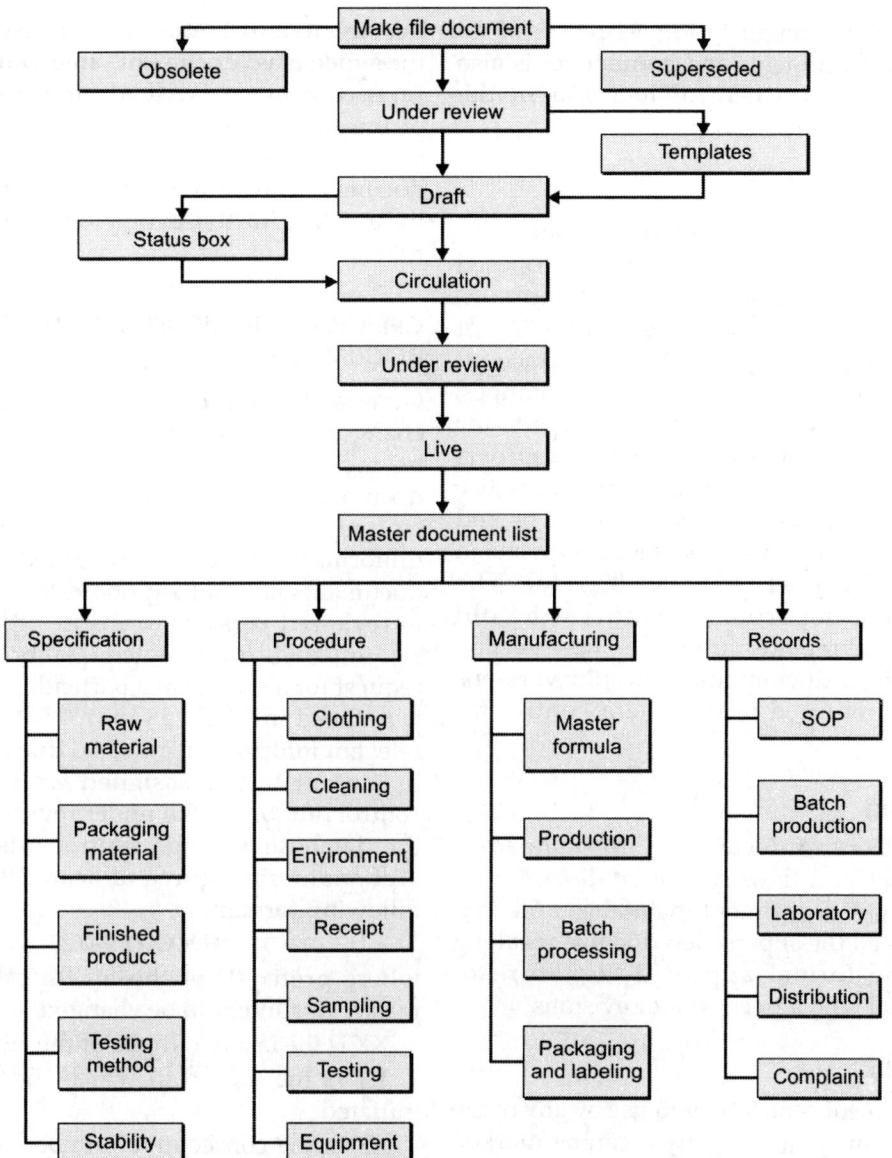

Fig. 6.2: Document database control system

departments get well informed before it becomes active (typically this is five days).

Distribution

Exactly on the effective date copies of the signed MASTER, document is routed to the affected departments.

Auditing

The document control personnel audit the binders on a periodic basis to assure that they contain the correct versions. Each document binder has a table of contents and contains only those documents that pertain to the functions the department, and it is responsible for. QA department holds a full set of all approved documents and another set is also maintained in a central location in the company.

Reviewing

Document review starts with circulation of a Change Control Form listing all the proposed changes to be made to the document, justification for the changes and a list of personnel who needs to review. Once all affected parties have agreed to the changes, the document control department prepares the revised version of the document for approval incorporating all changes. In common practice a new documents the version will be 00 and for each revision of a document the version number increases (01, 02, 03, etc). The respective department removes the old version and replaces it with the new version (for revised documents). The old versions must be returned to document control for archival.

Archiving

Old versions of documents are stamped as *superseded*, and these cannot be discarded or altered. QA department maintains a file that contains all the superseded documents along with the formal approval signature of personnel who agreed to the revisions.

Obsolete

If a document is no longer in use by any of the departments of a company it can be marked as obsolete. This particular document is stamped as *obsolete*, and previously distributed copies are removed from all document binders.

Superseded

The superseded *master* copy is retained with the *obsolete* copy stamped in black color for future reference, and the controlled and display copies are destroyed. Record of

documents issue, retrieval, and destruction of the superseded documents are maintained. A revised document is issued only after retrieval of the superseded control copy and display copy from concerned departments. All documents are retained for at least one year in addition to the expiry date of finished products.

CREATION AND MODIFICATION OF DOCUMENTS

General format and styles should not be changed in the template. The body layout may be modified to suit the purpose of the document, i.e. flowcharts, visual aids, tables, etc. may be added. The header's and footer's uniformity should be maintained for all the documents and not supposed to be changed in reviewed versions to ensure conformance to company's documented quality system. A request for a change in a particular document is initiated in Change Control Form with all relevant information attached due for change in the document, assigned with a change control number in the under review folder of the database. Change control numbers are alphanumeric figures allocated using the following format:

$$ID\text{-}XX\ YY\text{-}ZZ$$

where prefix ID is chosen for the type of master document to be changed

XX is the last two digits of the current year

YY is the month in which the change is initiated

ZZ is the consecutive number of changes for the specified document

Ensure that document number, and the change control number does not interchange. When the revised version of the document is ready, remove the original electronic version from the live folder of the database to the superseded folder. Replace it with the changed file with appropriate version number from the draft folder and update master document list. Retrieve the hard superseded copy from the master document file, stamp with "Superseded" and place it in the superseded master document file. File one changed and approved hard copy in the master document file.

Document Issuing and Maintaining

1. During issue of a document the necessary entries are made in the respective document control register with details like document name, document number, issued by, received by, retrieved document no (if any), number of copies retrieved, destroyed by, date, checked by and other relevant details (Fig. 6.3).

2. Photocopies of master copy are issued for regular production and filed in BMR/BPR. All sheets of photocopies should be signed and dated by QA personnel.
3. The completed batch record should come back to QA for review.
4. Validation protocol/Report/Summary: All validation protocols/reports/summary to be prepared by QA and issued to respective department.
5. The validation protocols, reports along with the QC results and summary reports are prepared and filed in respective validation records by the QA department after completion of validation.

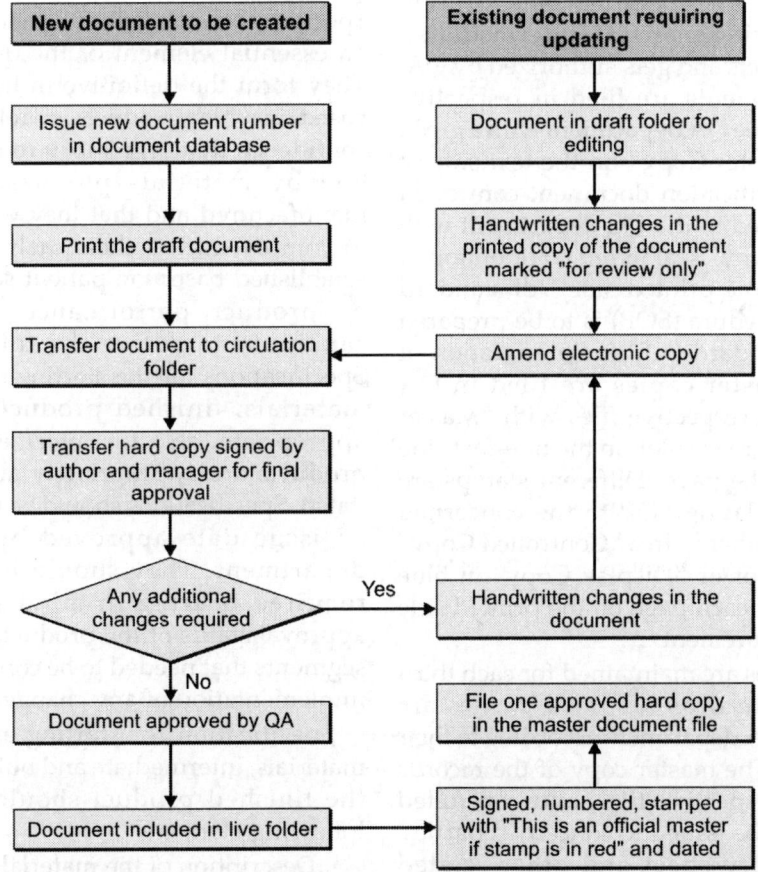

Fig. 6.3: Quality document management and change control system

6. Protocols and reports of cleaning validation with the QC analytical reports filed in the cleaning validation file.
7. Equipment qualification protocols and reports are issued by QA to the respective department.
8. QA compile all completed equipment qualification protocol and reports in individual qualification files:

Note: If the document is printed at any stage without the red stamp on it, it must be identified as an Uncontrolled Copy and must be destroyed within one day.

DOCUMENT MAINTENANCE

QC prepares all specifications of raw material/packing material/intermediate/finished products and gets authorized by QA. Original documents are filed in respective master files in the QA department with a green color seal "Master Copy" on the text side of the page. Specification document controlled copies are issued to the QC department with "Controlled Copy" seal in red color on top of each page on the printed side. All standard operating procedure (SOP) is to be prepared as per the standard SOP for preparation of SOP. SOP master copies are filed in QA department in respective files with "Master Copy" seal in green color on the non-text side (backside) of the page. Different stamps are used for circulating SOP to the concerned departments either with a "Controlled Copy" seal in red color or "Display Copy" in blue color on top of each page on the printed side as per the requirement.

Separate files are maintained for each third party. Batch records for third parties are prepared by QA department according to their requirement. The master copy of the records are filed in respective files, and controlled copies should be issued to concerned parties. Batch summary sheet and other related documents are collected, reviewed and filed by QA. All documents related to approval of artwork and the sample specimens are filed and controlled by both QC and QA department. Specification of stability samples is maintained by QC department separately.

DOCUMENTATION GUIDELINE FOR DIFFERENT SECTIONS

This section provides a comprehensive guideline on the documents required to be developed and maintained by different sections of pharmaceutical manufacturing company along with the details that are to be included in a particular document.

Specifications

Specifications for materials and products are an essential element of the quality system. They form the definitive in-house standard based on which products are released with the confidence that regulatory requirements are met by materials purchased, products manufactured and that they would continue to comply during their shelf life. They are established based on patient safety, material or product performance and process capability to define the tolerance limit. Specifications for the starting and packaging materials, finished products and where appropriate, also for intermediate or bulk products are appropriately authorized and dated. Specifications should be in writing with an issue date approved by the quality department. They should be updated as required bearing in mind the licensing approval status of the products in all market segments that needed to be considered before implementation of any change.

Specification for starting and packaging materials, intermediate and bulk product and the finished product should include the following elements:

- Description of the material.
- Designated name with company reference code.

- Names of approved manufacturers and suppliers.
- Specimen of printed materials.
- Sampling procedure, testing and retesting requirements and shelf life.
- Qualitative and quantitative requirements with acceptance limits.
- Storage conditions.
- Special precautions.
- Details of any factorization procedure if applicable.
- Requirements for reference samples.
- Drawings with dimensions.

Specification for purchasing procedure should be agreed with the supplier and include the following elements:

- Designated supplier and material manufacturer.
- Supplier and company reference code.
- The physical, chemical and wherever applicable microbiological parameters with limits and the test methods to be used.
- Sampling plans, quality levels, and acceptance/rejection criteria.
- The method to be used for packaging the material, e.g. container type, quantity per container, number of containers per pallet and labeling requirements. Documentation procedures
- Special conditions, when applicable for transport and storage.
- The documentation requirements of the supplier, including safety information booklets and certificates of analysis or conformity.

Analytical documents containing the results of analysis and testing of all starting materials, intermediates, bulk, and finished products should be recorded. There is also requirement for a policy and/or procedure to define retesting and investigation of out of specification results.

Starting materials testing records include:

- Date of receipt.
- Name of material, (in-house name).
- The batch number.
- The results of all tests carried out, including those obtained from a supplier's certificate of analysis, which should be identified as such.
- Identity of the person carried out the tests.
- Signed decision of the QC department on the status of the material, e.g. released, rejected or other status.
- Where potency is known to be variable, a clear statement of the values.
- Status decision and status review date or expiry date of the material.

Packaging components testing record should include:

- Date of receipt.
- Date of testing.
- Name of the component (in-house name).
- Batch number.
- Results of all tests carried out, including those provided by the supplier.
- Identify the person who carried out the tests.
- A signed decision by the quality department on the status of the component, released, rejected or other.

Intermediate, bulk, and finished product testing records should include:

- Date of manufacturing of the stage.
- Date of sampling and testing.
- Batch number.
- Name of the product (in-house name)

Specifications for Starting and Packaging Materials

Starting and primary or printed packaging materials Specifications should include:

a. Description of the materials, including;
   - The designated name and the internal reference code.
   - The reference to particular pharmacopoeial monograph.
   - The approved suppliers and the original producer of the products.
   - Specimen of printed packaging materials.
b. Procedures for sampling and testing or reference to the standard procedure.
c. Qualitative and quantitative acceptance limits requirements.
d. Storage conditions and handling precautions.
e. The maximum permissible storage period before retesting and reuse.

Specifications for Intermediate and Bulk Products

Specifications for intermediate and bulk products should also be available when purchased from external sources, or if data obtained from intermediate products are used for the evaluation of the finished product. The specifications should be similar to starting materials or for finished products, as appropriate.

Specifications for Finished Products

Specifications for finished products include:

a. The designated name of the product and the reference code where applicable.
b. The formula or a reference to the formula.
c. A description of the pharmaceutical form with the package details.
d. Procedure for sampling and testing or a reference to the standard procedure.
e. The qualitative and quantitative requirements, with the acceptance limits.

f. The storage conditions and special handling precautions, where applicable.
g. The shelf-life.

Specifications for the Testing Procedures

Specifications are developed for all raw materials, active pharmaceutical ingredients, excipients, in-process samples, packaging components, and finished products along with shelf life stability. The specification may include physical, chemical microbiological and functional attributes based on customer, company and regulatory requirements. For compendial items, compendial specifications are a minimum. SOPs must be there in place to ensure appropriate justification for specifications, approval of appropriate departments, including the quality unit and change control. Specifications for the testing procedures include the following:

a. A qualitative statement about the state (e.g. size, shape, solid, liquid) and color of the drug substance or product. If any of these characteristics changes during storage period, it should be investigated, and appropriate action is taken. The acceptance criteria specification includes the final approved acceptable appearance.
b. Identification tests should be specific for a drug substance, for example, identification solely by single chromatographic retention time is not regarded as being specific. However, the use of at least two chromatographic procedures, where the separation is based on different principles or a combination of tests into a single procedure, such as HPLC/UV diode array, HPLC/MS, or GC/MS is generally acceptable. The identification testing should be specific for the individual ions when the drug substance is in salt form. An identification test that is specific for the salt itself should suffice. Identification testing should optimally be able to discriminate between compounds of

closely related structure which are likely to be present.

c. Optically active drug substances need specific identification testing or performance of a chiral assay. Specific stability-indicating procedures are included to determine the content (strength) of the drug substance, though, in many instances, it is possible to employ the same procedure (e.g. HPLC) for both assays of the drug substance and quantitation of impurities. In cases where a non-specific assay method is employed, it is to be justified with other supporting analytical procedures to achieve overall specificity. For example, where titration is adopted as assay method for the drug substance, a suitable test for impurities should be used in combination of the assay.

d. Organic and inorganic impurities and residual solvents are included in impurity profiling.

Drug substances

In addition to the comprehensive tests listed above, the following tests can also be considered on a case to case basis for drug substances and/or drug products. Individual tests/criteria are to be included in the specification when the tests have an impact on the quality of the drug substance and drug product for batch control.

a. *Physicochemical properties:* These properties are as pH of an aqueous solution, melting point/range, refractive index, etc. The tests required to be performed in this category are decided based on the physical nature of the new drug substance and by its intended use.

b. *Particle size:* Particle size determination is necessary for some new drug substances intended to be used in solid or suspension drug products as it has significant effect on dissolution rates, bioavailability, and/ or stability.

c. *Polymorphic forms:* Some drug substances exist in different crystalline forms that differ in physical properties. Polymorphism may also include solvation or hydration products (also known as pseudopolymorphs) and amorphous forms.

d. *Tests for chiral form:* When drug substance is predominantly one enantiomer, the opposite enantiomer is excluded from the qualification and identification thresholds.

e. *Water content:* This test is essential when the drug substance is known to be hygroscopic or degraded by moisture or when the drug substance is known to be a stoichiometric hydrate. The acceptance criteria are justified with data on the effects of hydration, or moisture absorption using specific detection procedure for water (e.g. Karl Fischer titration) is preferred.

f. *Inorganic impurities:* Inclusion of tests and acceptance criteria for inorganic impurities (e.g. catalysts) are mostly based on knowledge of the manufacturing process studied during development stage. Procedures and acceptance criteria for sulfated ash/residue on ignition should follow pharmacopoeial precedents. Other inorganic impurities may be determined by appropriate non-pharmacopoeial procedures, e.g. atomic absorption spectroscopy.

g. *Microbial limits:* Total count of aerobic microorganisms, the total count of yeasts and molds, and the absence of specific objectionable bacteria (e.g. *Staphylococcus aureus, Escherichia coli, Salmonella, Pseudomonas aeruginosa*) are performed as per the specific need of drug substances using pharmacopoeial procedures. In microbiological terms, pharmaceutical products can be divided into two groups: Sterile and non-sterile. The type of microbial test(s) and acceptance criteria are based on the nature of the drug substance, method of manufacture and the intended use of the drug product. For example, sterility testing is appropriate for drug substances manufactured as a sterile product and endotoxin testing is appropriate for drug substances used to formulate an injectable drug product.

Drug products

Additional tests and acceptance criteria generally depends on the nature of particular drug product. The following selection presents the representative tests to be performed on sample of the drug products and the types of tests and acceptance criteria which may be appropriate. The specific dosage forms addressed here includes solid oral drug products, liquid oral drug products and parenteral (small and large volume).

Solid dosage form

The following tests apply to tablets (coated and uncoated) and hard capsules. One or more of these tests are also applicable to soft capsules and granules.

  a. *Dissolution:* The specification for solid oral dosage forms typically includes this test to measure the release potential of drug substance from the drug product. Single-point measurements are normally considered suitable for immediate-release dosage forms. Appropriate test conditions and sampling procedures are to be established for modified-release dosage forms. For example, multiple time point sampling are performed for extended-release dosage forms, and two-stage testing (using different media in succession or parallel, as appropriate) may be appropriate for delayed-release dosage forms.

  b. *Disintegration:* Disintegration may be substituted for dissolution for rapidly dissolving (dissolution >80% in 15 minutes at pH 1.2, 4.0 and 6.8) products

containing highly soluble drugs throughout the physiological range (dose/solubility volume <250 ml from pH 1.2 to 6.8). Disintegration testing is most appropriate when a relationship dissolution parameters has been established or when disintegration is shown to be more discriminating than dissolution. In such cases, dissolution testing may not be necessary.

  c. *Hardness/friability:* It is usually appropriate to perform hardness and/or friability testing as an in-process control. It is not necessary to include these attributes in the specification unless the hardness and friability characteristics have a critical impact on drug product quality (e.g. chewable tablets). For such cases acceptance criteria should be included in the specification.

  d. *Uniformity of dosage units:* This term includes both the mass of the dosage form and the content of the active substance in the dosage form and generally, the specifications include one or the other but not both. If appropriate, these tests may be performed in in-process material also. A pharmacopoeial procedure should be used, and the acceptance criteria should be included in the specification. When weight variation is applied for drug products exceeding the threshold value to allow testing uniformity by weight variation, adequate homogeneity of the product should be verified during drug development.

  e. *Water content:* Test for water content is included when appropriate, but the acceptance criteria is justified with data on the effects of hydration or water absorption on the drug product.

  f. *Microbial limits:* Microbial limit testing is an attribute of both GMP regulation as well as quality assurance. In general, it is advisable to test the drug product unless its components are tested before manufacture. It is not mandatory when the manufacturing process is known, through validation studies, not to carry a significant risk of microbial contamination or proliferation. These are applicable to excipients as well as to new drug products.

Oral liquids

One or more of the following specific tests are applied to oral liquids and powders intended for reconstitution as oral liquids.

a. *Uniformity of dosage units:* This is applied to both single-dose and multiple dose packages. The dosage unit is considered to be the typical dose taken by the patients, measured either directly or calculated based on the total measured weight or volume of drug divided by the total number of doses taken per day. When dispensing equipment (droppers or dropper tips for bottles) is an integral part of the packaging, this equipment is used to measure the dose. Otherwise, standard volume measures are used. Testing for uniformity of mass is generally considered necessary in case of powders for reconstitution.

b. *pH:* Acceptance criteria for pH are provided where applicable and the proposed range justified.

c. *Microbial limits*: Non-sterile oral liquid products must satisfy the appropriate microbiological purity criteria as set out in pharmacopoeial monographs for the microbiological specifications, criteria and the methods for the microbial examination of non-sterile products.

d. *Antimicrobial preservative content:* Acceptance criteria for preservative content should be established for oral liquids containing an antimicrobial preservative. Acceptance criteria for preservative content are based upon the levels of antimicrobial preservative necessary to add in the formulation to maintain microbiological quality of the product at all stages throughout its proposed usage and shelf-life. The lowest specified concentration of antimicrobial preservative used in the formulation should be demonstrated to be effective in controlling microorganisms by using a pharmacopoeial antimicrobial preservative effectiveness test. Testing for antimicrobial preservative content is normally performed at release.

e. *Antioxidant preservative content:* Release testing for antioxidant content is normally performed, but under certain circumstances, release testing may suffice when justified by developmental and stability data, and in-process testing. The acceptance criteria remain as a part of the specification when antioxidant content testing is performed as an in-process test, but when it is done only as release testing, this decision of reinvestigation depends on any changes in part of manufacturing procedure or the container/closure system.

f. *Extractables:* Tests and acceptance criteria for extractable from the container/closure system components (e.g. rubber stopper, cap liner, plastic bottle, etc.) are considered appropriate for oral solutions packaged in non-glass systems, or glass containers with non-glass closures. Test of extractable can be eliminated when developmental, and stability data showed evidence that extractable from the container/closure systems are consistently below levels that are demonstrated to be acceptable and safe. This is required to be reinvestigated if the container/closure system or formulation changes.

g. *Alcohol content:* The alcohol content should be quantitatively specified on the label in accordance with pertinent regulations.

h. *Dissolution:* For oral suspensions and dry powder products for resuspension, it may be appropriate (e.g. insoluble drug substance) to include dissolution testing along with acceptance criteria. Dissolution testing is mostly performed at release stage but may also be performed as an in-process test as required justified by product development data. The testing apparatus, media, and conditions should be Pharmacopoeial or otherwise justified and should be validated. Acceptance criteria are set based on the observed range of variation and also take into account the dissolution profiles of the batches showing acceptable *in vivo* performance. Developmental data should be considered when determining the need for either a dissolution procedure or a particle size distribution procedure.

i. *Particle size distribution:* Quantitative acceptance criteria regarding the percent of total particles in given size range. moreover, the adoption of procedure for the determination of particle size distribution is appropriate for oral suspensions. Acceptance criteria should be set based on the observed range of variation taking into account the dissolution profiles of the batches that showed acceptable performance *in vivo*, as well as the intended use of the product. The mean level of upper and/or lower particle size limits are to be well defined. The potential for particle growth should be investigated during product development, and the acceptance criteria should take the results of these studies into account. Particle size distribution testing can be proposed in place of dissolution testing with valid justification.

j. *Redispersibility:* Acceptance criteria for redispersibility is appropriate for oral suspensions with a tendency to settle on storage (produce sediment). Shaking before use is an appropriate procedure for patients but must be indicated in the labeling. The time required to achieve resuspension by the indicated procedure should be clearly defined.

k. *Rheological properties:* For relatively viscous solutions or suspensions, it is appropriate to include rheological properties (viscosity/specific gravity) in the specification with test procedure and acceptance criteria.

l. *Reconstitution time:* Acceptance criteria for reconstitution time are provided for dry powder products which require reconstitution with the justification of choice of diluent.

m. *Water content:* For oral products requiring reconstitution, test and acceptance criterion for water content are proposed when appropriate. When the effect of absorbed moisture versus water of hydration has been adequately characterized during the development of the product, determination of loss on drying is generally considered sufficient.

Parenteral drug products

The following tests apply to parenteral drug products.

a. *Uniformity of dosage units:* This test is applied to both single-dose and multiple-dose packages, especially on powders for reconstitution, uniformity of mass testing is generally considered acceptable using a pharmacopoeial procedure.

b. *pH:* Acceptance criteria for pH is to be provided where applicable with the proposed range justified.

c. *Sterility:* All parenteral products must have a test procedure and acceptance criterion for the evaluation of sterility. Parametric release approach may be proposed for terminally sterilized drug products, justified based on data generated during development and validation.

d. *Endotoxins/Pyrogens:* Test procedure and acceptance criterion for endotoxins, using the Limulus Amoebocyte Lysate test is typically included in the specification of parenteral products. Pyrogenicity testing may be proposed as an alternative to endotoxin testing where justified.

e. *Particulate matter:* Parenteral products must have appropriate acceptance criteria for particulate matter. This will generally include acceptance criteria for visible particulates and/or clarity of solution, as well as for sub-visible particulates as appropriate.

f. *Water content:* Test procedure and acceptance criterion for water content is proposed when appropriate for products requiring reconstitution and non-aqueous parenterals.

g. *Antimicrobial preservative content:* Parenteral products containing antimicrobial preservative, acceptance criteria for preservative content should be established based on the levels of antimicrobial preservative necessary to maintain microbiological quality of the product throughout its proposed usage and shelf life. The lowest specified concentration of antimicrobial preservative effective in controlling microorganisms is established by pharmacopoeial antimicrobial preservative effectiveness test.

h. *Antioxidant preservative content:* Release testing for antioxidant content is usually performed, if testing is performed as an in-process test, the acceptance criteria should remain part of the specification.

i. *Extractables:* Control of extractables from container/closure systems is considered significantly important for parenteral products compared to oral liquids. However, the test can be eliminated when development and stability data showed evidence of the consistently low level of extractables that demonstrated to be acceptable and safe. Acceptance criteria for extractables from the container/closure components are considered appropriate for parenteral products packaged in non-glass systems or glass containers with elastomeric closures where data demonstrate the need. The components of the container/closure system (e.g. rubber stopper, metal closure, etc.) are listed, and acceptance criteria data are collected for these components early in the development process.

j. *Functionality testing of delivery systems:* Parenteral formulations packaged in pre-filled syringes, autoinjector cartridges or equivalent should have test procedures and acceptance criteria related to the functionality of the delivery system. These include control of syringeability, pressure and seal integrity (leakage), and/or parameters such as tip cap removal force, piston release force, piston travel force and power injector function force.

k. *Osmolarity:* When tonicity of a product is declared in its labeling, appropriate control for its osmolarity should be performed.

l. *Particle size distribution:* Quantitative acceptance criteria and procedure for the determination of particle size distribution is appropriate for injectable suspensions and can also be used in place of dissolution testing when development studies demonstrate that particle size is the primary factor influencing dissolution. The acceptance criteria should include acceptable particle size distribution with well-defined mean, upper and/or lower particle size limits based on the observed range of variation, *in vivo* performance and intended use.

m. *Redispersibility:* Acceptance criteria for redispersibility is considered appropriate for injectable suspensions that can settle on storage (produce sediment).

n. *Reconstitution time:* Acceptance criteria for reconstitution time are provided for all parenteral products that require reconstitution with choice of diluents.

MANUFACTURING, FORMULAE, PROCESSING AND PACKAGING INSTRUCTIONS

Master Formula Record

Master Formula Record is a product specific document complied, checked, authorized and approved by competent technical personnel from different, but interlinked departments including formulation development, production, packaging, and QC. Master formula record is a written procedure dated and signed by competent technical staff and independently checked, dated and signed by authorized person. To assure batch to batch uniformity, master formula record for each drug product, including batch size is prepared.

Master formula record contains batch manufacturing record (BMR), batch packing record (BPR), intermediate/packing material/finished product specification and a specimen of printed packaging material. All documents of master formula record is stamped as Master Copy in green at the non-text side (back side). Like other documentation, master formula Record is also processed for review and changes, if any, approved by designated persons responsible for production and QC.

Master formula record shall include:

a. Patent/proprietary name of the drug product and its strength.

b. Pharmacopoeial/generic name of the drug product and its strength

c. Dosage form (e.g. tablet, ampoule) and physical characteristics (e.g. bi-convex tables, fill volume of the ampoule, printing on a capsule, etc.) of the drug product.

d. Detailed information on drug product containers, closures, primary and secondary packaging materials.

e. The name and weight/measure of active ingredients per dosage unit or unit weight/measure of the product and total weight/measure of any dosage unit.

f. Identity, quality, and quantity of every ingredient, including overages/assay value based quantities, if any.

g. Complete list of all the ingredients used in the manufacturing of the drug product indicating unique quality characteristics, if any.

h. A statement of theoretical weights/measures and practical (expected) yields at appropriate stages of processing including permissible limits beyond which investigation is required.

i. Brief description of all vessels, equipment, machinery used for manufacturing of the drug product.

j. Broad outlines of the stepwise manufacturing process as a flow chart and packaging process.

k. Critical in-process checks and controls, including limits, thereof to be exercised during processing and packaging.

l. Precautions to be taken during manufacture and storage of the semi-finished product.

m. Complete manufacturing control instructions, sampling/testing procedures, specifications, special notations and precautions to be followed.

n. Sufficient details of precautions to be taken during manufacturing to ensure both product quality and personal safety.

o. All analytical controls including limits, thereof applicable to the finished product.

p. Stability test results covering the assigned shelf life.

q. Product history data giving references for changes in manufacturing/packaging introduced over the years (preferably).

r. Samples of printed packaging components (preferably).

Master Production Record

Master production record is a product specific document complied, checked, authorized and approved by competent technical personnel. Master production record describes the manufacturing, packaging and control details of a particular product in a written procedure. To get uniformity in master production and control record, it should be prepared, dated and signed by one person and independently checked, dated and signed by at least a second person for each and every batch. Master formula record should be open for review. Changes if any should be approved by designated persons responsible for production and QC. The master manufacturing records should clearly state:

a. Name of equipment to be utilized with a code number.
b. Manufacturing process from step to step with time, temperature, speed and sequence of adding ingredients.
c. Critical in-process checks and controls with their limits.
d. Possibilities of any hazardous conditions what may exist, and special precautions and the necessary safety measures to be adopted.
e. Actual and theoretical yields.
f. Space for signature and date of the operator, supervisor performing or checking each significant step.
g. Description of the drug product containers, closures, and packaging materials, including a specimen copy of each label and all other labeling and inserts. This is signed and dated by the person responsible for approval of such labeling.

The master production record contains:
a. The name and strength of the drug product and description of the dosage form.
b. Physical characteristics of a product.
c. The name and weight of each active ingredient per dosage unit or unit weight of the drug product, and a statement of the total weight of the dosage unit.
d. The name of other ingredients besides active ingredients indicating any unique quality characteristics and code number to solve the complexity of chemical name should be utilized.
e. An accurate statement of the weight of each component using the same weight system.
f. Any excess of components should be justified in the master records, e.g. overages to be added and the actual quantities approved by QC. Inclusion of a generic calculation in the master batch record can minimize the potential for calculation error.
g. Statement of theoretical and practical (expected) yields at different stages of manufacturing with minimum and maximum limits beyond which investigation is required should be included. Acceptable actual yields (action levels) should be calculated.
h. Statement of expected duration (time lapse) permitted for each stage of manufacture with minimum and maximum limits.
i. It should also include complete manufacturing and control instruction, sampling and testing procedures, specification, special notations and precautions to be followed.
j. Name of persons authorized for processing along with date and sign.

Batch Manufacturing/Processing Records

Batch processing record is a product and batch-specific document designed to give a complete and reliable picture of the manufacturing history of each batch of every product. Batch processing record is primarily based on the master formula record and is compiled, checked, approved and authorized by competent technical persons responsible for production and QC. Batch processing Record is a mandatory requirement and thus should comply with Schedule U of Drugs and Cosmetics Act & Rules, 1945. Batch Processing Record document is intended to be used on the shop-floor and shall thus be designed giving clear, precise information and instruction. For example, batch processing Record for tablet should consist of the following:

- A manufacturing work order,
- A coating work order,
- Stage-wise processing details,
- In-process checks and tests,
- Compression and coating details,
- Deviation (if any).

Before batch processing begins, recorded check procedure is followed to confirm that the equipment and workstation are clear of previous products or products of the previous batch and any document or material not required for the planned batch process (line clearance). During processing, the following information should be recorded at the time each action has taken place, and after completion, the record is dated and signed in agreement by the person responsible for the processing operations. The following issues should be taken into consideration:

a. It is a product and batch-specific document designed to give a complete and reliable picture of the manufacturing history of each batch of every product.
b. All entries must be made correctly and promptly be the person(s) performing the task(s)
c. Operating staff must be trained to appreciate its importance.
d. This record should be compiled, checked, approved and authorized by competent technical persons responsible for production and quality control.

e. Every batch should have specific control number in a numeric or alphanumeric indicating year, month or week and internal manufacturing identifier.
f. This record provides a detailed description of all the processing operations and controls, when they are performed, by whom and where.
g. The record should provide the information on which ingredients were added, which control measures were exercised for in process and final assay of the drug product and the entire aspect of information produced during the manufacturing cycle.
h. It is mandatory to keep retain sample from the finished product from unpacked and packed portions of the batch under control by the authorized person (s), usually in QC.
i. It shall be reviewed by an independent authority, such as QC before a finished product is cleared for distribution and/or sale.
j. The batch record is kept safely under control of the authorized person (s), usually in QC and shall be conveniently retrievable.
k. It shall be retained for a period not less than the shelf life of the product for which the record has complied. (It is, however, a common practice to keep all the records for 5 years, which is the stipulated maximum shelf life, according to the regulations, for any individual chemical/drug and /or formulation (s) thereof). In exceptional cases, such as pending disputes in the Court of Law, the relevant records may have to be retained until the dispute is finally settled.

Batch processing record should include:
a. The name of the drug product.
b. Dates of the original functionality and dates and times of commencement, of

significant intermediate stages and completion of production.

c. A statement of the processing location and the major equipment and lines to be used.

d. Specific identification code and quantities of all materials used, whether or not the material appears or tested in the finished product. The batch number and/or analytical control number as well as the quantities of each starting material weighed (including the batch number and amount of any recovered or reprocessed material added).

e. The methods or reference to the methods used for preparing the critical equipment (e.g. cleaning, assembling, calibrating, sterilizing).

f. Detailed stepwise processing instructions (e.g. checks on materials, pre-treatments, the sequence for adding materials, mixing times, temperatures, etc.).

g. In processing and laboratory control results.

h. Any special precautions to be followed.

i. A statement of the actual yield and percentage theoretical yield at appropriate phases of processing.

j. Statement of actual duration (time) consumed for each stage of manufacturing.

k. The instructions for the in-process controls with their limits.

l. Identification of the persons performing and directly supervising each significant step in the operations.

m. Signed authorization for any deviation, if occurs, during processing, from the master formula record and or batch manufacturing records.

n. The requirements for bulk storage of the products in any intermediate stage including the container, labeling, and special storage conditions.

o. Description of finished drug product containers and closures system.

p. Complete labeling control record, including the specimens copies of all labeling used.

q. Reconciliation of materials received, used, rejected and/or destroyed and returned/delivered to a warehouse or in any other pro-designated location.

r. Quantity and source of recovered/reworked materials used, provided, however, it is in accordance with relevant Master formula.

s. If a single lot of bulk manufactured product is utilized in more than one packaging order, a record should exist which shows
   i. Each packaging order to which the bulk was assigned.
   ii. Packaging control numbers
   iii. Quantity utilized in each order
   iv. Date of each packaging operation.

Packaging and Labeling Records

Packaging and labeling operations are performed following written procedures designed to assure that correct labels, labeling, and packaging materials are used for drug products and are adequately controlled. These procedures shall incorporate the following features:

a. Inspection of the packaging and labeling facilities immediately before operation to assure clearance of all previously processed drug products. The inspection shall also assure removal of packaging and labeling materials not suitable for subsequent operations. Results of inspection are documented in the batch production records.

b. Examination of packaging and labeling materials for suitability and correctness before commencement of packaging operations, and documentation of such examination in the batch production record.

c. Identification and handling of filled and finished drug product containers that are set aside and held in unlabeled condition for future labeling operations, to preclude chances of mislabeling of individual containers, lots or portions of lots. Identification need not to be applied on each container but shall be sufficient to determine name, strength, the number of contents and lot or control number of each container.

d. Identification of the drug product with a particular lot or control number enabling tracing of manufacturing history and control of the batch.

e. Prevention of mixups and cross-contamination by physical or spatial separation from operations of other drug products.

Batch packing records consists of the packing work order, overprinting details, packing details, in-process checks, bottle washing and filling (liquid orals), bottle cleaning and filling (dry syrup), shipper or cartoon weight unit profile and deviation record (if any).

Packaging and labeling operations record shall include the following:

a. Identity and quantity of each shipment/lot of components, drug product containers, closure, labeling.

b. The name of the supplier and the supplier's lot number.

c. Specification of receiving the code.

d. Date of receipt.

e. The name and address of the primary manufacturer if different from the supplier.

f. An individual inventory record of each component should be maintained along with its utilization for various batches.

g. Record of labels, labeling document examination, and review, should be documented and kept to establish conformity as per the established specifications.

h. Documentation of rejected components, drug product containers, closure, and labeling should be done.

i. Documented record of test results, conclusions reached and dispositions.

Packaging Instructions

Formally authorized packaging instructions should be prepared for each product, pack size and type.

This generally includes the following:

a. Name of the product.

b. Description of the pharmaceutical form, and strength where applicable.

c. The pack size expressed regarding the number, weight or volume of the product in the final container.

d. Complete list of all the packaging materials required for standard batch size, indicating quantities, sizes, and types, with the code or reference number related to the specifications of each packaging material.

e. A reproduction of the relevant printed packaging materials, and specimens indicating the batch number allocation, space references, and shelf life of the product.

f. Special precautions to be observed, including a careful examination of the area and equipment in order to ascertain the line clearance before next operation begins.

g. Detailed description of the packaging operation, including any significant subsidiary operations, and equipment to be used.

h. Details of in-process controls with instructions for sampling and acceptance limits.

Batch Packaging Records

A batch packaging records are prepared and maintained for each batch or part batch processed as a relevant part of the packaging instructions (records). The method for preparation of such records is designed in a standardized way to avoid transcription errors. The record carries the batch number and the quantity of bulk product to be packed, as well as the batch number and the planned quantity of finished product that is to be processed for packing.

Before any packaging operation begins, checks are to be done for line clearance. All the information should be entered at the time each action has taken place, and after completion, the record should be dated and signed in agreement by the person(s) responsible for the packaging operations. The record contains the following:

a. The name of the product.

b. The date(s) and time of packaging operation performance.

c. The name of the person responsible for carrying out the packaging operation.

d. The initials of all the operators performing the different significant steps.

e. Identity and conformity checks with the packaging instructions including the results of in-process controls are recorded.

f. Details of the packaging operations carried out indicating equipment references and the packaging lines used.

g. Samples of printed packaging materials used as specimens indicating batch code, expiry date and other additional overprinting are retained

h. Notes on any particular problem or unusual event including details, with a signed authorization in case of any deviation from the manufacturing formula and processing instructions.

i. The quantities and reference number or identification of all printed packaging materials and bulk product issued, used, destroyed or returned to stock and the quantities of obtained product, in order to provide for an adequate reconciliation.

Review and release of batch records: All manufacturing control records are reviewed and approved by the QC unit to determine compliance with approved written procedures before a batch is released or distributed. Any unexplained discrepancy or failure of a batch or any of its components to meet any of its specifications should be investigated. The investigation should extend to other batches of the same drug product and should include the conclusions and follow up.

A checklist is customarily maintained defining the specific documents that should be in the batch record and what is to be checked on each document. If the release criteria are not stated on the batch record, they should be included on the checklist.

Items to be entered on the checklist may include:

a. Batch record in the current format and approved as an accurate copy.

b. Components which are authentic and released by QC were used in manufacturing.

c. Correct quantities of components were used in manufacturing.

d. All components were within the retest dating period.

e. Manufacturing control documents are correctly completed.

f. Yields and accountability are within action levels.

g. Only correct product was packaged.

h. Correct packaging components were used.

i. The labeling bears the correct control numbers.

j. Packaging control document was properly completed.

k. In-process and finished products QC laboratory test result values were within specification.

l. If any deviation has occurred in the production stage, it must be documented, investigated, and appropriate levels of management must be involved in the review and any decision making.

m. Written investigation of any deviation from the procedure was maintained and approved. The follow-up and corrective actions are required to minimize the potential for reoccurrence, retaining and revalidation.

n. Control samples have been taken.

PROCEDURES

Receipt

Written procedures and records are maintained for the receipt of each starting, primary and printed packaging material.

The records of the receipts should include:

a. Date of receipt.

b. The name of the material on the delivery note and the containers.

c. Manufacturer's batch or reference number

d. The 'in-house' name and/or code of the material if different.

e. Supplier's name and manufacturer's name.

f. Total quantity and number of containers received.

g. The batch number assigned after receipt.

h. Any relevant comment (e.g. state of the containers).

Written procedures are made available for the internal labeling, quarantine, and storage of starting materials, packaging materials and other materials received as appropriate.

Sampling

Written procedures for sampling including the person(s) authorized to take samples, the methods, and equipment to be used, the amounts to be taken and precautions to be observed to avoid contamination of the material or any deterioration in its quality are maintained. Special sampling instructions are prepared and followed for antibiotics, steroids, sterile, radioactive or any other hazardous products.

Testing

Written procedures are maintained for testing of materials and products at different stages of manufacturing describing the equipments to be used. All the tests performed along with results and final QC decision (approved/rejected) are recorded. Written release and rejection procedures are prepared and made available for materials and products in particular for the release of the finished product for sale in accordance to the requirements of Schedule U. Records are maintained for distribution of each batch of a product in order to facilitate immediate tracing in case recall of the batch is necessary.

Other Departmental Documents

Clear operating procedures should be available for major manufacturing and test equipments. Records are kept for major or critical equipment recording as appropriate, for validations, calibrations, maintenance, cleaning or repair operations, including the dates and identity of people who carried these operations. Log books are recorded in chronological order of use for principal or critical equipment and the areas where the products have been processed. Written procedures and the associated records are maintained for:

- Validation.
- Equipment assembly and calibration.

- Maintenance, cleaning, and sanitation.
- Personnel clothing, hygiene and training.
- Environmental monitoring.
- Pest control.

The following is a comprehensive list of log books recommended to be maintained by the various departments of a pharmaceutical manufacturing unit:

Production department
- General housekeeping
- Temperature and humidity
- Air pressure differential
- All equipment calibration
- All equipment operation log
- Equipment cleaning
- Planned preventive maintenance of equipment
- Issue and control of materials
- Intermediate log
- Overprinting of packaging materials
- Transfer pump and transfer line log

Utility department
- Demineralized water plant operation
- Demineralized water plant maintenance
- Planned preventive maintenance of air handling units
- Compressed air
- Steam generators
- Filters

QC department
- Volumetric solutions
- Reference standards
- Working standards
- Reserve samples
- Control samples
- Calculation sheet
- Glassware calibration

- Distilled waterlog
- Instrument operation
- Autoclave calibration
- Media preparation
- Media stock
- Growth promotion test
- Plate exposure test
- Subculturing and destruction of sub-culture
- Media destruction
- Fumigation and de-fumigation log
- UV lamp log

Training record
- Annual training schedule
- Training modules
- Individual training records
- General training record
- Material/visual aids/literature used for training

QA department
- Technical change procedure
- Raw material and finished product specification
- Packing specification
- Validation register (cleaning, process, and method)
- Change control
- Instrument calibration (External agency)
- Line clearance register
- Deviation record
- Out of specification records
- Monthly report
- Annual report
- Audit report
- Training record
- Medical checkup record
- Pest control record
- Market complaint record

RECORDS

Standard Operating Methods and Records

Standard operating procedure (SOP) provides step-by-step instructions for carrying out a particular operation or task. The SOP is a procedure document which mostly describes the regular recurring operations appropriately to comply with quality guidelines. SOP aims to achieve quality output maintaining uniformity of performance and efficiency while reducing miscommunication and failure to comply with pharmaceutical regulations. Written SOPs are maintained and followed for:

- Receipt of materials
- Sampling
- Batch numbering
- Testing
- Records of analysis
- Equipment assembly and validation
- Analytical apparatus and calibration
- Maintenance, cleaning, and sanitation
- Personnel matters including qualification, training, clothing, hygiene
- Environmental monitoring
- Pest control
- Complaints
- Recalls

Equipment Cleaning and Use Record

Record of all major pieces of equipment cleaning, maintenance (except routine maintenance such as lubrication and parts adjustment), and use are maintained in written with individual equipment logs that must show the date, time, product and lot number of each batch processed. If equipment is used only for one product, then individual equipment logs are not required, batches of such product follow a numerical order and manufactured batches are numbered in numerical sequence. For such dedicated equipment, the records of cleaning maintenance and use are

part of the batch record. The cleaning record entries should be done with special care to comply with the following facts:

a. Equipment should be classified as major and minor.
b. Only approved (trained) and authorized personnel are permitted to perform a process.
c. Processing can be prevented until any prior steps or checks are performed.
d. The person responsible should enter the date and sign while performing and double-checking the cleaning and maintenance.
e. The logbook should have the entry in chronological order.
f. Computerized systems are preferred for having advantages of more consistent control. This also enables to incorporate electronic signature/initials that frequently involve a personal password or a personal magnetic card with a secure system to manage allocation and review.
g. Operational timing should be recorded precisely.

Laboratory Record

Laboratory record includes the complete data derived from tests that are necessary to assure compliance with established specification and standards, including examination and assays.

a. Identification of sample received for testing with the description, quantity, lot no. or other distinctive code, date of sampling and the date when the sample was received for testing.
b. Cross-referencing the samples regarding the bulk containers from which they are taken should be done. The amount of sample taken is recorded to allow effective reconciliation.
c. While testing the sample, each method used for testing should be documented. Methods used should meet the proper standard of accuracy and reliability as

applied to the product. If the test method is pharmacopoeial, its reference should be given.

d. Monograph reference number and issue date should be documented. Copies of superseded monographs for the released products must be retained.

e. Records regarding testing, i.e. all raw data, graphs, charts, spectra generated from laboratory instrumentation are appropriately identified to show the specific components, drug product container, closure, in-process material or a drug product and its lot tested.

f. Data calculation details of all tests carried out in connection with the test, including units of measure, conversion factors and equivalency factors should be appended.

g. Result statement should be comparative with the standards of identity, strength, quality, and purity of the component, drug product container, closure, in press material, or drug product tested. Action levels should be based on historical data. Confirmation that results lie within the action levels are delegated to a responsible analyst.

h. Results outside the action level, but inside specifications, are usually referred to a more senior individual and require evaluation for the possible cause of deviation before deciding on status. Standard written methodology or procedures should identify these action levels and the review process.

i. Records must indicate the person who has performed each test. Since initials and signatures of many people are similar, it is better to mention names printed or typed.

j. Following recent advances, methodologies can be modified, but they should be validated. Method modified along with the valid reason for modification should be maintained, and validation document of a new method for accuracy,

consistency, etc should be kept. A standard assay method should only be changed when it becomes essential.

k. Complete records of standardization of laboratory working standards, reagents, and solutions are maintained. Record of periodic calibration of laboratory instruments, apparatus, gauges and recording devices should be kept.

Distribution Records

Before distribution or dispatch of a given batch of a drug product, it is mandatory to ensure that the batch has been duly tested, approved and released by the QC personnel. The predispatch inspection shall be performed on each consignment on a random basis to ensure that only the correct goods were dispatched. Detailed instruction for warehousing and stocking of parenterals, biologicals, and vaccines should comply with guidelines (e.g. cold chain maintenance) even after the batch is released for distribution. Periodic audit of warehousing practices followed at the distribution level are to be carried out and records thereof maintained. SOPs are developed for warehousing of products. Records for distribution are maintained in a manner to facilitate prompt and complete recall of the batch.

The distribution record should contain the following particulars:

a. Name and strength of the product.

b. Description of the dosage form.

c. Name and address of the consignee.

d. Date and quantity shipped.

e. Lot or control no of the drug product.

f. Distribution record includes invoice, bills of lading, customers receipts, internal warehouse, storage and inventory records.

Recording of the batch number of each order consignment is to accomplish the purpose of immediate tracing of a specific lot of product distributed to the particular clearing and forwarding agent (C & Fs), wholesalers, retails and in turn customers receiving the product.

Complaint files

All complaints concerning product quality are carefully reviewed and recorded according to approved written procedures. Each complaint is investigated/evaluated by the designated personnel of the company and records of investigation and remedial action taken thereof are maintained. Reports of serious adverse drug reactions resulting from the use of a drug along with comments and documents are compulsorily needed to be reported to the concerned licensing authority within specified timeline. Written procedures describing the action taken after the recall of the defective product is prepared and maintained by the QA department.

Effective product recall is based on the following fundamentals:

a. A prompt and effective product recall system for defective products recall are developed and kept updated to ensure timely information sharing from all concerned stockists, wholesalers, suppliers up to the retail level within a shortest determined period. The effectiveness of the arrangements for recalls is evaluated from time to time. The licensee should make sure the effectiveness of both print and electronic media in this regard.

b. An established written procedure in the form of SOP is maintained for effective recall of products distributed by the licensee. Recall operations must be capable of being initiated promptly to reach at the level of each distribution channel in the shortest possible time.

c. Distribution records are readily made available to the persons designated for recalls.

d. Designated person check for record reconciliation between the delivered and the recovered quantities of the products.

e. Recalled products are to be stored separately in a secure segregated area while pending final decision.

f. The need for a recall is decided by a number of complaints received from consumers, customers, traders, and professionals.

g. Each complaint is evaluated by knowledgeable and responsible personnel.

h. Validity and seriousness of complaint are judged by cross-checking the records of production, packaging, and distribution of drug product and testing the retained samples.

i. A complaint number is assigned to start the recall action plan. Complaint file also contains investigation report suggesting modification if any required to be incorporated in the manufacturing process and storage condition adversely affecting drug stability at various places.

j. A written record of each complaint is maintained in a file designated for drug product complaints.

k. Complaint file must provide a clear cut picture whether the similar complaint is received for other batches of the same product.

Complaint record should include:

a. The name, batch number, manufacturing date and other relevant details related to the identification of the product

b. The dosage form and strength of the product

c. Details of product complaint

d. Details of product investigation

e. Corrective and preventive action taken against the complaint

f. Finding of the investigation and follow up.

The records relevant to the investigation of product complaint are maintained in the

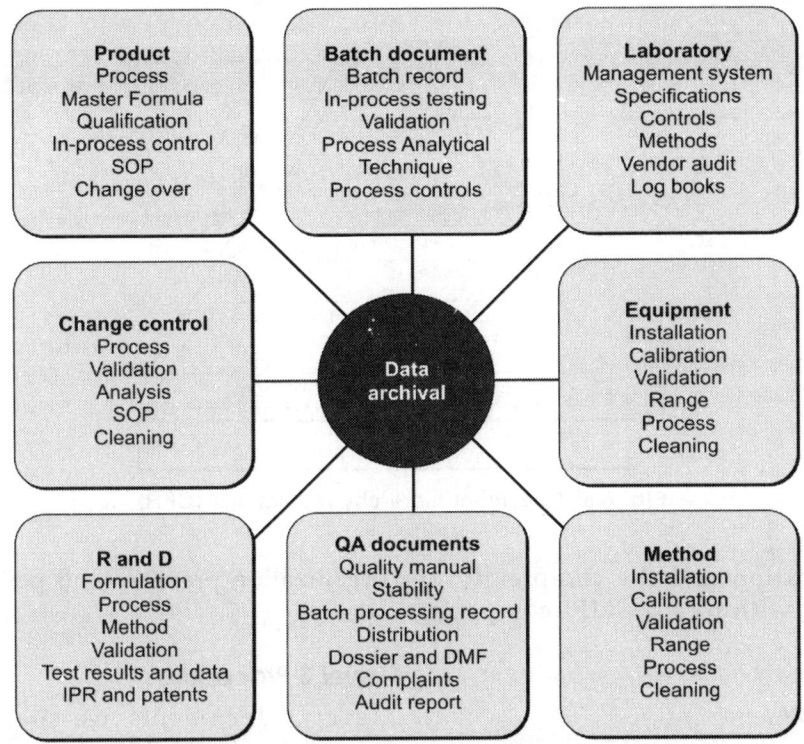

Fig. 6.4: Documentation archival control system

establishment where the investigation was carried out. If in case investigation against complaint was found not to be necessary its records should also be kept, and persons involved in all decisions related to product complaint handling, investigation, and referral action must sign the record.

DOCUMENT HIERARCHY

Pharmaceutical companies establish and maintain the required GMP documents also called quality management system documentation (QMS) in a hierarchical manner starting with the general regulations and working followed by downward to more specific documents such as related quality records for convenient archival. QMS documentation provides a clear framework of the operations in an organization, allowing consistency of processes and a better understanding of the quality system, and also provides evidence of objectives and goals achievement (Fig. 6.5).

Level 1 Manual

Level 1 documents mostly include quality manual, quality objectives, organizational chart, qualification and responsibilities of all personnel, etc., which defines companies approach and responsibility. The manual includes the QMS scope, exclusions from the standard, references to relevant documents and the business process model. These documents establish overall principles and guidelines that are required to be implemented on future development plans, documentation and implementation of cGMP compliant quality system. These top-level documents are nonspecific in nature, and content of the manual depends on the size of

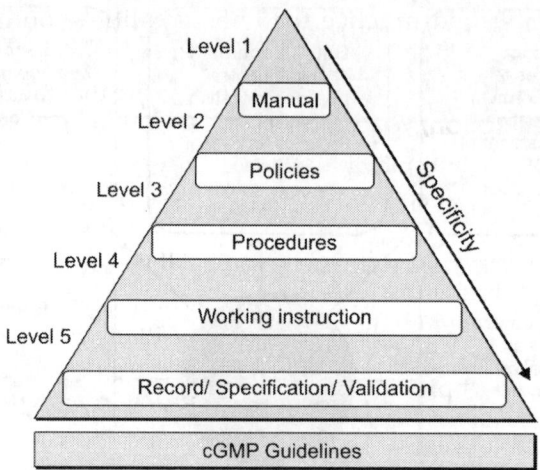

Fig. 6.5: Document hierarchy regulations (CFR)

the organization and the complexity of operations within a cGMP compliant company.

Level 2 Policy

Level 2 documents are the quality policy and quality goals of an organization. The quality policy defines the quality objectives of an organization, and the quality goals are defined by quantifying the quality objectives. The policy represents a declarative statement by an organization stating the commitment of the organization to quality and continual improvement. Company quality policies establish guidelines to which all subsequent level documents must comply to ensure consistency across departments that is equally applicable with all departments within a GMP compliant company. These documents are not meant to provide specific working instructions for documenting data but rather provides overall intentions and guidelines governing critical programs or systems along with explanations of the rationale and program designs. The quality policy should be clear and short as usual. It is used by the company for promotional purposes and is displayed in the organization premises and posted on websites.

Level 3 Procedures

Level 3 documents are specific quality procedures in the form of descriptive text, tables, flow charts or combination that defines what to perform, who will perform and when. These documents are mostly developed in the form of SOP for specific functions within a department. These practical instructions documents provide specific step-by-step instructions to perform the operational tasks or activities that are generally devised in the previous levels.

Level 4 Working Instructions

Level 4 documents are the blank documents used to record data generated during the testing, inspection and other processes. These working instruction documents include the elements like; the title of procedure, purpose describing the rationale, scope explaining the aspects to be covered, responsibilities and authorities of personnel involved, description of activities, results of the activities described in the procedure and relevant document control as per the established practice for document control.

Level 5 Records/Specification/Validation

The last level of documents in a hierarchical document structure is the most specific, (e.g. batch record, test methods, validation procedures, etc.) and apply to a specific department, product, equipment or process. Level 4 document provides a template for the recording of all production and quality related tasks and activities as well as provide means for documenting such tasks in data sheets, labels, forms or test reports. The details outlined in the level 5 documents may override directions given in other level documents. The document hierarchy pyramid is an example of documents organization system. More or fewer levels can be added/ subtracted to meet specific needs. Training of personnel makes them competent which can decrease the need for maintaining highly detailed working instructions. Properly structured documentation make operations much easier, while incorrect documentation can bring noncompliance.

DOCUMENT CHECKLIST

QA develop a comprehensive checklist for the policies, procedures, and guidelines (PPGs) documents that are required to be fulfilled before formal release and distribution:

1. The SOP is to be written in an instructional language and should not contain any ambiguous phrases.
2. All details related to document identification should be entered in the header and footer sections.
3. Appropriate document code should be obtained from the quality facilitator.
4. SOP numbering should be consistent with the sequence of numbering within the relevant department.
5. The title should reflect the topic of the PPG.
6. Ensure that the revision number is correct (i.e. that it is 0 if the PPG is new, and should increase by one from the previous revision number whenever a change been made to the PPG).
7. All pages are sequentially numbered.
8. The current date of PPG data entering/ written is being included.
9. The routing details of the document have been completed and signed.
10. The names of the writer/reviewer, approver with designation has been included.
11. The appropriate personnel should approve the PPG's at management level.
12. If the document is an SOP, it should be stated throughout the header/footer if guideline in all the headings throughout the document.
13. All required headings as per template have been completed (e.g. purpose, scope, responsibility, etc.) with additional headings as and where required.
14. Literature supporting a particular guideline must be indicated ensuring proper appraisal.
15. The evidence supporting PPGs are being referenced in the documents.
16. The PPGs should mention due time frame of revision (mostly it is stated at the beginning of the PPG folder that it will be revised on an annual or biannual basis as acceptable).
17. A process of identifying that the PPG has been read or received by the relevant recipients is in place.
18. Distribution list must mention wherever a particular document has been attached as relevant to the master copy of the PPG.

Form 1: Document Creation and Change Control Form

1. Form initiator			
Date		Area	
Initiator name		Position	
Line managers name			
2. Create a new document			
Document type (SOP, Form, etc.)		Ref No.	
Title			
Reason for change			
3. Cancel document			
Document type (SOP, Form, etc.)		Ref No.	
Title			
Reason for cancellation			
Comments			
4. Approval of line manager			
Name			
Sign		Date	
5. Approval of QA manager			
Name			
Sign		Date	
6. Document control officer (DOC)			
Initiator informed		Name	
Sign		Date	

Form 2: Master Document Change Control Form

Change control No: ID-DD-MM-YY		
1. Request information		
Name of requester		
Department	Contact:	
Urgency of change	Date:	
2. Change information		
Action		
Document to be changed		
Document number to be changed		
Raw material/finished product/ packaging material	Code	
Other related information	Description	
3. Details of changes		
Reason for change		
Current text		
Comments		
QC Manager	Name	
	Date	Sign
Comments		
QA Manager	Name	
	Date	Sign
Comments		
Other associated manager	Name	
	Date	Sign
Comments		

Form 3: Goods Receipt Form

Supplier/Manufacturer Name							
Consignment No.	Address						
Receipt date.							
Purchase order no.	No. of pallets/cartoons						
Vendor receipt no.	No. of containers						
Receiving section	No. of ID level						
In general condition of container:							

Item No.	Material name	Material code	Mfg batch no.	Quantity	Quantity after samples	Date	Date of re-sampling

Receiving staff name:		Sign	Date	
Sampling staff name:		Sign	Date	
Storage type	Location bin		Date	Sign
Quarantine/bulk/under test				

Form 4: Sample Request Form

Sample Type (tick): Raw material/packaging material/bulk drug/finished Goods

Product/material name: ....

Product/material code: ....

Initial GRS number: ....

Lab. Batch no.: ....

Quantity required: ....

Location of transfer: ....

Requested by: ....

Released by: ....

Date: ....

Description of product/material ....

Comment: ....

Prepared by:	Sign:	Date: ....
Approved by:	Sign:	Date: ....

Form 5: Raw Material/Packaging Material/Bulk Drug Lab Test Data Entry Form

Material (Name/code no.)	Lab batch no.	Test #1 Method No. Specification	Test #2 Method No. Specification	Test #3 Method No. Specification	Result	Test pass/fail	Test starting date	Test finish date	Test performed by	Test approved by	Date

Form 6: Monthly Production Schedule Form

Date:

Process line:

Dosage form:

P&P name/generic name:

Day	Date	Batch no.	Strength/ description	Production quantity	Start time	Finish time	Units	Packs	Comments

Prepared by:	Sign:	Date:
Approved by:	Sign:	Date:

Form 7: Raw Material Log

Material name	Material code	Mfg's lot no.	Mfg/supplier name/address	Purchase order no.	Goods receipt slip no.	Lab batch no.	Pack-aging box	Storage condition/location	Status (Quarantine under test/passed/rejected)	Date of receipt	Expiry date	Ware-house incharge sign	Date

Prepared by:	Sign:	Date:
Approved by:	Sign:	Date:

Form 8: Finished Good Log

Product name	Product code	Descrip-tion	Batch no.	Batch size	Container/ packaging	Manufac-turing date	Expiry date	Storage condition/ location	Status (under test/passed/ rejected)	Person respon-sible	Sign

Prepared by: Sign: Date:

Approved by: Sign: Date:

Form 9: Raw Material Retention Sample Log

Material name	Material code	Description	Lab batch no.	Primary/ secondary packaging/	Expiry date	No. of samples	Sampling date	Storage condition/ location	Date of dispersal	Person responsible	Sign

Prepared by:		Sign:	Date:
Approved by:		Sign:	Date:

Form 10: Finished Good Log

Product name	Product code	Descrip-tion	Batch no.	Expiry date	Secondary packaging/ box	Primary packaging/ units	Person respon-sible	Date of sampling	Date of dispersal	Storage condition/ location	Sign

Prepared by:		Sign:	Date:
Approved by:		Sign:	Date:

Form 11: Expired Raw Material Information Form

Raw material name		
Raw material code no.	Lab batch no.	
Manufacturer batch no.	Expiry date	
Original quantity received	Original date of receipt	
Date issued	Quantity remaining	
Any previous extension of shelf life	Yes	No	If yes, last testing date
Is this quantity worth for testing		

Testing details

Amount to be sampled	Storage Bin
Packing condition	
Warehouse incharge	Sign Date

Raw material specification no.

Test	Result

Decision

Passed/Rejected: _____ If passed new expiry date: _____

Tested by: _____ Sign: _____ Date: _____

QC Lab Manager: _____ Sign: _____ Date: _____

Form 12: Deviation Report Form

Deviation report no.	Date
Reported by	Responsible section/division

Deviation report type (fill in applicable information)

Material complaint deviation

Vendor Name/no.	Material name
Material code	Purchase order no.

Process / Procedural Deviation

Product name/code.	Batch no.
Process line	Master formula no.

Audit deviation

Audit type	Audit ref. No.

Description (Must be filled in for all deviation types)

Production/warehouse/Area Manager Response Tasks (Describe the facts, corrective actions taken, if preventative action is necessary to list in the follow-up tasks. Sent the report to QC management response tasks)

Name	Sign	Date

(Contd.)

Form 12: Deviation Report Form (*Contd.*)

QC management response tasks (Review production/warehouse/area manager's response and justify the efficacy of corrective actions taken, if preventative action is necessary to list in the follow-up tasks. Sent the report to QA management response tasks)

Name		Sign	Date

Follow-up task

Task 1

Assigned to			Due date of submission
QA manager approval		Sign	Date

Task 2

Assigned to			Due date of submission
QA manager approval		Sign	date

List all follow-up tasks. Attach extra sheets, if necessary

Form 13: Process Failure/Laboratory Error Investigation Report Form

Description of event and details: Process Line(s), Product Name(s), Product Code(s) and Batch No.(s) to be added here.

Investigation type: Type of investigation (e.g. Process Failure, Operator Error, Lab Error, etc.)

Conditions	Indication		
Cleaning of vessel	Yes	No	NA
Quantity of raw material	Yes	No	NA
Weighing	Yes	No	NA
Blanding time/condition	Yes	No	NA
Reagent preparation	Yes	No	NA
pH adjustment	Yes	No	NA
Instrument calibration	Yes	No	NA
Approved change over	Yes	No	NA
Approved line clearance	Yes	No	NA
Others			

Suspected causes and rationales: Enter rationale for a suspected cause. Categorize as Primary/Contributing/Unlikely.

Risk Analysis: Potential impact on other processes: Outline whether this event could have an impact on any other equipment or processes and rationale behind this conclusion.

Corrective and preventive actions to be taken: State corrective and preventive actions, which need to be taken and the reasoning behind decisions made.

Name/Position	Sign	Date
Prepared by:		
Checked by:		
Authorised by:		
Approved by:		

Executive Summary: The executive summary should contain a brief description of the event, root cause found during the investigation and a final summary on product disposition to be entered here.

List of Attachments (As applicable)
Investigation meeting minutes
Supporting Batch Documentation/Log Books
Deviation Report/s
Supporting Facilities Data
Supporting Analytical Data
Validation Data
Evidence of actions completed
SOP Updates
Employee Awareness Forms
Training/Assessment Updates
Summary of Investigation Tasks
Summary of Corrective Actions Tasks
Summary of Preventative Actions Tasks

Form 14: Complaint Investigation Report Form

Complaint identification	
Complaint receipt no.	
Date of complaint receipt	
Complaint receipt mode	
Name and other details of complainant	
Product details	
Product name	
Product code no.	
Product batch no.	
Date of manufacturing	
Date of expiry	
Packaging type	
Processing line	
Nature of complaint	
Complainant identification details	
Complaint as described by the complainant	

(Contd.)

Form 14: Complaint Investigation Report Form (Contd.)

Investigation detail	
Review of document	
Review of logbook	
Feedback from the operator, manager	
Testing of the defective product	
Determination of validity of the complaint	
Complaint investigation outcome	
Identification of potential causes with justification	
Identification of control points	
Identified changes in processes	
Previous occurring	
Corrective action (Enter details of actions required urgently to correct the assignable causes)	
Preventive action (Enter details of actions required to prevent recurrence when the complaint is determined to be valid)	
Outcome and feedback	
Investigated by	Sign	Date
Reported by	Sign	Date
QA manager approval	Sign	Date

Form 15: Document Review Check Sheet

Sl. No.	Policy, SOP or guideline number and name	Date review date	Date review carried out	Change required before review date? Y/N	Next review date	Document changed due to review Y/N	If changes made: New revision no. of document	
							Done by: (Name/ Designa- tion/ Date)	Approved by: (Name/ Designa- tion/ Date)
1.								
2.								
3.								
4.								
5.								

* All concerned departments should prepare and maintain the document review checklist.

Table 6.1: List of documents maintained in the production unit with purpose and scope

Sl. No.	Document title	Purpose	Scope
1.	Document control	Control of the issuance of document, including number of copies issued and access control	All internal documents pertaining to the manufacturing facility and premises
2.	Integrated quality management	Quality management systems for the organization	Quality policy in the company
3.	Organization chart and job descriptions	Job description and authority levels	All key personnel
4.	Quality manuals	Quality statement and quality policy	Company's policy and commitment to quality
5.	Site master file	Compliance to GMP of Pharmaceutical Inspection Convention (PIV)	All manufacturing plants
6.	Good laboratory practice manual	Guidelines of QC, R&D staff for GLP	All quality and R&D personnel
7.	Good manufacturing practice manual	Guidelines to production staff on cGMP	All quality and R&D personnel
8.	Instrument and equipment operating procedures	Standard procedures for instruments and equipment	All devices, equipment and instruments
9.	Validation master plan	Master plan for all validations—analytical, water systems process, AHU, etc.	All processes requiring validation
10.	Standard operating procedures (master SOP list)	Standard procedures for functioning	All departments SOPs
11.	Master formula record	Standard procedures for manufacturing	All product stages for APIs and intermediates
12.	Material specifications	Specifications for raw material, packing materials	All ingredients
13.	Testing methods, general analytical methods	Analytical methods and procedures	All methods—physical, chemical, microbiological, instrumentation
14.	Product review system	Standard procedures for a product review	QA documentation, control, and validation of product review
15.	Deviation and change control system	Standard procedures for deviation and change control	Production, QC and QA documentation, control and validation and change control
16.	Training records	All training	All personnel concerned with different departments, instruments, facility management
17.	Product complain and recall system	Standard procedures describing complaint and recall system	QA for optimization and audit of complaint and recall system
18.	Water management system	Water supply facility of the manufacturing unit	QC water quality control and validation system

(Contd.)

Sl. No.	Document title	Purpose	Scope
19.	Cleaning and sanitation system	Guideline to store, manufacturing, QC and R&D departments regarding the standard procedure of cleaning and sanitation	All departments like production, QC, R&D facility, devices, equipment and instruments
20.	Pest control system	Standard procedures describing pest control of the premises	All facilities and premises building
21.	Waste management system (effluent treatment and pollution control)	Waste management systems for all the facilities like production, QC, R&D and store	All the operational facilities generating waste and effluents
22.	Audit management system	Quality management systems for the organization	Audit management and implementation policy of the company
23.	Maintenance and operational management	Management and maintenance of all the operational facility and the equipment	All the operational facilities and the equipment
24.	Emergency management system	Management of incidents, accidents, hazards in the facility	Covers all the processes currently operational in all facility

Table 6.2: Document location and maintenance system

Sl. No.	Document type	Location
1.	Control method, instrument, and equipment operating procedure, testing methods, general analytical methods, sampling, RM & PM specification, finished goods specifications, stability specifications, all test report	QC Section
2.	Production control method, finished goods specifications: Test report, raw material specification: Test report, IPQC record, change over and change control reports, master formula record	Production
3.	Site master file, annual product review, quality policy, training programme, meeting minutes, audit management system, maintenance and operational management, emergency management system	Regulatory
4.	Raw material specification: Test report, packaging material specification test report	Warehouse
5.	Organization chart and job descriptions of personnel, training records receipt, bill of material	Planning/Accounts
6.	Batch record, stability study record, audit report, validation master plant, validation record, quality manual, GLP and GMP manual, SOPs, forms, product complaint/returned/recall record, retain sample record, displays, vendor audit, calibration report, deviation and change control record, product review record, water management record, cleaning and sanitation record, pest control record, waste management record	QA Section

Table 6.3: Approval matrix and review period of quality documents

Sl. No.	Document type	Prepared by	Checked by	Approved by	Review period
1.	Quality policies	Officer QA	Executive QA	Top Management	As per company policy
2.	Organization chart and job descriptions of personnel	Officer QA	Executive QA	Top Management	Annually
3.	Site master file	Officer QA	Executive QA	QA Head	Annually
4.	Technical files	Officer QA	Executive QA	QA Head	Annually
5.	Forms	Officer QA	Executive QA	QA Head	As per requirement
6.	Displays	Officer QA	Executive QA	QA Head	As per requirement
7.	Quality template (manual)	Officer QA	Executive QA	QA Head	As per requirement
8.	Vendor audit report	Officer QA	Executive QA	QA Head	Annually
9.	Quality audit report	Officer QA	Executive QA	QA Head	Annually
10.	Testing methods	Officer QC	Executive QC	QC Head	As per requirement
11.	Analytical methods	Officer QC	Executive QC	QC Head	As per requirement
12.	Specification of RM, PM and finished goods	Officer QC	Executive QC	QC Head	Annually
13.	Stability specifications	Officer QC	Executive QC	QC Head	As per requirement
14.	Instrument and equipment operating procedure	Officer QC	Executive QC	QC Head	Annually/As per requirement
15.	Master formula	Officer production	Executive production	Head production	Annually
16.	SOPs	Officer production	Respective department executive	Respective department executive	Annually
17.	Production control method	Officer production	Executive production	Head production	Annually
18.	IPQC record	Officer QA	Executive QA	QC Head	Annually
19.	Batch record	Officer production	Executive production	Head production	Annually
20.	Deviation and change control report	Officer QC	Executive QC	QC/QA Head	Annually
21.	Stability study record	Officer QC	Executive QC	QC Head	Annually

(Contd.)

Sl. No.	Document type	Prepared by	Checked by	Approved by	Review period
22.	Maintenance, operational and procedural manuals	Officer maintenance	Executive Maintenance	Head maintenance	Annually
23.	Change over and change control reports	Officer QC	Executive QC	QC Head	Annually
24.	Validation and calibration report	Officer regulatory	Executive Regulatory	QA Head	Annually
25.	Annual product review record	Officer QA	Executive QA	QA Head	Annually
26.	Product complaint/Returned/Recall record	Officer QA/QC	Executive QA/QC	QC/QA Head	As per requirement
27.	Dispatch report	Officer Store	Executive store	Plant Head	Financial year
28.	Retain sample record	Officer QC	Executive QC	QC Head	Annually
29.	Training record	Respective department Officer	Respective department executive	Respective department executive	Annually/As per requirement
30.	Meeting minutes	Respective department officer	Respective department executive	Respective department executive	Monthly/As per requirement
31.	Receipt, Bill of material	Officer store	Executive Store	Production Head	Annually
32.	Cleaning and sanitation record	Respective department officer	Respective department executive	Respective department executive	Annually
33.	Pest control report	Respective department officer	Respective department executive	Respective department executive	Annually
34.	Water management record	Officer QC	Executive QC	QC Head	Annually
35.	Waste management record	Officer QC	Executive QC	QC Head	Annually

Table 6.4: Document retention time schedule

Sl. No.	Document type	Retention time	Responsible department
1.	Site master file	30 years after superseded by new version	QA
2.	Quality manual	30 years after superseded by new version	QA
3.	Organization charts and job descriptions	30 years after superseded by new version	QA
4.	Employee personal file	30 years after employment ends	QA
5.	Manufacturing facility record	7 years after life of facility, premises, utility	QA
6.	SOPs	7 years after superseded by new version	Respective departments
7.	Specification of RM, PM and finished goods	7 years after superseded by new version	QC
8.	RM, PM test record	3 years after batch is completely distributed	QC
9.	Manufacturing process validation record	1 year after last manufactured batch expires	QC
10.	Master formula record	20 years after superseded by new version	Production
11.	Batch records	Expiry period of the product with additional 1 year	Production
12.	Packaging and labeling record	Expiry period of the product with additional 1 year	Production
13.	IPQC record	Expiry period of the product with additional 1 year	QA
14.	Finished product QC record	Expiry period of the product with additional 1 year	QC
15.	Deviation records	Expiry period of the product with additional 1 year	Production
16.	Laboratory record	Not less than 10 years	QC
17.	Stability records	Expiry period of the product with additional 1 year	QC
18.	Validation records	7 years after life of equipment	QA
19.	Calibration record	7 years after life of equipment	QC
20.	Log books	Not less than 10 years	Respective departments
21.	Environment, health and safety management records	Not less than 10 years	QA
22.	Maintenance, operational and procedural manuals	7 years after superseded by new version	QC
23.	Instrument and equipment maintenance record	7 years after life of equipment	Maintenance department

(Contd.)

Sl. No.	Document type	Retention time	Responsible department
24.	Cleaning and sanitation record	Not less than 10 years	Respective departments
25.	Pest control records	Not less than 10 years	QA
26.	Employee training records	30 years after employment ends	HR and Training department
27.	Employee health record	40 years after employment ends	QA
28.	Inspection record	7 years after closure of inspection	QA
29.	GMP audit report	10 years after closure of audit	QA
30.	Vendor audit report	7 years after discontinuation of vendor	QA
31.	Receipt and bill of material	Not less than 10 years	Store
32.	Receipt and bill of equipment	7 years after life of equipment	Store
33.	Dispatch/distribution record	Expiry period of the product with additional 1 year	Store
34.	Retain sample record	Expiry period of the product with additional 1 year	QC
35.	Annual product review	Expiry period of the product with additional 1 year	QC
36.	Other GMP records	7 years after superseded by new version	QA
37.	Water management record	Not less than 10 years	QC
38.	Waste management record	Not less than 10 years	QC
39.	Clinical/preclinical drug development record	30 years from initial approval	QA
40.	Product development record	10 years after expiry of all contractual obligations	QA
41.	Documents, dossiers submission record	7 years after life of product line	QA
42.	Adverse event record	7 years after expiry period of the product	QA
43.	Product complaint/recall record	6 years after closure of case	QA
44.	Returned goods records	6 years after closure of case	QC
45.	Computer system documentation	30 years after life of system	QA
46.	Import and export record	Not less than 8 years	QA
47.	Intellectual property records	6 years after life of copyright, patent or trademark	QA

Table 6.5: Master documentation list

Sl. No.	Title

Administration
1. Housekeeping and sanitation
2. Pest control
3. Organization chart and staff welfare
4. Medical records of employees
5. Employee training
6. Uniform distribution
7. Visitor entry

Engineering and Maintenance
1. Work order
2. Organization chart and responsibilities of engineering persons
3. DM water regeneration
4. Steam generation and supply system
5. Sanitation of pipes carrying distilled water/de-ionized water
6. Numbering of gauges and measuring devices
7. AHU filter cleaning procedure
8. Calibration of pressure gauge
9. Calibration of TIC/temperature gauge
10. Calibration of vacuum gauge
11. Preventive maintenance of blender
12. Preventive maintenance of centrifugal pump
13. Preventive maintenance of centrifuge
14. Preventive maintenance of micronizer
15. Preventive maintenance of multimill
16. Preventive maintenance of vacuum pump
17. Preventive maintenance of premises electricity supply
18. Preventive maintenance of reactor
19. Preventive maintenance of sifter
20. Preventive maintenance of filter
21. Preventive maintenance of steam tray dryer
22. Preventive maintenance of vacuum tray dryer
22. Preventive maintenance of all concerned equipment

Warehouse
1. Receipt and storage of incoming materials
2. Handling of rejected raw material/packing material
3. Issuance/dispensing of material
4. Sampling procedure for raw material/packing material
5. FIFO inventory management

Purchase
1. Vendor selection and approval
2. Vendor audit
3. Material procurement
4. Vendor reapproval

(Contd.)

Sl. No.	*Title*
5.	Vendor validation
6.	Continuous vendor evaluation

Production
1. Organization chart and responsibilities of production personnel
2. Entry into manufacturing area
3. Equipment/instruments log book
4. Housekeeping and sanitization
5. Portable/DM/DI water
6. Steam supply
7. Master formula
8. Batch manufacturing procedure
9. Filling of batch processing records
10. Blending batches of API/intermediates
11. Operation and calibration of weighing balances
12. Operation of all manufacturing equipments
13. Entry and exit from production area
14. Utility record
15. Operation of ejector system
16. Operation of filter
17. Operation of sifter
18. Operation of blender
19. Operation of micronizer
20. Operation of multimill
21. Operation of centrifuge
22. Operation of steam tray dryer
23. Shutdown of the plant
24. Starting up of the Plant
25. Batch change over
26. Shift change over
27. Product change over
28. Deviation and change control

Microbiology
1. Cleaning and sterilization procedure of laboratory
2. Entry into clean room
3. Fumigation
4. General microbiological procedures
5. Cleaning procedure for colony counter
6. Media preparation
7. Culture maintenance
8. Culture transfer
9. Maintenance and sub-culturing of standard cultures
10. Operation of laminar flow bench
11. Operation of autoclave
12. Sampling procedure for microbiological examination of personnel working in the clean and aseptic room

(Contd.)

Sl. No.	Title

13. Sampling procedure for microbiological examination of air
14. Sampling procedure for microbiological examination of sterile products
15. Sampling procedure for microbiological examination of APIs
16. Sampling procedure for microbiological examination of intermediates
17. Sampling procedure for microbiological examination of water
18. Effluent treatment

Quality Control
1. Organization chart and responsibilities of QC personnel
2. Entry into QC section
3. Housekeeping and sanitization
4. Equipment/instrument codification
5. Allotment of analytical report numbers
6. Calibration of laboratory equipment/instrument
7. Cleaning of glassware.
8. Analyst validation
9. Analytical method validation
10. Preparation and standardization of volumetric solutions
11. Preparation of Reagents
12. Operation and cleaning of double distilled water unit
13. Operation and calibration of analytical balance
14. Operation and calibration of melting point apparatus
15. Operation and calibration of pH meter
16. Operation and standardization of conductivity meter
17. Operation and calibration of bulk density apparatus
18. Operation and calibration of hot air oven
19. Operation and calibration of muffle furnace
20. Operation and calibration of particle size analyzer
21. Operation and calibration of polarimeter
22. Operation and calibration of vacuum over
23. Operation of kart fisher titration, standardization and determination of moisture in materials
24. Operation of ultraviolet fluorescence viewing cabinet
25. Operation and calibration of UV-visible spectorophotometer
26. Operation and calibration of FT-IR spectrophotometer
27. Operation and calibration of gas chromatography
28. Operation and calibration of high pressure liquid chromatography instrument
29. Operation and calibration of stability test chambers
30. In-process analysis all concerned products
31. Preventive maintenance of laboratory equipment/instrument.
32. Recording and calibration of wet and dry bulb hygrometer.
33. Releasing the raw materials, packing material, intermediates, and finished batches
34. Retesting of materials
35. Sampling plan
36. Stability studies of finished products and intermediates
37. Validation of working standard, impurity standards and reference standards

(Contd.)

Sl. No.	Title

Quality Assurance

1. Site Master File
2. Organization chart and responsibilities of quality assurance
3. Authorized signatories
4. Allotment of batch and lot numbers to APIs/intermediates
5. Approval and clearance of finished product APIs/lots
6. Packaging and Labeling of APIs/intermediates
7. Control of external origin documents
8. Release of finished product
9. Control of records
10. Document control
11. Control samples
12. Procedure of procedure
13. Process validation
14. Water system validation
15. AHU system validation
16. Sewage disposal system validation
17. Environmental monitoring
18. Equipment assembly and validation
19. Out of specification results
20. Corrective action, preventive action
21. Nonconforming material review
22. Planned and unplanned deviations
23. Product recalls and returns
24. Reprocessing/reworking of rejected finished APIs
25. Annual product review
26. Internal audit
27. Management review
28. Marketing complaints
29. Contract analysis
30. Organization assessment
31. Product complaint
32. Product returned
33. Product recall
34. Rejected product disposal
35. Training record

Research and Development

1. Organization chart and responsibilities of R&D
2. Entry into R&D unit
3. Project implementation and reporting
4. Experimental plan
5. Laboratory record keeping
6. Operation of all equipment and instrument
7. All experimental record maintenance
8. All equipment and instrument calibration validation
9. All equipment and instrument log book
10. All chemical and reagent record
11. Safety measures R&D laboratory
12. Technology transfer

Sampling Control

CHAPTER OVERVIEW

KEY POINTS

- In contrast to the traditional approach, the total quality control (TQC) concept has a goal of zero defective product in the manufacturing process, though unrealistic to be able to achieve permanently. Based on statistical methods, a small number of representative samples from the finished products are tested to reach a conclusion concerning the acceptability of an entire batch of drug product.
- As it is not practical to do acceptance testing on 100% of the product, sampling choice becomes crucial. The cGMP requires that the samples be a true representative of the population based on sampling plans of appropriate statistical criteria. The statistical quality control criteria include appropriate acceptance levels and/or appropriate rejection levels.
- Probability sampling is the mathematical approach of sampling that includes random, systematic, stratified and cluster sampling. The nonprobability sampling is a non-mathematical method where samples are selected in a nonrandom manner like convenience, quota, judgment and snowball sampling. Sampling error can be calculated in probability sampling but not in nonprobability sampling where results are reported as plus or minus in respect to sampling error.
- The sample size is the number of items selected for the test from a batch. Cochran formula for statistical sample size determination depends on batch size, confidence interval, standard deviation and confidence level.
- Sampling by attributes are used when a batch is accepted or rejected based on the number of defective products detected in the sample and sampling by variables is used when a quantitatively measured quality variable is used as a quality indicator.
- Attribute sampling is based on the sampling tables prepared following the acceptable quality level (AQL).

TOTAL QUALITY CONTROL

The traditional concept of quality control in pharmaceuticals typically involves compliance of drug products manufactured with designated standards (specifications) ensuring that the facility and personnel perform in accordance with the design. Sampling and statistical methods are commonly applied to accept or reject batches of products to ensure quality compliance. Batch rejection is based on non-conformance or violation of the relevant specifications. The implicit assumption in the traditional quality control practice is widely based on *acceptable quality level* which is an allowable fraction of defective items. Raw materials received from suppliers and the finished products manufactured by the production department is tested and passed as acceptable if the estimated percentage of defective items are within the acceptable quality level.

In contrast to the traditional approach of quality control, the concept of *total quality control* is not to allow any defective product in the whole production process with a goal of zero defect. Although the zero defects realistic goal can never be permanently achieved, organizations have to strive continuously for the goal and eventually the defects can be reduced by substantial amounts year after year. This concept and approach of quality control were first developed in manufacturing firms of Japan and Europe and later on was widely accepted by companies worldwide. The best known formal certification for quality commitment is the ISO 9000 standard. ISO 9000 emphasizes good documentation and quality practices with a series of planning cycle for the implementation of quality goal and review.

Total Quality Control (TQC) is a commitment to quality expressed by all counterparts of an organization and typically involves many elements. *Quality by design specification* is adopted to ensure product quality as a major element. Other elements include extensive training for personnel, expending the responsibility of defects detection between quality control inspectors to floor workers and continual maintenance of equipment. Involvement of the staff in quality control can be formalized in *quality circles concept* in which groups of workers meet regularly to make suggestions for quality improvement. Material vendors are also required to assure supply of no defect goods. All raw materials delivered by the suppliers are inspected, and batches of goods with any defective items are returned. Suppliers with good track records are thus audited, certified and are subject to complete inspection subsequently.

Nowadays companies have realized the substantial economic benefits of commitment towards total quality control that was long unappreciated in traditional approaches. Expenses associated with inventory management, rework, scrap disposal and warranties are eventually reduced with acceptance of TQC concept. With betterment of quality aspects in the working atmosphere, workers enthusiasm and commitment also got improved. Customers always appreciate products with higher quality, and as a result, total quality control became a competitive advantage. Commitment to best quality maintenance even without endorsing the goal of zero defects can pay real dividends to manufacturers. In most instances, finished product testing invariably causes destruction of sample material, due to this, exhaustive testing of every single unit of finished pharmaceutical product is not possible. As a result, a small number of representative samples are tested to establish the basis of accepting or rejecting a particular product batch or shipment of drug material. Based on statistical methods the results of tests done on a small sample number are considered to interpret and reach a conclusion concerning the acceptability

of an entire lot or batch of drug product. Acceptance inspection is performed at many stages in the pharmaceutical process, from testing raw materials to the final packaging stage. Acceptance testing is necessary since 100% inspection is not practical and would be very costly. Sampling is a regulatory requirement in the pharmaceutical industry. The cGMP requires sampling plans to be defined as well as samples to be representative of the population and based on appropriate statistical criteria. The statistical quality control criteria include appropriate acceptance levels and/or appropriate rejection levels. Pharmaceutical quality control unit mathematically decides the acceptance criteria for the sampling and testing conducted. These criteria must be adequate to assure that batches of drug products meet the appropriate specification of quality control based on these the approval and release conditions are finalized.

STATISTICAL QUALITY CONTROL

An ideal quality control program must test all materials coming out of a particular facility. Statistical methods are essential for interpretation of the results of testing done on a small sample size superimposed as representative for the whole batch. Interpretation of quality status based on tests done on a small sample fraction can be quite misleading without adequate statistical analysis. As an example, if there are ten defective pieces of material in a batch of one hundred the QC department might not find *any* defective pieces or might have *all* sample pieces defective while taking a sample of five pieces for analysis. If as in the case, none of the samples are found defective drawing a direct inference that none of the batch products are defective would be incorrect. Application of statistical sampling methods has the best chances of identifying a justified quality representative sample that is to be tested from a big batch.

Two types of statistical sampling are commonly used for quality control of material batches:

1. *Sampling by attributes,* when acceptance or rejection of a batch is based on the number of defective or non-defective products detected in the sample.
2. *Sampling by variables,* when instead of using classification based on defective and non-defective the measured variable of quantitative quality or value is detected in the sample.

Whatever sampling plan is used for testing, it always assumes that samples are the representative of the entire batch under consideration. Samples are chosen randomly so that each member of the batch has an equal chance to be chosen. Convenient sampling plans like withdrawing every twenty-fifth piece or after every 25 minutes or picking a few pieces at random from finished product batch may be adequate to ensure a random sampling. Random nature of sample selection process can substantially modify test results interpretation.

SAMPLING BY ATTRIBUTES

Sampling by attributes is a widely practiced sampling method to determine whether or not a particular batch or batch of products is acceptable. This process assumes that each item in a batch can be tested and classified as either acceptable or rejected based on the mutually acceptable testing procedure and acceptance criteria. Each batch is tested to determine suitability to minimum acceptable quality level (AQL) mostly expressed as the maximum percentage of defective items allowable in a batch or process. Sampling by attributes process tests a pre-defined number of samples from a batch. If the number of defective items is higher than a trigger level, the batch is rejected or otherwise accepted.

This type of sampling plan development requires consideration of probability, statistics and acceptable risk levels on the part of the supplier and also a consumer. If in case the number of defective items is greater than the pre-defined number, then additional sampling and testing can be done rather than an immediate rejection of the batch. In many cases, the trigger level is the identification of a single defective item out of the collected samples. The result of sample testing is interpreted based on the mathematical calculation in this type of sampling plan.

A batch is defined as acceptable if it contains a fraction of p_1 or less defective items and is defined unacceptable if it contains a fraction of p_2 or more defective units. Usually, the acceptance fraction is less than or equal to the rejected fraction, $p_1 \leq p_2$, and the two fractions are often equal so that there is no ambiguous range of batch acceptability between p_1 and p_2. These are the probabilities that acceptable batches might be incorrectly rejected (termed *producer's risk*), or deficient batches might be incorrectly accepted (termed *consumer's risk*) given sample size and a trigger level for batch rejection or acceptance.

For mathematical interpretation let's consider a batch of finite number N, in which m items are defective, and the remaining $(N - m)$ items are non-defective. If a random sample of n items were taken from this batch, the probability of having different numbers of defective items in the sample could be determined with a pre-defined acceptable number of defective items. To determine the probability of accepting a batch as a function of the sample size, the allowable number of defective items and the actual fraction of defective items is to be calculated. The number of possible samples with exactly x defectives is the combination associated with obtaining x defectives from m possible defective items and $n - x$ non-defective items from $N - m$ non-defective items. With these given possible numbers of samples, the probability of having an exactly x defective item in the sample is given by the ratio as the hypergeometric series:

$$P(X = x) = \frac{\binom{m}{x}\binom{N-m}{n-x}}{\binom{N}{n}}$$

With this equation, the probability of obtaining different numbers of defectives in a sample of a given size is calculated. Assumably if that the actual fraction of defectives in the batch is p and the actual fraction of non-defectives is q, then p plus q is one resulting in $m = Np$, and $N - m = Nq$. The function $g(p)$ represents the probability of having r or less defective items in sample size n is obtained by substituting m and N and summing over the acceptable defective number of items. When the number of items in the batch N is larger in comparison with the sample size n, then the function $g(p)$ is approximated by the binomial distribution:

$$g(p) = \sum_{x=0}^{r} \binom{n}{x} p^x q^{n-x}$$

or

$$g(p) = 1 - \sum_{x=r+1}^{n} \binom{n}{x} p^x q^{n-x}$$

Given the sample size is n and the number of allowable defective items in the sample is r, the function $g(p)$ specifies the probability of accepting a batch. This function $g(p)$ can be represented graphically for each combination of sample size n and number of allowable defective items r, where the curve is referred to as the operating characteristic curve (OC curve). Considering a special case of sample $n = 1$, the function $g(p)$ can be simplified:

$$g(p) = \binom{1}{0} p^0 q^1 = q$$

So the probability of accepting a batch is equal to the fraction of acceptable items in the batch. For example, a batch has fifty percent chances of being accepted from a single sample test even if the batch is defective when the probability is 0.5.

Acceptance Probability Calculation

Assume that sample size is five ($n = 5$) from a batch of one hundred items ($N = 100$). The batch of materials is to be rejected if any of the five samples is defective, so $r = 0$. As a function of the actual number of defective items the probability of acceptance can be computed considering $x = 0$, for $r = 0$, $N = 100$ and $n = 5$ following the equation

$$P(X = x) = \frac{\binom{m}{x}\binom{N-m}{n-x}}{\binom{N}{n}}$$

For a 2% defective fraction ($p = 0.02$), the acceptance value is:

$$g(p) = \frac{\binom{2}{0}\binom{98}{5}}{\binom{100}{5}} = \frac{\dfrac{98!}{93!.5!}}{\dfrac{100!}{95!.5!}} = \frac{98!.95!}{93!.100!} = 0.9020$$

The probability of having defective items calculated using the binomial approximation is:

$$g(p) \approx \binom{5}{0} p^0 q^5 = q^5 = (0.98)^5 = 0.9039$$

This is a difference of 0.0019 or 0.21 percent from the actual value of 0.9020 found above. If the acceptable defective proportion is 2% ($p_1 = p_2 = 0.02$), the chances of an incorrect rejection or the producer's risk is $1 - g(0.02) = 1 - 0.9 = 0.1$ or 10%. When the actual proportion of defective item is 1%, the producer's risk is only 5%. The manufacturer must ensure higher than minimum acceptable quality products to reduce the probability of rejection practicing this sampling plan.

SAMPLING BY VARIABLES

Sampling by attributes is based on an item classification as non-*defective* or *defective*, whereas sampling by variables is for application to continuously measurable quantities, where a particular level of a variable quantity is defined as acceptable quality. In a sample, the measured values of an attribute are used to determine the overall acceptability of a batch or lot. Sampling by variables come out with more information from tests since it is based on actual measured values rather than simple classification.

Compared to the sampling by attributes, the acceptance sampling by variables is more efficient which requires testing of fewer samples for obtaining the desired quality control level. Following the concept of sampling by variables, the quality of an acceptable batch is defined with an upper limit **U**, a lower limit **L** or both. An acceptable quality level is defined as a maximum allowable fraction of defective items, **M** complying with these boundary conditions. Figure 7.1 illustrates the probability distribution of the item attribute as **x**.

Defective item is equal to the area under the distribution function, with an upper limit of **U** ($x \geq U$). This fraction of defective items is compared to the allowable fraction **M** to determine the acceptability of a batch. Following the concept of a lower and an upper limit of acceptable quality, the fraction of defective item would be the fraction of items greater than the upper limit or less than the lower limit. The limits are also valued to be imposed upon the acceptable *average* level of the variable. In this process, the fraction of defective items is estimated by using measured values from a sample of items compared to sampling by attributes, which measures a random number of samples of a given size obtained from a lot or batch. The resulting distribution of values approximates the normal distribution when the source of variations is a large number of little but independent random effects. In case the distribution of measured values does not approximate normal distribution, sampling by

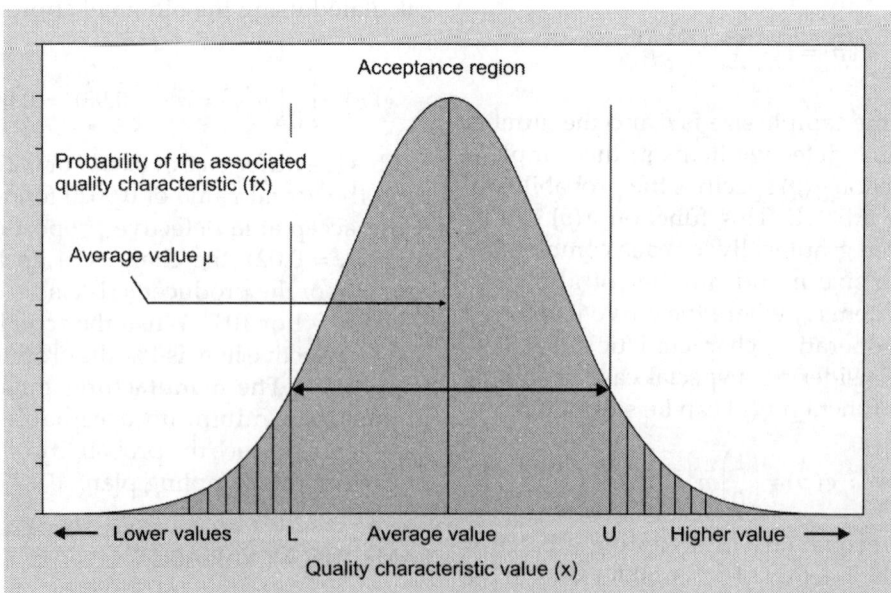

Fig. 7.1: Variable probability distributions and acceptance regions in a quality characteristic distribution curve

attributes is adopted. Deviations from normal distributions can appear as skewed or non-symmetric or as distributions with fixed upper and lower limits.

SAMPLING METHODS

The sample is withdrawn from a population or batch to conduct quality control tests. There are different methods of choosing the respondent samples classified as *probability* or *nonprobability* sampling. A mathematical approach to sampling is called probability sampling, and non-mathematical approach is simply called nonprobability sampling. In probability sampling, each member of the batch has a known non-zero probability of being selected. The types of probability sampling method include random, systematic, stratified and cluster sampling. Sampling error is the probability of a sample to differ from the batch. Sampling error can be calculated easily in probability sampling. In nonprobability sampling, samples are selected in a nonrandom manner from the batch which includes types like convenience, quota, judgment and snowball sampling. Sampling error cannot be calculated in nonprobability sampling thus results are reported as plus or minus in respect to that of sampling error.

Factors that commonly influence the choice between the sampling designs are:
- Nature, quality and other characteristics of the representative batch
- Lot/batch diversification
- Availability of auxiliary information about sub-groups of the batch
- Level of accuracy requirements and the need to measure accuracy
- Required detailed of analysis of the sample
- Multiple variables of selection criteria
- Required sampling frequency
- Cost/operational concerns
- Time limit

Probability Sampling

Probability methods are the best group of methods that gives powerful statistical analyses on the results.

1. **Random sampling:** Random sampling is the unadulterated form of probability sampling. Each item of the batch has an equal and known chance of being selected, but with a very large batch, it is often difficult to identify every item of the batch so the pool of available items can become biased.

   Simple random sampling: In this method, every item in a batch has the same probability of being selected. In simple random sampling, all items of the batch are given an equal probability of selection. Batches are not required to be subdivided or partitioned as this can minimize bias and simplify result analysis. The occurrence of variation between individual results within a sample group is an indicator of variation in the overall batch. Simple random sampling is cumbersome and tedious when sampling needs to be done from large target batches. Random sampling can be done with or without replacement where the sampled item is not returned to the batch after it is selected. Though in the case of pharmaceutical products all sampling is meant to be without replacement.

   Matched random sampling: In matched random sampling each item is measured twice for the same attribute or variable under different circumstances, commonly called repeated measures. Matched random sampling is a method of assigning individual members/participants a group, in which pairs of members/participants are first matched on some common characteristic and then individually assigned randomly in groups. For example, the run times of a group of athletes for 1500 m before and after a week's special training; the milk yields of cows before and after feeding particular diet for 15 days. In pharmaceuticals, this type of sampling is applied at pilot stage R&D studies and in preclinical and clinical studies.

2. **Systematic sampling:** Systematic sampling is used as a replacement for random sampling called an **n**th selection technique. In this method, every **n**th item from a list or series is selected as the sample, starting with a sample item randomly from the first **k** elements. Systematic sampling relies on arranging the target batch according to an ordering scheme and then selecting items at regular intervals following that ordered scheme. The required sample size is calculated prior, and sampling starts with the selection of the first item randomly and then proceeding with the selection of every **n**th item from then onwards (n = batch size/sample size). It is crucial to set the starting point automatically in the list which is randomly chosen from the first item to the **n**th item in the list, e.g. on a batch of 1000 items let the sample size needed is 100, then k is 1000/100 = 10, so the first sample should any from 1st to 10th item, let it be 6th now following that every 10th item (16th, 26th, …, 996th) will be selected from the batch. This type of sampling procedure is frequently followed in process quality control sampling of pharmaceutical products.

3. **Stratified sampling:** The statistical stratified sampling method is used when representatives from each subgroup within the batch need to be represented in the sample. Stratified sampling (random within target groups) uses a probability method which is superior to random sampling as it reduces sampling error. In stratified sampling, batch is divided into subgroups (strata) based on mutually exclusive criteria. A stratum is a subset of the batch that shares at least one common characteristic. This method implementation requires first to identify the relevant stratum and their actual representation in the batch. Random sampling is then used to select *sufficient* number of items from each stratum. Random or systematic samples are also used to take samples from each subgroup. The sampling fraction for each subgroup can be taken in the same proportion as the subgroup is represented in the batch, e.g. in customer satisfaction survey a large batch of customers are subdivided into strata based on job category, i.e. 60% private, 20% corporate and 20% government employee. The sample size selected from each stratum is to be in proportion to the number of customers in each stratum in the batch, so then 6 private, 2 corporate, 2 government employees were randomly selected. Stratified sampling is often used when one or more of the stratum in the batch have a low incidence rate relative to the other stratum. An equal number of items from each subgroup can also be selected in stratified sampling case based. In the pharmaceutical field also this type of sampling is used for market survey and brand promotional activities.

4. **Cluster sampling:** The cluster sampling method is also called block sampling. In cluster sampling, the batch is divided into groups called clusters that are based on criteria as heterogeneous as possible, unlike stratified sampling which is based on homogeneous selection criteria. In cluster sampling, instead of considering all the items from the entire batch right off, the researcher takes several steps in gathering the sample population. A simple random sample of clusters is selected from the lot, and random samples are then taken from the selected

clusters. Cluster sampling is a type of 'two-stage sampling' or 'multistage sampling'; in the first stage, a sampling area is chosen and in the second stage sample of respondents *within* those areas are selected. Clusters can be chosen from a cluster-level frame (common property) or with an element-level frame (common criteria). Cluster sampling in general increases the variability of sample estimates higher than that observed in random sampling, depending on how the clusters differ in between as compared to within-cluster variation.

Nevertheless, disadvantages of cluster sampling are the reliance of sample estimate precision correlated to the actual basis of clusters selection. In case the clusters chosen are biased in some certain way, inferences drawn about batch parameters from these sample estimates cannot be expected to be accurate. Cluster sampling represents a lot about the particular clusters, but as the clusters are selected randomly and every cluster has not been sampled, generalizations cannot be made about the entire batch.

Multistage sampling: Multistage sampling is a composite form of cluster sampling in which two or more levels of items are embedded in one another. The first stage is the formation of the clusters for sampling, and in the second stage, a sample of primary items are randomly selected from each cluster (rather than using all units contained in all selected clusters). In the following stages, from each of those selected clusters, additional sample items are selected and so on. All ultimate items selected at the last step of this procedure are then tested. Multistage sampling is used frequently when complete detail of all items of the batch is not available and is inappropriate.

Moreover, by avoiding the use of all sample units in all selected clusters, multistage sampling avoids the large and unnecessary costs associated with traditional cluster sampling, e.g. a pharmaceutical manufacturer wants to survey the performance of an OTC medicine is marketed all over India. The entire population of India is divided into different clusters (Delhi, Mumbai, Kolkata, and Chennai). Then the researcher selects a number of clusters that are from 2 cities depending on simple or systematic random sampling. Then, from the randomly selected clusters (Delhi and Chennai) the researcher can either include all the subjects or can further select a number of subjects from each cluster through simple or systematic random sampling.

Non-Probability Sampling

1. **Convenience sampling:** Convenience sampling (sometimes known as opportunity sampling) involves sampling from the part of the batch which is readily available and convenient. Convenience sampling is commonly used in exploratory research where a researcher is interested in getting a reasonable approximation of truth. This sampling method is inefficient to make any generalizations about the total batch as it is not representative enough but is quick and cheap. The nonprobability method is mostly used during preliminary stages research studies to get gross estimate of the results without incurring more cost or time. This type of sampling is useful for pilot testing. Convenience sampling is typically quicker and uses smaller sample sizes than other sampling techniques. The main disadvantage of convenience sampling is that since it is not statistically based, generalizations about the total batch cannot be made.

2. **Quota sampling:** Quota sampling is the nonprobability sampling method equivalent to stratified sampling. Like stratified sampling, stratum are first identified following their due representation of proportions in the batch. Then convenience or judgment sampling procedure is followed to select the required number of items from each stratum. This method differs from stratified sampling only in the manner that here the stratum is sampled by random sampling, whereas in quota sampling the selection of the sample is non-random. For a particular analysis and valid results, the number of units needed to be sampled from a batch is determined. The batch is first segmented into mutually exclusive sub-groups then convenience or judgment sampling is used to select the units from each segment based on a specified proportion. If the number of items in different sub-groups is small, then equivalent numbers are required to enable for substantial analysis and conclusions. The subtypes are:

Proportionate quota sampling (in proportion to batch sub-groups)

Non-proportionate sampling (minimum number from each sub-group)

Dimensional quota sampling (representing a maximum number of characteristic).

For example, in a survey blood pressure patients of 50–60 ages were sample out of 50 females and 80 males.

3. **Judgment sampling:** Judgment sampling is a common nonprobability/non-statistical method where sampling is done based on knowledge and experience of researcher involved, e.g. based on experience, an auditor may decide the type of samples which are more apt to have non-conformances or which types of items have had problems in the past with higher quality risk to the organization. This is an extension of convenience sampling, e.g. in market survey, a researcher may decide to draw the entire sample from one 'representative' city, even though the batch includes all cities. When using this method, the selector must be confident that the chosen sample is indeed representative of the entire batch.

4. **Snowball sampling:** Snowball sampling (also called chain-referral sampling) is a particular type of nonprobability sampling method used when the desired sample characteristic is rare. It may be extremely challenging or cost prohibitive to locate respondents that represent a particular rare characteristic. Snowball sampling depends on referrals from initial stage subjects to generate additional subjects. Though this technique can dramatically lower search costs, it comes at the expense of introduction of bias because the technique itself increases the likelihood that the sample may not be a representative of a right cross-section of the batch. Mostly used in social science studies where existing study subjects are used to recruit more subjects as a sample.

To summarise, between two broad sampling frames, probability and nonprobability, there are eight types of sampling methods, all with particular advantages and disadvantages and unique characteristic features.

SAMPLE SIZE

The sample size is the part of the batch selected for testing targeted to assess quality control attributes in pharmaceutical manufacturing, e.g. to determine the assay value of drug in a batch of finished tablet with 1 lakh tablets, some tablets need to be tested that constitutes the sample size representing the batch. The sample size here will represent all tablets of this batch, the test results of which will decide conformance or non-conformance of the batch with predefined specification and ultimately its market release. Testing only a small number of samples from the batch may create doubt on the result precision. Hundred percent assurance cannot be achieved by testing a certain percentage of the material of the actual batch. This uncertainty is called sampling error and is usually measured by a confidence interval. This uncertainty on the test results can be ruled out by determining the sample size needed for an experiment following the principle of statistics.

SAMPLE SIZE DETERMINATION

The statistical process of appropriate sample size determination takes into account factors like total size of the batch, the margin of error allowable (confidence interval), reliability on the data collected (standard deviation) and the probability that margin of error is accurate (confidence level).

Population size: Finding a sample size can be one of the most challenging tasks in statistics. The sample size is typically denoted as n, positive integer. Large sample sizes are needed for statistically to be accurate and reliable with larger pollution or batch size. Typically, precision is directly proportional to sample size for an estimated parameters in a batch when all addition parameters are equal.

The margin of error (confidence interval): The sample size is also directly related to the test process margin of error. The margin of sampling error is the confidence interval in the percentage that it expresses the probability that the data received is accurate. The confidence interval statistically measures the

number of chances for the results expected to be within a specified range out of 100 times. If the confidence interval of a method is 90%, then it can be expected that 90% of the test results will be similar if the test is repeated.

The margin of sampling error is calculated

as $= \dfrac{1}{\sqrt{n}} \times 100$ (n = sample size).

Standard deviation: Standard deviation measures how much individual pieces of data vary from the average data measured.

Precision (confidence level): The probability of accuracy of the margin of error also called the level of precision or the confidence level depending upon the attributes of the target batch under consideration. The degree of variability differs considerably when the batch is more heterogeneous. Larger sample size is required to get an optimum level of precision in such cases. It is expressed in the plus-or-minus figure usually reported in the result values.

Sample size determination is the act of selecting an appropriate number of items to include in statistical sampling. The sample size required in a study is determined based on the paradigm of data collection and the necessity of sufficient statistical power. Large sample sizes usually lead to increased precision as per the well-known statistical phenomenon of the law of large numbers and the central limit theorem. Repeated measurements and replication of independent samples are often required in measurement and experiments to reach the desired precision.

Cochran Formula for Sample Size Determination

The Cochran formula is used to calculate an ideal sample size given a desired level of precision, confidence level and the estimated proportion of the attribute present in the population, especially appropriate with large batches.

Cochran formula for large batch:

$$n = \left(\frac{z}{e}\right)^2 \times pq \qquad (7.1)$$

where n = sample size

z = confidence interval (find the z-value in a Z table that converts percentage to a representative value)

e = desired level of precision (i.e. the margin of error),

p = estimated proportion of the batch which has the attribute in question

$q = 1 - p$.

Cochran formula for a small batch: If the batch size is small a modified version of the above formula is used for calculation:

$$n = \frac{n_0}{1 + \dfrac{(n_0 - 1)}{N}} \qquad (7.2)$$

where, n_0 = Cochran's sample size recommendation by using Eq. (7.1)

N = population size

n = the new adjusted sample size.

This is to find a sample size with a given confidence interval and confidence level (margin of error or weight) but unknown population standard deviation (SD).

The sample size for a known confidence interval and confidence level, and unknown SD:

$$n = \left[\frac{\text{substituted } Z\text{-value of } z/2}{e}\right]^2 \times pq \qquad (7.3)$$

To find a sample size with a given confidence interval and confidence level (margin of error or weight or e) and also known as population standard deviation.

The sample size for a known confidence interval, confidence level, and SD:

$$n = \left[\frac{\text{substituted } Z\text{-value for } z/2 \times \text{SD}}{e}\right]^2 \qquad (7.4)$$

where, SD or σ = standard deviation for the population

For calculation of sample size using these formulas estimation of batch proportion with a required attribute is to be calculated, e.g. to estimate the proportion (p) of residents in a community who are at least 65 years old, the batch proportion $p = X/n$. Where X is the number of 'positive' observations, e.g. the number of the person at least 65 years old out of the n sampled people. In case of pharmaceutical quality control test of drug formulation batches, the observation batches are independent of proportional attribute distribution, like all the items in a batch of tablet formulation is assumed to be similar in respect to drug content. In such cases, this estimator batch proportion is assumed to have a (scaled) binomial distribution and is also a form of the sample mean (from a Bernoulli distribution which has a maximum variance of 0.25 for parameter p of 0.5). Here the sample means X/n has maximum variance $0.25/n$, which occurs when the true parameter value for $p = 0.5$. Practically, since p is unknown, the maximum variance is often used for sample size assessments. For sufficiently large n (usually with atleast 10 positive and 10 negative response observations, the p distribution will closely approximate a normal distribution with same mean and variance. Using this approximation, it can be shown that ~95% of this distribution's probability lies within 2 standard deviations of the mean:

$$(\hat{p} - 2\sqrt{0.25/n}, \hat{p} + 2\sqrt{0.25/n}) = (\hat{p} - B, \hat{p} + B)$$

When the sampling error is bound to be less than B; the equation will be:

$$\varepsilon \approx B = 2\sqrt{0.25/n} = 1/\sqrt{n}$$

To give, $1/\varepsilon^2 \approx 1/B^2 = n$.

This will form a 95% confidence interval for the true proportion when this interval needs to be no more than z units wide

$$4\sqrt{0.25/n} = N \qquad (7.5)$$

In some special cases batch or population mean can be used to calculate sample size when the population proportion is arbitrary.

Sample size can be calculated based on the population mean with a known confidence level (z) or standard deviation (σ).

Sample size based on batch mean:

$$n = 4\sigma^2 / e^2 \qquad (7.6)$$

with known standard deviation

or $\qquad n = (z/e)^2$

with known confidence level

Batch means estimated using an independent and identically distributed sample of size n, where each data value has a variance or standard deviation σ^2, the standard error of the sample mean μ is: $\sigma^2/\sqrt{n}$. This equation quantitatively describes that the estimate becomes more precise with the increase in sample size. Using the central limit theorem, approximating the sample mean with a normal distribution yielding an 95% confidence interval is justified, where $Z = 4\sigma/\sqrt{n}$ is units in width, that yields the sample size $n = 16\,\sigma^2/Z^2$. This fact is proved mathematically in the central limit theorem. The central limit theorem explained when sample size n was taken from any arbitrary population (with any arbitrary distribution) to calculate the overall batch mean $\bar{x}$, then sampling distribution of $\bar{x}$ will approach the standard normal distribution as the sample size n increases with mean μ and standard error will be $\sigma/\sqrt{n}$. So, the margin of error $e = z_{\alpha/2} \times \sigma/\sqrt{n}$. Here $z_{\alpha/2}$ is known as the critical value, the positive z value that is at the vertical boundary for the area of $\alpha/2$ in the right tail of the standard normal distribution curve as in Fig. 7.2.

The Eq. (7.4) can be modified and used when σ is known and the sample size n is required to be established with a confidence of $1 - \alpha$, where the mean value μ lies within a specified limit of $\pm e$ value, so Eq. (7.6) is $n = (z_{\alpha/2} \times \sigma/e)^2$.

Based on this equation it is easy to show that as n becomes very large, this variability becomes small with greater statistical power and a smaller confidence interval. A typical statistical aim is to demonstrate with 95% certainty that the true value of a study parameter is within a distance of B which is the error range (e) that decreases with increasing sample size (n). Based on Eq. (7.5), it can be

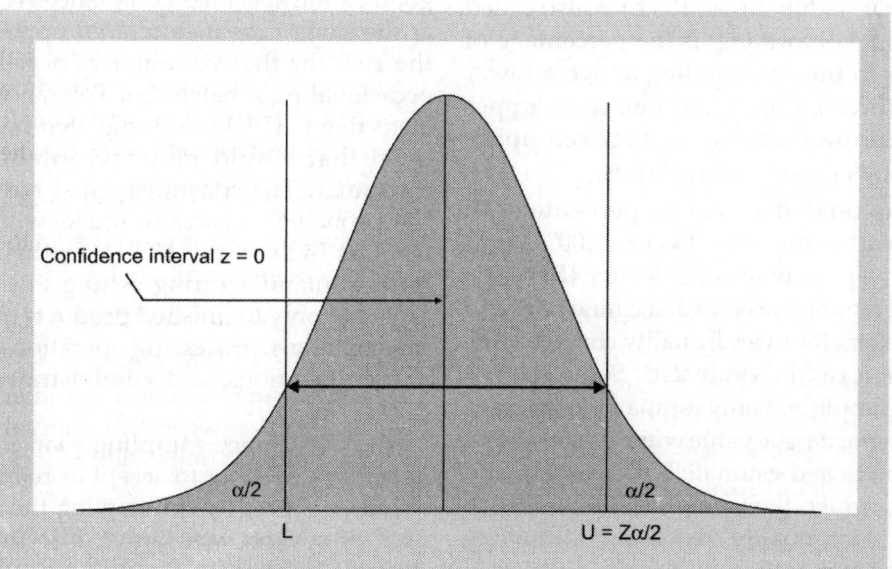

Fig. 7.2: Normal standard quality distribution curve with a confidence interval

solved for n, yielding $n = 1/B^2 = 4/z^2$ where B is the error bound of the estimate. Estimate is usually given as within $\pm B$, so, for $B = 10\%$ required $n = 100$, for $B = 5\%$ required $n = 400$ and while for $B = 1\%$ the sample size $n = 10000$ is required.

SAMPLING PLAN

Quality level goals depend on the defined measure of an acceptable quality limit (AQL) and a rejectable quality limit (RQL). AQL is the minimum level of actual quality limit at which a material batch is considered fully acceptable. RQL is the maximum level of quality defects at which a material batch is considered unacceptable and thus, rejectable. Quality of a product is thus simply defined as the fraction of the total batch items that follow the overall quality characteristic distribution and lies within specification limits. It is usually expressed as either:

- Percent Defective (PD) is also called percent nonconforming, is the percentage of items in the batch falling outside specification limits.
- Percent within limits (PWL) is also called percent conforming, is the percentage of items in the batch falling above a lower specification limit and below an upper specification limit or in between upper and lower specification limits.

PWL is related to PD as percentage of product within the limit (PWL) = 100% items in a batch – percentage of defective (PD). The statistical model is used to determine how and to what extent the overall quality characteristic distribution can be estimated. Some models are quite simple and only estimates an average quality characteristic value while other models are complete and estimate both average and variation, which then provides the ability to estimate batch quality. Batch overall quality is expressed as PWL which is the fraction of the batch that falls within specifications.

Acceptable Quality Level (AQL)

The AQL provides the maximum percent of defective products that are permitted as the lower limit of the baseline requirement for the quality control of the product batches. The primary purpose of setting an acceptabl-equality limit is to decide whether or not the batch under test is likely to be acceptable, but not to estimate the quality of the batch. The manufacturer is required to develop and design a sampling plan in a way such that permits a *high probability of accepting* a batch that has a defect level less than or equal to the AQL.

ISO 2859 (sampling procedure for inspection) is designed to encourage manufacturers to have the batch process quality averages consistently better than the AQL; otherwise, it can impact the risk of switching to tighter regulatory supervision concerning pharmaceutical products. For the health care products, the designation of an AQL does not imply that the manufacturer has the right to supply any nonconforming items that fall below AQL. The aim to instruct the manufacturer to maintain a process average at least as good as the specified acceptance AQL, while at the same time maintain an upper limit to the risk for the consumer of accepting the occasional poor batch. Lot Tolerance Percent Defective (LTPD) is a designated high defect level that would be unacceptable to the consumer. The consumer must have a very low probability of accepting a lot with a defect level as high as the LTPD. In the pharmaceutical manufacturing setting this is applicable not only to finished products but also to raw materials, processing operations, maintenance operations, and administrative procedures.

The acceptance sampling plan is used to determine whether to accept or reject a batch of material produced following the standard quality control technique. The in-process controls implied to the manufacturing and packaging of pharmaceutical products done in a controlled manner ensuring that the resultant products comply with its predefined specification. Control aspects applied to environment and equipment is also considered as a part of in-process control, i.e. in the case of tablet manufacturing, the in-process quality control (IPQC) factors like weight variation, friability and hardness are the most important one that in turn affects the performance of the finished products. Injectables and ophthalmic solutions must undergo inspection for container filling, presence of glass particles in the vials, presence of foreign particles of dust, fibers, etc.

As per acceptance sampling plan, a random sample is taken out from a large number of items and tested in respect to the quality characteristic of interest. The entire batch is declared acceptable when the sample passes the test, but if the sample fails the test, either (a) the entire batch is subjected to 100% inspection so that all defective items can be repaired or replaced; or (b) the entire batch is rejected. In the case of pharmaceutical manufacturing, the latter process is followed to comply with cGMP guidelines.

For statistical IPQC spot checking of production batch, samples are randomly taken out according to the sampling table and inspected. If the number of defectives is found to be exceeding the acceptance number given in the table, the batch is re-inspected and further processed if the number of defective items are below the acceptance number, it is passed/accepted.

Types of the Acceptance Sampling Plan

In acceptance sampling plan a set of rules are set out in the form of specifications for making decisions of conformance and nonconformance. There are two major acceptance classification plans; by attributes (accept or reject) and by variables. The attribute sampling is the most common for acceptance

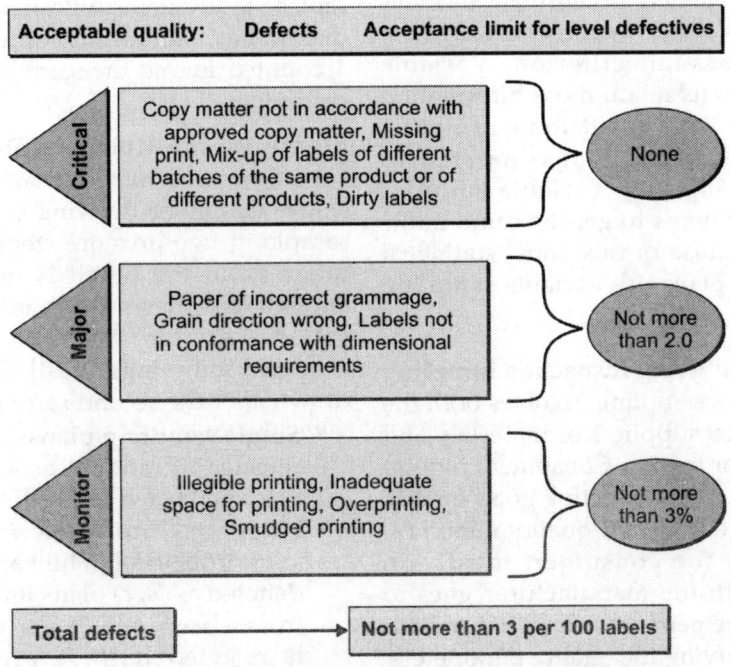

Fig. 7.3: Acceptable quality limit for samples

sampling in the pharmaceutical manufacturing field.

Attributes vs. variables sampling plan: When inspection of items in a batch leads to a binary result (either the item is considered conforming or nonconforming) or the number of nonconformities in a batch are counted, it is with sampling by attributes, but if the inspection of item leads to a continuous measurement, then it is sampling by variables.

- **Attribute sampling:** As per attribute sampling, each sample is inspected for the presence or absence of one particular or several attributes (often called quality characteristics or compliance to specifications). Testing is done to detect these quality characteristics compared to standard and then recorded as either passed or failed.

- **Variable sampling:** As per variable sampling, measured quality characteristics are used as continuous variables. Unlike attribute sampling, measurement values are retained. Because these values are retained rather than converted into a discrete pass-fail criterion. Variable sampling plans retain more information per sample than do attribute sampling plans. This means that compared to attribute sampling, variable samples takes fewer items to get the same information. Because of this, most statistical acceptance plans use variable sampling plan.

Incoming vs. Outgoing inspection sampling plan: Acceptance sampling involves both the manufacturer (or supplier) of materials and the consumer (or buyer). Consumers require this to limit the risk of rejecting good quality materials or accepting bad quality materials. Consequently, the consumer, mostly in conjunction with the manufacturer goes to contractual agreements as it is called written guarantee, specifying the quality parameters. A company can be both a producer of goods purchased by another company and a consumer of goods or raw materials supplied by another company. When the batches are inspected before the product are released for shipment to consumers, it is called an outgoing inspection. Inspection done by the consumer after they receive material from the supplier is called an incoming inspection.

Rectifying vs. non-rectifying sampling plans: A rectifying sampling plan is applicable if the defects that are found in the tested sample items can be corrected immediately. This plan is similar to attributes sampling plan, but it ensures release of a batch with highest quality after inspection as in case of sample failure the whole batch is reinspected and rectified. This applies to nondestructive testing methods of samples, which had a predetermined plan on what to be done with nonconforming items found during the inspection. Most of the pharmaceutical quality testing destroys the sample itself. In pharmaceutical quality control sampling plan it is not permitted to replace faulty items with new ones as it will disrupt batch uniformity or reworking can be accounted for, so the sampling plan is non-rectifying.

Single vs. multiple sampling plans: The sampling procedure consists of drawing a single sample or drawing of more than one sample in two or more steps. If the sample taken from the batch is not informative enough, another sample is taken which is called a double sampling procedure. In multiple sampling, additional samples are drawn after the second sample.

- **Single sampling plans:** Only one item is selected at random as a sample from a batch and batch disposition is determined based on information of this single sample testing. The sampling plan is denoted as (n, c) plans for a sample size n from a batch of N items, where the batch is rejected if there are more than c defectives. This is the most common and easiest sampling plans used although not efficient enough regarding the average number of samples needed.

- **Double sampling plans:** Testing of the first sample here gives three possibilities:
  1. Accept the batch
  2. Reject the batch
  3. No decision—resample the batch

  If it is the no-decision case, a second sample is taken, and the final decision is taken based on the combined result of both the samples.

- **Multiple sampling plans:** As an extension of the double sampling plan here more than two samples are withdrawn and tested to conclude.

- **Sequential sampling plans:** This is the utmost extension of multiple sampling where from a batch, items are selected one at a time, and after inspection of each item decision is made about acceptance or rejection the batch or to select another unit for testing.

- **Skip lot sampling plans:** In skip batch sampling process only a fraction of items from the batch under consideration are inspected.

Single vs. double stage sampling plans: This sampling procedure also consist of drawing of samples in one or more stages, but in contrast to previous one in place of taking a single sample at a time this process follows the statistical analysis to withdraw a specified number of sample to follow the standards of AQL.

- **Single-stage sampling plan:** A certain number of sample items (n) are drawn and inspected. That number n depends mainly on the size of the batch as per statistical analysis. The batch is passed if the number of defects found is under the AQL limit.

- **Double-stage sampling plan:** This sampling process starts with taking a smaller number of sample (n_1, n_2 .... to reach a total number of n) stage wise unlike taking a total number of n at a time. When the number of defects in n_1 is above certain limits, more samples are picked.

DESIGNING A SAMPLING PLAN

Sampling by Attributes Plan

Attribute sampling plans are often used to inspect the effectiveness of the process and to determine the rate of compliance with established criteria. Attributes sampling plan follows an acceptance system that provides tightened but reduced sampling plans based on tables to be applied for attributes inspection for percent nonconforming or nonconformities per 100 units. In acceptance testing by attributes sampling, a sample is randomly taken and inspected against established specifications, and if the number of defects exceeds the allowable number of defects, then the entire lot is rejected. Acceptance sampling tables are prepared for attribute sampling based on the AQL designation as specified in the company standard operating procedure (SOP). Different AQLs may be designated for different types of defects (critical, major, and minor). AQL is the maximum percent defective or the maximum number of defects allowed per hundred units as a process average. The inspection level determines how the lot size and the sample size are related, special and general inspection level correlating the batch size with respective sample size code letters as illustrated in Table 7.1.

Attribute sampling plans are based on n, c for a sample size n from a batch of N items, where the batch is rejected if there are more than c defectives. This process is based on the sampling plan tables that provide the exact number of sample required for a particular batch size with a sample size code in respect to that exact acceptance or rejection numbers are also mentioned depending on AQL. Accept and reject number in Table 7.1 signifies the

Table 7.1: Acceptance level of the attribute sampling plan

Sample size code letter	Sample size	Critical defect 0.01% Accept	Critical defect 0.01% Reject	Major defect 0.65% Accept	Major defect 0.65% Reject	Minor defect 4.00% Accept	Minor defect 4.00% Reject
A	2	0	0	0	0	0	0
B	3	0	0	0	0	0	0
C	5	0	0	0	0	0	1
D	8	0	0	0	0	0	1
E	13	0	0	0	0	0	1
F	20	0	0	0	0	1	2
G	32	0	0	0	1	2	3
H	50	0	0	0	1	3	4
J	80	0	0	0	1	5	6
K	125	0	0	1	2	8	9
L	200	0	0	2	3	12	13
M	315	0	0	3	4	18	19
N	500	0	0	5	6	18	19
P	800	0	0	8	9	18	19
Q	1250	0	0	12	13	18	19

upper limit for the number of defective items (c) found in the respective sample size withdrawn and tested. AQL for critical defect is c = 0 for a maximum number sample size 10,000. Determination of sample size and accept/reject levels of items are based on:

- Type of sampling plan
- Size of lot
- Acceptable quality level
- Application type, i.e. incoming, in-process or final inspection
- The inspection feature and critical level
- Defect history

The rejection criteria marked as defects are classified into three major categories: Critical, major, and minor based on criticality to product quality attributes. Each defect category is assigned a different AQL level as the customer's risk associated with different defects categories are not of the same level. Critical defects compromise with product safety, purity or identity that may be potentially harmful to the consumer. A major defect jeopardizes the integrity or function of the item or product, whereas minor defect does not affect product safety, purity, identity or functional integrity of the product. These defects categorization are defined based on the product attribute.

Different types of attribute sampling plans are single, double and multiple sampling. Sampling tables are development taking concern for the recommended sampling plan, inspection level, types and accept/reject criteria as per the inspection procedure. Acceptance levels for attribute sampling plan as per the inspection level and types of sampling plan are given in Table 7.3 to Table 7.7. In an expected batch size of 25,000 tablets, it would be impossible to test all units, so a representative sampling size should be selected. When the inspection sample size is to be determined as per sampling by attributes plan, general inspection, level III based on a single sampling plan. A batch of 25,000 tablets corresponds to code letter M in general inspection level III plan as per Table 7.5. The sample size for code letter M corresponds to

315. When the AQL level desired is specified as 0.65%, a major defect like creaking or chipping of the tablet surface, it means that 315 samples are needed to be inspected and should not have more than 4 defective items to pass the batch.

The sampling tables are used for selecting the sampling plan instead of developing a sampling plan based on complex statistics. Details of attribute sampling table bears the lowest sample size which makes it the most economical. It is the easiest to setup and track because of the lower sample size required. In processes with destructive testing, it is more practical to use this type of sampling plan. This sampling also saves documentation time. The common mistakes of an attribute sampling plan are the selection of incorrect sampling size, selection of incorrect acceptance criteria or attribute plan used for variable data.

Applying the concept of sampling by attributes, suppose the target is to ensure zero defective items in a batch with 5,000 items. With an AQL of no defective items ($p_1 = 0$) in the sampling plan, the allowable defective items in the sample are zero ($c = 0$). As a function of the fraction of actual defective items the probability of accepting the 5,000 items using the binomial approximation shows the sample size:

$$g(p) = (1-p)^n$$

To ensure ninety percent chance of rejecting a batch with 1% (p = 0.01) actual defective items the required sample size is calculated as:

$$g(p) = 1 - 0.90 = 0.1 = (1 - 0.01)^n$$

Then $n = \dfrac{\ln(0.1)}{\ln(0.99)} = \dfrac{-2.30}{-0.01} \approx 229$

It is evident from the sample number (n = 229) that large sample size is required to ensure relatively high probabilities of zero defective items.

Sampling by Variables Plan

Sampling by variables plan assumes that the measured characteristic is virtually always normally distributed as illustrated in Fig. 7.1. The normal distribution is a reasonably good assumption for measured characteristics such as drug content or dissolution or disintegration time of tablets. Applying the concept of sampling by variables the fraction of defective items in a sample is estimated from the batch mean ($\bar{x}$) and standard deviation (s). Mathematically, n is the number of items in the sample and $\bar{x}_i$ where, $i = 1, 2, 3, ..., n$ is the measured values for the variable characteristic x. The sample mean μ is an estimate of the overall batch mean $\bar{x}_i$:

$$\mu \approx \bar{x} = \frac{1}{n}\sum_{i=1}^{n} x_i$$

An estimate of the batch standard deviation is s, the square root of the sample variance statistic:

$$s^2 = \frac{1}{n-1}\left(\sum_{i=1}^{n} x_i^2 - n\bar{x}^2\right)$$

Based on the estimated values of the sample mean ($\bar{x}$), standard deviation (s) and the desired limits the various fractions of interest for the batch can be calculated. The acceptable batch quality t distributed curve is defined with an upper limit U and lower limit L with $n-1$ degrees of freedom. The t distribution is similar in appearance to a standard normal distribution, though the variability in the function *decreases* as the degrees of freedom *increases* and with very large degrees of freedom, the t distribution coincides with the normal distribution. The probability that the average value of a batch is greater or lower than a particular lower or upper limit is calculated as:

$$t_L = \frac{(\bar{x}-L)\sqrt{n}}{s}, \quad t_U = \frac{(U-\bar{x})\sqrt{n}}{s}$$

The sum of the probabilities of being above the upper limit or below the lower limit is calculated as estimated upper (T_U) and lower (T_L) limits. The fraction of items above the upper limit or below a lower limit are estimated similar to that of batch average with the only difference that the square root of the sample number does not appear in the formulas:

$$t_{AL} = \frac{\bar{x} - L}{s}, \quad t_{AU} = \frac{U - \bar{x}}{s}$$

Here t_{AL} is the test statistic for all items with a lower limit and t_{AU} is the upper limit. This procedure follows specifications regarding the allowable test statistic value instead of using sampling plans that specify an allowable fraction of defective items. This procedure requires the sample average to be a pre-specified number of standard deviations away from an upper or lower limit. Application of sampling by variables requires specification of sample size and the relevant upper or lower limits along with either. The allowable fraction of items falling outside the designated limits or the allowable probability that the batch average falls outside the designated limit. Random samples are drawn from a pre-defined batch and tested to obtain measured values for variable attributes. From these values, the sample means, standard deviation and quality control test statistic are calculated. Finally, the test statistic of the batch is compared to the allowable quality level and is either accepted or rejected. The manufacturer can adopt two general strategies for meeting the required specifications while the following sampling by variables strategy, first, can ensure that the average quality level is quite high even with large variability and second, can meet the desired quality target by reducing the variability within batches. Sampling by attributes is based on binomial distribution, thus the performance is measured by the operating characteristic (OC) curve. The OC curve shows the probability for an accepted batch with any given fraction defective item.

Sequential Acceptance Sampling Plans

Sequential sampling is different from single, double or multiple sampling. Sequential acceptance sampling plans are statistically the most efficient type of sampling plan. Though it has a multistage sampling, it does not need to take more sample items than that is necessary but provides enough data to make a decision. For each decision, it allows the operator to increase the sample size one item at a time, or to form into groups to match the logistics of the situation. The sequence sampling can be one sample at a time, usually called item-by-item sequential sampling or can be in sample sizes greater than one, referred to as sequential group sampling. Item-by-item sequential sampling is more popular where the cumulative number of observed defectives are plotted on the graph as in Fig. 7.4. The x-axis is the total number of items thus far selected, and the y-axis is the total number of observed defectives in a batch. If the plotted point falls within the parallel lines, the process continues by drawing another sample. As soon as a point falls on or above the upper line, the batch is rejected. Moreover, when a point falls on or below the lower line, the batch is accepted. The process can theoretically last until the lot is 100% inspected, but as a rule of thumb, sequential-sampling plans are truncated after the number inspected reaches three times the number that would have been inspected using a corresponding single sampling plan.

Regarding direct method of sampling without replacement, general sequential sampling plans can be assumed where, Sn = the number of defective items after n inspected items (random variable), An = the acceptance number at stage n, Rn = the rejection number at stage n. For $n = 1, ..., n_{max}$, the $n_{max} \leq N$ is the truncation sampling number and N is the size of the lot to be inspected.

Here the sequential sampling plan for attributes is defined by:

The acceptance regions = $Sn \leq An$

The rejection regions = $Sn \geq Rn$

The continuation regions = $An < Sn < Rn$

Both acceptance numbers and rejection numbers must be integers. For $n = 26$, in an

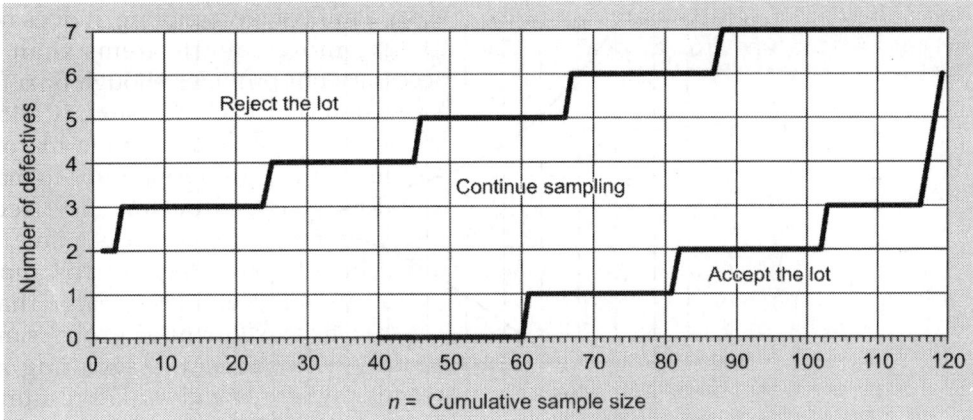

Fig. 7.4: Attribute sequential sampling plan

attribute, sequential sampling plan with the acceptance number 0 and the rejection number is 3. Here for $n = 2 ... 15$ the An ≥ 2 and for $n = 16 ... 26$ the An ≥ 3. The efficiency of the sequential sampling scheme is measured by the average sample number (ASN) required for a given set of Type I and Type II errors. The number of samples needed for the sequential sampling scheme varies from trial to trial, and the ASN represents the average of what might happen over many trials with a fixed incoming defect level.

Two kinds of the sequential plan for variables are sequential **probability ratio (SPR)** and **truncatable single sample** (TSS). Abraham Wald developed the SPR test, that is widely used in quality control in manufacturing and detection of anomalies in medical trials. SPR test was initially developed as an inspection tool to determine whether a given batch meets the desired quality requirements.

As in classical hypothesis testing, the SPR test starts with a pair of hypotheses, say H_0 for the null hypothesis and H_1 for alternative hypothesis respectively.

$$H_0 : p = p_0$$
$$H_1 : p = p_1$$

Here the SPR test for sequential sampling plan for attributes is defined by:

The acceptance regions $H_0 = Si \leq a$

The acceptance regions $H_1 = Si \geq b$

The continuation regions $= a < Si < b$

Si = the number of defective items after n inspected items (random variable), a = the acceptance number at stage n and b = the rejection number at stage n, where a and b depends on the type I and type II errors desired, α and β value. The values are as of a $\cong \log \beta / 1 - \alpha$ and $b \cong \log 1 - \beta/\alpha$, to set the thresholds appropriately, here α and β must be decided beforehand.

TSS for variables is a method to create fixed-n and sequential acceptance sampling plans and fixed-n and sequential hypothesis tests. TSS methodology is implemented in a fixed-n, or sequential way applied to variables sampling for percentage nonconforming items and hypothesis testing for the mean of a population. Sequential is the most efficient kind of decision because the rules allow stopping of data collection before reaching the calculated fixed-n if sufficient evidence to satisfy the risks of type I and II error has been gathered. The sample size of a TSS plan cannot exceed the sample size of the fixed-n plan whose operating characteristic it matches. The

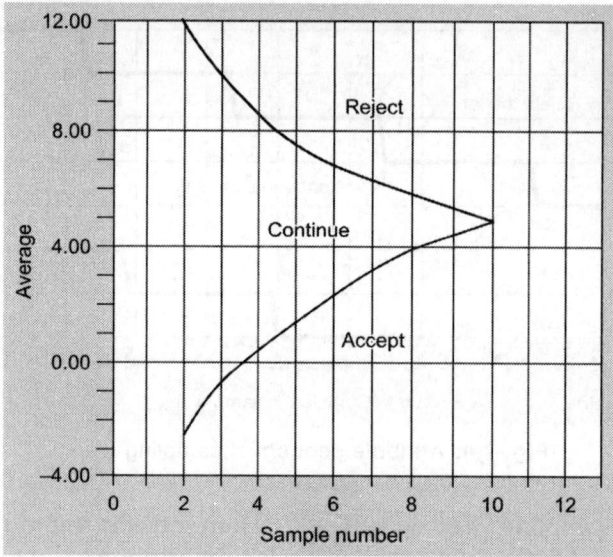

Fig. 7.5: Variables sequential sampling plan

OC-curves of TSS plans matches fixed-n OC-curves more closely than SPR. Generally, TSS plans are favored over SPR plans, though both offers sound statistical risk protection. The reason behind it is that in TSS method sample size limit of fixed-n which improves its acceptance among operators and inspectors, especially in manufacturing.

OPERATING CHARACTERISTIC (OC) CURVE

Product disposition decisions are essentially based on the sampling plans used for testing of each batch of product. In attribute sampling plans, the accept/reject decisions are based on the number of defects and defectives, while in variables sampling plans, it depends on sample average and standard deviation decisions based on measurements and calculations. Sampling plans that require only a single set of sample are known as single sampling plans, while double and multiple sampling plans require additional sample sets. For example, an attribute single sampling plan with a sample size n = 50 and an acceptance number c =1 requires sample of at least

50 units be inspected. If the number of defectives in that sample is one or zero, the batch is accepted or otherwise rejected. However, as the accept/reject decisions are based on a small sample size of the batch, there is always a chance of making an incorrect decision. Operating characteristic (OC) curve is a graphic display of the performance of a sampling plan that plots the probability of accepting a batch against the proportion of defective units. This curve plots the probability of accepting a batch in Y-axis versus the batch fraction or percent defectives in X-axis. The OC curve is the primary tool for displaying and investigating the properties of an acceptance sampling plan. The OC curve is a graph showing what any particular sampling plan can be expected to do regarding the acceptance and rejection of batches. An understanding of the implications of an OC curve also helps in understanding the risks to the manufacturer and consumer at the time of deciding the inspection levels and batch sizes. Each possible plan can have its OC curve. Horizontal scale shows the percentage of defective items in a batch and the vertical scale

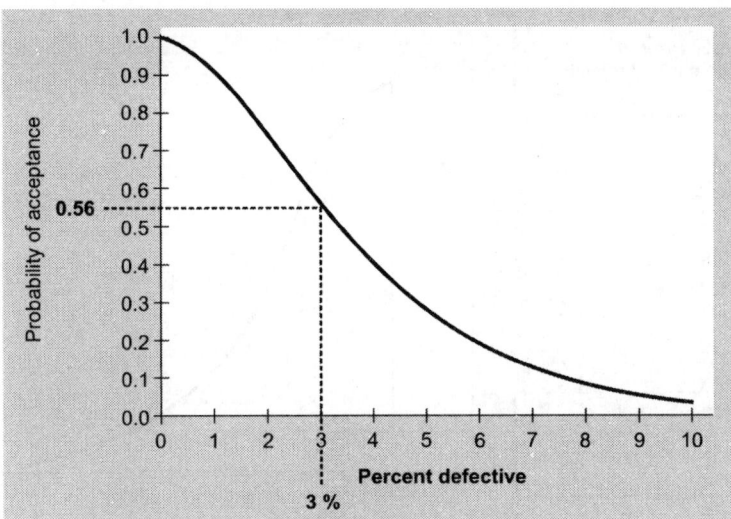

Fig. 7.6: OC curve of the single sampling plan

shows the probability of acceptance of the batch with a particular percentage of defects.

OC curve describes the efficiency of a sampling plan in discriminating between good and bad batches. The behavior of a sampling plan can be described by its OC curve, which plots percent defectives versus the corresponding probabilities of acceptance. Figure 7.6 shows the OC curve of the attribute single sampling plan described above. With that plan, if a batch is having 3% defective items, the corresponding probability of acceptance is 0.56. Similarly, the probability of accepting a batch that has 1% defective item is 0.91, and the probability of accepting batch with 8% defective is 0.07.

An OC curve is summarized by two points on the curve: The acceptable quality level (AQL) and the lot/batch tolerance percent defective (LTPD). The AQL defines the acceptance rate of the sampling plan, and mostly, it is a pre-decided percent of defective items with a 95% percent chance of acceptance. The LTPD describes what the sampling plan generally rejects, and it is that percent of defective items with a 10% chance of

acceptance. Manufacturer aspires to implement a sampling plan that must always accept the batches with quality level better than the AQL and reject the batches with a quality level below the AQL.

The two points on the OC curve logically corresponds to Type I and Type II errors. However, such ideal OC curve performance for a sampling plan can be achieved only with 100% inspection. A typical OC curve for a single-sampling plan shows the probability of rejecting a good lot (producer's risk) and the probability of accepting a bad lot (consumer's risk). Manufacturer chooses a sample size n and an acceptance number to achieve the level of performance specified by the AQL, α, LTPD and β as described in Fig. 7.7.

As shown in Fig. 7.8, the single sampling plan where $n = 50$ and $c = 1$. It has an AQL of 0.72% defective and an LTPD of 7.6% defective. The sampling plan routinely accepts batches that are 0.72% or better and rejects batches that are 7.6% defective or worse. Batches that are between 0.72% and 7.6% defective are sometimes accepted and sometimes rejected.

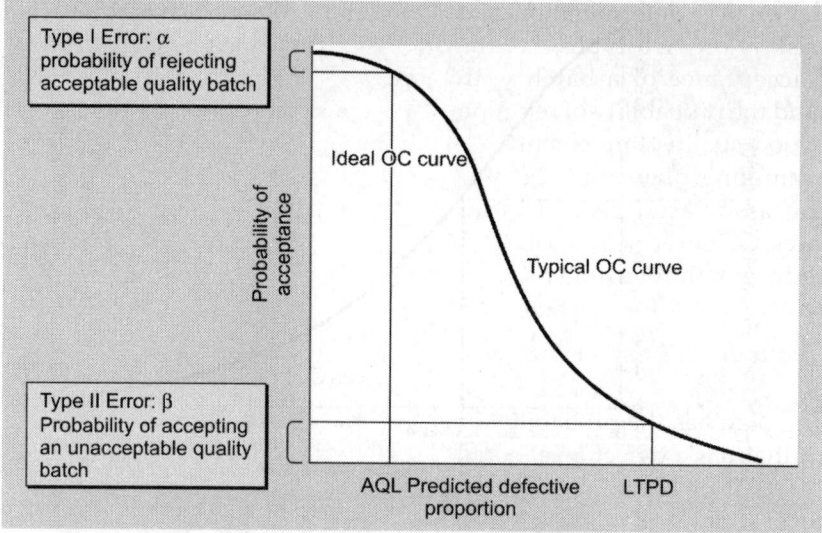

Fig. 7.7: Type I and type II errors

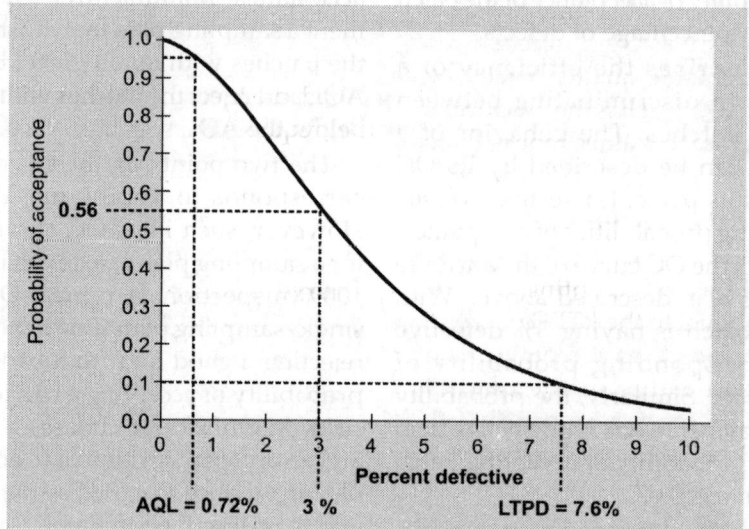

Fig. 7.8: The acceptable quality level and the batch tolerance percent defective

Error Estimation with Sampling Plan OC Curve

Sampling plan OC curves are used to estimates the quality of a substantial material batch that eventually involves risk. There is always some probability that a random sample may not be able to represent all the items of the whole batch and will thus be an incorrect estimate of batch quality. As the results drawn on the sample test is based on probabilities, there is always a chance of making an incorrect conclusion.

The risk is an inherent part of statistical acceptance plans. An incorrect estimate or error in material quality determination and its associated risk is off two types, i.e. the probability of acceptance of a batch with quality defects and the probability of rejection of a batch with good quality. Implementation of a statistical sampling plant must be able to calculate the associated risk of error occurrence chances. OC curve helps to address the risk form producer's and consumer's point of view visually.

Type I Error or α: Producer's risk or wrongful rejection

A given sampling plan has the probability of rejecting a batch that has a defect level equal to or below the AQL. Type I error is associated with the producer's point of view when a batch is rejected having true quality characteristic is AQL. The producer or manufacturer will eventually suffer when a batch with AQL level has been rejected that was having an acceptable quality level. The risk of rejecting an AQL batch is the producer's risk (α risk) and typical α values ranges from 0.2 to 0.01.

Type II Error or β: Consumer's risk or wrongful acceptance

This is the probability of accepting a batch with a defect level equal to the LTPD or more. Type II error corresponds to acceptance of a batch with the true value of the quality characteristic at RQL. The risk of accepting an RQL batch will eventually affect the customers. When such batch is released in the market, the consumer will suffer due to the products of a batch with unacceptable quality. The risk of accepting an RQL is called consumer's risk (β risk), and typical values range from 0.2 to 0.01.

The risks of these two errors are inversely related and determined by the level of significance and the power for the test. Error possibilities in a sampling plan are necessary to define the chances of risks on the consequences of the decision making of the batches. The OC curve sampling plans consist of sample size and a decision rule that involves the acceptance limit(s) and a description of how to use the sample test results to accept or reject the batch. As the two points in the OC curve defines the acceptable and unacceptable quality levels for acceptance sampling, it also determines the risk associated with the acceptance/rejection decision. The two-point method of developing acceptance sampling plans requires the specification of two points of the OC curve.

DRAWING AN OC CURVE

OC curve is useful for:

- Selection of optimum sampling plans
- Selection of a plan that can effectively reduce risks.
- Keeps inspection cost low.
- It estimates the type I and types II errors possibility associated with the sampling plan

Types of OC Curve

Type A: Anticipate the probability of acceptance of individual batches coming from limited production.

Type B: Provides the probability of acceptance for batches coming from a continuous process.

Type C: Present the long-run percentage of product accepted during the sampling phase.

Decision based on sample testing		Results of decision	
		Accept	Reject
Batch quality	Good (AQL)	Correct decision (probability = 1 − α)	Producer's point Type I Error Alpha (α) risk
	Bad (RQL)	Consumer's point type II Error Beta (β) risk	Correct decision (probability = 1 − β)

Fig. 7.9: Decision table for type I and type II error

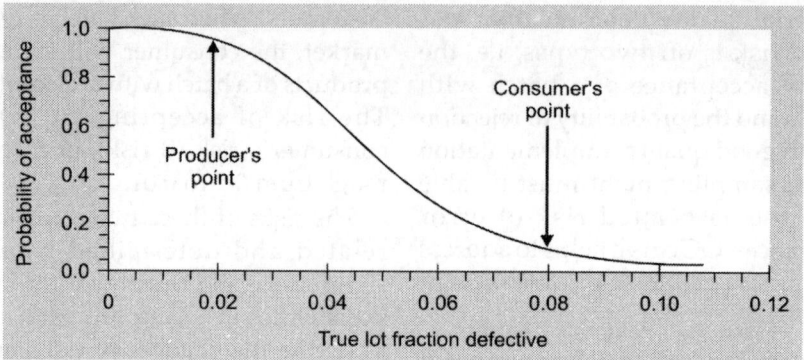

Fig. 7.10: The two-point method of sampling plan OC curve development

OC curve calculation:

The different methods for the OC curve calculations are:

1. Binomial Distribution
2. Poisson Formula

The single-sampling plan OC curve follows the binomial distribution as each item inspected is either defective (bad) or not (good). The probability of accepting the batch equals the probability of taking a sample of size n with a proportion defective of p while finding c or fewer defective items. When n is greater than 20 and p is less than 0.05, the Poisson distribution can be used as an approximation to the binomial by taking advantage of tables for drawing OC curve. To draw the Poisson distribution OC curve took up the probability of accepting the batch for a range of p values. For each p value, multiply p by the sample size n, to find the value of np in the left column of the table and move to the right until you find the column for c and record the value for the probability of acceptance, pa. When p = AQL, the producer's risk $\alpha = 1 - pa$ and when p =LTPD, the consumer's risk $\beta = pa$.

CHANGES IN THE OC CURVE

Sampling plan can be modified accordingly to reduce the probability of rejecting good batches and accepting bad batches. As

discussed above the sample number n and acceptance level c affect the shape of the OC curve. A better formulated single sampling plan will lower producer's risk with a lower consumer's risk.

Effect of Sample Size on the OC Curve

If n is increased while c is constant, a lower acceptance level is obtained with increasing n. As shown in Fig. 7.11, the probability of accepting a batch containing 2% defectives is 68% for $n = 50$, 24% for $n = 100$, 1% for $n = 200$, and 0% for $n = 400$ at $c = 1$. With more samples tested, the probability of accepting a batch with defects decreases. Thus when a manufacturer claims to accept zero defects and test a very small sample size, there is a high probability of accepting defects in the batch without being able to detect them. If the proportion defective in the batch is p = AQL = 0.01 while $n = 80$, then $np = 0.80$ and the probability of acceptance of the lot is only 0.809 (from cumulative Poisson probabilities table) while $c = 1$. Thus the producer's risk is 0.191. Similarly, if p = LTPD = 0.06, $np = 4.8$, the probability of acceptance or the consumers risk is 0.048. Thus *increasing n while holding c constant increases the producer's risk and reduces the consumer's risk.*

Effect of Acceptance Level on OC Curve

If sample size n constant with an increase in the acceptance level c, it lowers the probability

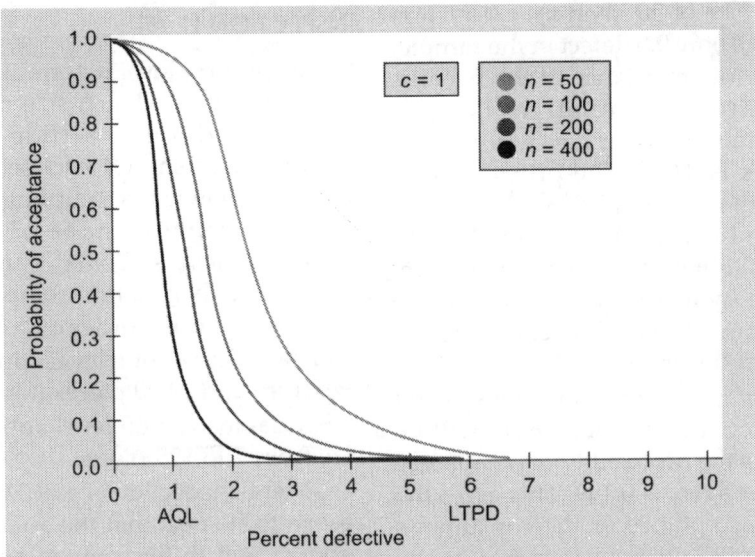

.**Fig. 7.11:** Effect of increasing sample size with a constant acceptance level on the OC curve

of finding defects, in turn, increases the risk of accepting a bad batch. As shown in Fig. 7.12, the probability of accepting a batch containing 2% defectives is 78% for $c = 4$, 60% for $c = 3$, 40% for $c = 2$, and 18% for $c = 1$ at $n = 50$. With the increase in acceptance level, the probability of accepting a batch with defects increases. Thus when a manufacturer claims to accept zero defects and set the acceptance level very low, there is a less probability of accepting defects in the batch without being able to detect them. If the batch has $p = $ AQL $= 0.01$

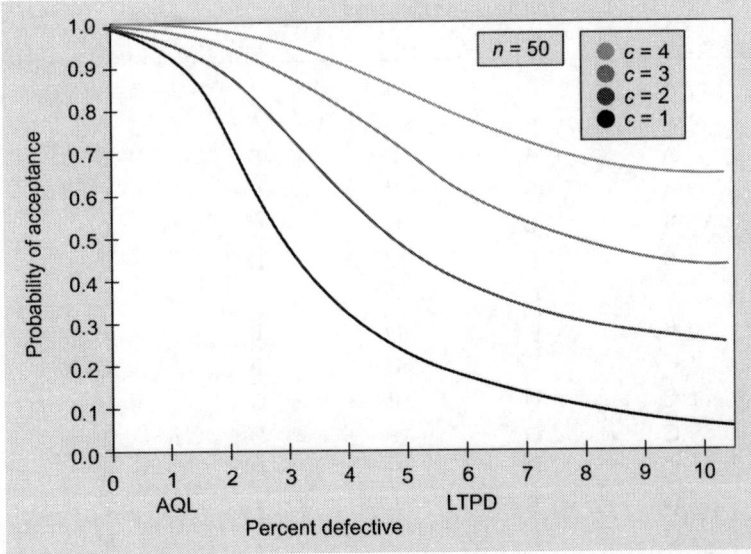

Fig. 7.12: Effect of increasing acceptance level with a constant sample size on the OC curve

with a sample size of 50, then $np = 0.50$, it is expected to have only 0.5 defect in the sample. The probability of acceptance of the batch is only 0.910 (from cumulative Poisson probabilities table) while $c = 1$, thus, the producer's risk is 0.090. The probability of acceptance of the batch is 0.986 while $c = 1$, thus, the producer's risk is 0.090. The probability of finding more than two defects can be reduced by increasing the acceptance number from one to two, thus consequently lowering the producer's risk.

Similarly, if $p =$ LTPD $= 0.06$, the expected number of defectives in the sample will be $np = 3$ that gives the probability of acceptance or the consumer's risk is 0.199. This gives the probability of acceptance or the consumer's risk equal to 0.423 with an increase in the acceptance number from one to two. This increases the probability of getting a sample with two or fewer defects and therefore increases the consumer's risk. Thus *increasing c while holding n constant decreases the producer's risk and increases the consumer's risk.*

INSPECTION LEVEL

The inspection level determines the relationship between the batch size and the sample size. In addition to setting the AQL, the manufacturer should choose the inspection level to implement a sampling plan properly. The AQL table is made of two different inspection levels, General and special that fundamentally differ on sample size requirement for a specific order quantity.

General inspection level applies for sample size from 2 to 2,000 pieces.

Special inspection level applies for sample size from 2 to 125 pieces.

General inspection is used when there is no reason to suspect that the quality level of the product will differ from an acceptable level. The general inspection level has three designates sublevels that are G-I, G-II, and G-III, as given in Table 7.2. Unless otherwise specified, level II is used as the default level. General level inspections are commonly done for an actual quality test of consumer goods.

Table 7.2: Sample size code letters

Batch size	Special inspection level				General inspection level		
	S-1	S-2	S-3	S-4	I	II	III
2–8	A	A	A	A	A	A	B
9–15	A	A	A	A	A	B	C
16–25	A	A	B	B	B	C	D
26–50	A	B	B	C	C	D	E
51–90	B	B	C	C	C	E	F
91–150	B	B	C	D	D	F	G
151–280	B	C	D	E	E	G	H
281–500	B	C	D	E	F	H	J
501–1200	C	C	E	F	G	J	K
1201–3200	C	D	E	G	H	K	L
3201–10000	C	D	F	G	J	L	M
10001–35000	C	D	F	H	K	M	N
35001–150000	D	E	G	J	L	N	P
150001–500000	D	E	G	J	M	P	Q
500001 over	D	E	H	K	N	Q	R

Reduced inspection (General level-I inspection): Level I may be used when less discrimination is required, so fewer samples are inspected. This inspection level is appropriate when the manufacturer is confident that the quality of the products is acceptable, when suppliers have a good quality background or where destructive testing is required to be performed. The G-I inspection level requires the smallest sample size of these three options.

Normal inspection (general level-II inspection): It is the default level, and it is chosen for 90% of inspections in quality control. Many manufacturers start with a G-II inspection level first following AQL for the inspection system.

Tightened inspection (General level-III inspection): The level is followed when greater discrimination is required, so more samples are checked. This inspection level is used for suppliers that recently had severe quality problems or for high-value products. This stricter inspection level allows for less risk of accepting a batch with excessive defects, which is especially important if one of the suppliers has a history of poor quality. Next, to 100 percent inspection, this general inspection level offers the largest scope and most assurance best quality status.

Four additional special levels, S-1, S-2, S-3, and S-4 are also given in Table 7.1 and are used where relatively small sample sizes are necessary and larger sampling risks can be tolerated. Special inspection levels are used where very few sample size can be checked. The special levels are used testing samples that either lengthy or destroy the samples. These special levels can also be used that are appropriate for container-loading supervision where supervision is done to ensure the materials inside the cartons, without spending too much time at that checking.

Sample sizes are designated by code letters; sampling table shall be used to find the applicable code letter for the particular batch based on batch size and the prescribed inspection level. The AQL and the code letter is used to obtain the sampling plan from the master table (Tables 7.3 to 7.5). If sampling plan is not available for a given combination of AQL and code letter, the tables direct the

Table 7.3: Acceptable quality level (AQL) in single sampling plans with inspection level I (general level)

Batch size	Code letter	Sample size	0.65	1.0	1.5	2.5	4.0	6.5	10	15
2–8	A	2	↓	↓	↓	↓	↓	1	↓	↓
9–15	B	3	↓	↓	↓	↓	1	↑	↓	2
16–25	C	5	↓	↓	↓	1	↑	↓	2	3
26–50	D	8	↓	↓	1	↑	↓	2	3	4
51–90	E	13	↓	1	↑	↓	2	3	4	5
91–150	F	20	1	↑	↓	2	3	4	5	6
151–280	G	32	↑	↓	2	3	4	5	6	8
281–500	H	50	↓	2	3	4	5	6	8	10
501–1200	J	80	2	3	4	5	6	8	10	13
1201–3200	K	125	3	4	5	6	8	10	13	↑
3201–10000	L	200	4	5	6	8	10	13	↑	↑
10001–35000	M	315	5	6	8	10	13	↑	↑	↑
35001–150000	N	500	6	8	10	13	↑			
150001–500000	P	800	8	10	13	↑				
500001 over	Q	1250	10	13	↑					

Table 7.4: Acceptable quality level (AQL) in single sampling plans with inspection level II (general level)

Batch size	Code letter	Sample soze	0.65	1.0	1.5	2.5	4.0	6.5	10	15
2–8	A	2	↓	↓	↓	↓	↓	1	↓	↓
9–15	B	3	↓	↓	↓	↓	1	↑	↓	2
16–25	C	5	↓	↓	↓	1	↑	↓	2	3
26–50	D	8	↓	↓	1	↑	↓	2	3	4
51–90	E	13	↓	1	↑	↓	2	3	4	6
91–150	F	20	1	↑	↓	2	3	4	6	8
151–280	G	32	↑	↓	2	3	4	6	8	11
281–500	H	50	↓	2	3	4	6	8	11	15
501–1200	J	80	2	3	4	6	8	11	15	22
1201–3200	K	125	3	4	6	8	11	15	22	↑
3201–10000	L	200	4	6	8	11	15	22	↑	
10001–35000	M	315	6	8	11	15	22	↑		
35001–150000	N	500	8	11	15	22	↑			
150001–500000	P	800	11	15	22	↑				
500001 over	Q	1250	15	22	↑					

Table 7.5: Acceptable quality level (AQL) in single sampling plans with inspection level III (general level)

Batch size	Code letter	Sample size	0.65	1.0	1.5	2.5	4.0	6.5	10	15
2–8	A	2	↓	↓	↓	↓	↓	↓	↓	↓
9–15	B	3	↓	↓	↓	↓	↓	1	↑	↓
16–25	C	5	↓	↓	↓	↓	1	↑	↓	2
26–50	D	8	↓	↓	↓	1	↑	↓	2	3
51–90	E	13	↓	↓	1	↑	↓	2	3	4
91–150	F	20	↓	1	↑	↓	2	3	4	6
151–280	G	32	1	↑	↓	2	3	4	6	9
281–500	H	50	↑	↓	2	3	4	6	9	13
501–1200	J	80	↓	2	3	4	6	9	13	19
1201–3200	K	125	2	3	4	6	9	13	19	↑
3201–10000	L	200	3	4	6	9	13	19	↑	
10001–35000	M	315	4	6	9	13	19	↑		
35001–150000	N	500	6	9	13	19	↑			
150001–500000	P	800	9	13	19	↑				
500001 over	Q	1250	13	19	↑					

user to difference letter (Tables 7.6 and 7.7) where the sampling size is given by the new code letter, but not by the original letter. If the procedure decides to test different sample sizes for different classes of defects, the code letter derived corresponding to the largest sample size may be used for all classes of defects. As an alternative to a single sampling plan with an acceptance number of 0, the plan with an acceptance number of 1 with its correspondingly larger sample size for a designated AQL, may be used.

Table 7.6: Single sampling plans (normal inspection)

Code letter	Sample size	0.010	0.015	0.025	0.040	0.065	0.10	0.15
					AQL			
					Ac Re			
G	32	↓	↓	↓	↓	↓	↓	↓
H	50							
J	80							01
K	125						01	↑
L	200					01	↑	↓
M	315				01	↑	↓	12
N	500			01	↑	↓	12	23
P	800		01	↑	↓	12	23	34
Q	1250	01	↑	↓	12	23	34	56
R	2000	↑	↓	12	23	34	56	78

Table 7.7: Double sampling plans (normal inspection)

Code letter	Sample	Sample size	Cumulative sample	1.5	2.5	4.0	6.5	10
						AQL		
						Ac Re		
G	First	20	20	02	03	13	25	36
G	Second	20	40	12	34	45	67	910
H	First	32	32	03	13	25	36	59
H	Second	32	64	34	45	67	910	1213
J	First	50	50	13	25	36	59	711
J	Second	50	100	45	67	910	1213	1819

The **producer's point** controls the acceptance of batches that are at an acceptable quality level. The goal is to prevent good batches from being rejected.

The **consumer's point** controls the rejection of batches that are at a rejectable quality level. The goal is to prevent bad batches from being accepted.

Setting an AQL does not guarantee the customer a batch of worse quality will not get accepted. When the average quality of a batch submitted for testing is little worse than the AQL, it can probably get accepted if a tightened inspection is not called for. In general, the customer gets the product quality, which is on average better than the AQL level decided by the manufacturer. The tables are arranged to provide an economic incentive as the manufacturer cannot afford to have more than a small proportion of batches manufactured to get rejected and will surely improve the quality if this proportion is exceeded.

SAMPLING PROCEDURE

The procedure for selection of samples in all stages of manufacturing from the receipt of raw materials through bulk intermediates to final packed stocks are to be described in written standard operating procedures. Since the results obtained after testing the samples determine whether a batch or delivery is acceptable or not, it is essential to provide clear instructions to the sampler to ensure that appropriate representative samples have been taken. The sampling SOP should include the following elements:

- Designation of persons responsible for sampling.
- The appropriate sampling plan that specifies the size and quantity of the required sample calculated according to the batch/delivery size, the number of containers to be sampled, absolute numbers of samples required and their destination.
- The external checks and inspections to be performed before sampling, i.e. verification of material and batch codes or bar codes, conditions of containers, condition, and appearance of the material.
- Precautions to be observed to avoid contamination of the material or deterioration of quality. Specific precautions to be observed, especially concerning the sampling of sterile and hazardous materials.
- Safety precautions adopted to protect the sampler and product.
- To ensure sampling of one container only at a time from a batch.
- Techniques and equipment required for sampling, including sterile methods where appropriate.
- The type of sample container to be used for a particuler function and proper labeling.
- Instructions for any required sub-division or pooling of the samples.
- To provide a sampling checklist, that is to be completed by the sampler for QA documentation purpose.
- Identification marking to be made on all the original sampled containers.
- Specific cleaning and storing instructions for sampling equipments.
- In case of non-compliance reporting details on why material does not meet the samplers acceptance criteria.

- Re-secure method of original containers after sampling which should take care not to contaminate the material.

The extent of record keeping as per SOP at the sampling stage is the responsibility of the sampler and the store persons who undertake receipt inspection of the container and contents. However, as a minimum, a record should be made of all external checks and inspection performed before and during sampling.

Specific Sampling Instructions

During manufacturing and packaging sampling is done to ensure compliance of the resultant product with its predefined specifications. The quality of a batch of raw or packaging materials procured from a vendor is assessed by withdrawing and testing a representative sample. As specified in a sampling plan the number of samples needed to be taken for preparation of a representative sample size is determined statistically. The number of individual samples which are to be blended to form a composite sample is also defined, taking into account the nature of the material, knowledge of the supplier and the homogeneity of the composite sample. In-Process Quality Control (IPQC) tests are performed for quality assurance of products with consistent performance while manufacturing of pharmaceutical dosage forms like tablet, capsule, syrup or injection. Quality attributes such as injectables and ophthalmic solutions must undergo inspection of filled containers and vials for contamination with any glass or foreign particles, specks of carbon formed during sealing of ampoules, particles of dust, fibers, etc. Use of automatic or semi-automatic machines for inspection is advisable, but trained human eye is also considered up to a certain extent. Random statistical sampling is also to be performed as per AQL sampling plan for spot checking of IPQC materials following sampling table. Similarly, sampling of finished products is done depending on the batch size to undertake final quality check for market release of a batch.

Sampling of Raw Material

Pharmaceutical raw materials are the Active Pharmaceutical Ingredient (API) and excipients like additives, preservatives, coloring and flavoring agents that used for manufacturing of formulations. Most of the pharmaceutical manufacturers procure these items from audited vendors and suppliers. Identity and quality checks are must to do before approving the use of these ingredients for dosage form manufacturing. The identity of a complete batch of multi-container starting materials can only be ensured when individual samples are taken from all the containers and identity tests are performed on each sample. A proportion of the containers is permissible to sample only where a validated procedure has been established to ensure that all containers of starting material of a single batch have been correctly identified on its label. The following are some critical factors that should be taken into consideration while sampling of raw material.

1. Both active and inactive pharmaceutical materials are to be sampled from all the containers as a general rule.
2. The total quantity of material to be sampled is the total of the quantity required for analysis and test along with quantity required to be kept as a control sample and for microbiological analysis.
3. On receipt of goods received note (GRN) from stores, enter the details of the GRN into raw material inward register as per the batch Analytical Reference No. (A.R. No)
4. Thorough checking of the GRN of a material to be sampled and if any entry is missing in GRN, get it rectified by stores personnel.
5. Ensure proper recording of the observations while sampling in the sampling checklist.

6. Prepare 'UNDER TEST' labels with relevant details in sufficient quantity equivalent to the number of containers as stated in the GRN and two additional labels for affixing on the status card and on retain sample identification bag.
7. Check for the required quantity of self-sealing polythene bags.
8. Check the sampling thief for cleanliness.
9. Check for safety apparels that are required to be used during sampling of material.
10. Check for the cleanliness of the sampling kit.
11. The sampling kit must contain 'UNDER TEST' labels, self-sealing polythene bags, safety apparels, GRN, and checklist.
12. The quantity of material required to be sampled from each container is calculated, e.g. Starch BP material: Total quantity required to be sampled (as per the attached index) is 32 gm, and no. of containers as per GRN is 8. Quantity to be withdrawn from each container = Total quantity required/no. of containers = $32/8 = 4$ gm.
12. A minimum of 2 gm of material should be sampled from each container if the quantity required to be withdrawn from each container is less than 2 gm.
13. Put 'ON' the power switch and air flow of the sampling booth.
14. **Sampling procedure**
    i. Check and ensure that the sampling booth is clean.
    ii. Assure operation of sampling booth follows relevant SOP.
    iii. Check for the pressure differential of the booth. Ensure the pressure differential is within the set limits.
    iv. Check for the calibration of the balance.
    v. Check for the consignment details as given in the checklist and record.

vi. Check the cleanliness of the container to be sampled and bring all the containers of the identified batch near the sampling booth.

vii. Take one container at a time into the sampling booth and check for the following on the container label.
  a. Name of the material
  b. Pharmacopoeia Grade
  c. Batch no
  d. Date of mfg./date of expiry
  e. Manufacturer.

viii. After ensuring the correctness of the supplier label as per the GRN, open the container.

ix. Check the physical appearance of the material. If any foreign particles are found to be present, note it down on the checklist.

x. Seal the polythene bag immediately after sampling.

xi. Reseal the material and close the container. If poly bag/paper bag are pierced for sampling purpose, the pierced portion should be covered with LDPE sheets (10 × 10 cm) and pasted outside with Bopp tape.

xii. Affix 'UNDER TEST' label on the container. The label should be pasted on the right side of the manufacturer label.

xiii. Shift the container outside and bring another container into the sampling booth.

xiv. Follow step 14.7 to 14.13 for all the containers. In case of such raw materials prone to have microbiological contamination, samples are drawn-aseptically. For sampling sterilized bottles, scoop, nose mask, and hand gloves are to be used.
The sterile jars/bottles are marked with a marker pen about the type of sample:
  • Laboratory sample (LS)
  • Micro status sample (MS)
  • Outside testing sample (OS)
  • Secondary standard sample (SS)

xv. After all the containers have been sampled, shift the containers back to the quarantine area and affix 'UNDER TEST' label on the status card, sampled bag, and microbiology sample if any.

xvi. Put 'OFF' the airflow and power switch.

xvii. Enter the details in the sampling log.

xviii. Inform stores personnel to get the area cleaned and to make entries in the log book after cleaning.

xix. For liquids/solvents liquid sampler are used. Sampleis taken from all the containers in to clean dry bottles. Incase of microbiology test sterilized bottles are used.

xx. Place all the sampled materials and checklist into the sampling kit and bring it back to QC.

xxi. Ensure final dispersal of the sampling bag and sampling thief to the store quarantine area. Place the sampling thief back into the polythene cover and send for washing.

xxii. Enclose the sampled materials into another dry polythene bag.

xxiii. Attach the checklist to the GRN and stamp the GRN with 'SAMPLED' seal with sign and date.

Sampling of Packaging Material

Primary and secondary packaging materials are used for packaging of final medicinal products. Primary packaging is the component that is or may be in direct contact with the dosage form, and secondary packaging components are not and will not be in direct contact with the dosage form. Typically packaging materials are containers (ampoules, vials, bottles), closure (screw caps, stoppers), over wraps (aluminum and PVC foils. blister packs), administration accessories and container labels. The following are some important factors that should be taken into consideration while sampling of packaging material.

1. In the quarantine area, identify the material pack to be sampled following the quarantine label affixed by the warehouse staff.

2. Check for the total number of packages as mentioned in GRN.

3. Check packing condition of the material and details mentioned on the labels.

4. The packs should be cleaned externally and are opened only after ensuring proper cleaning. Materials are observed for any abnormalities, and if any, is record it on the Sampler's Check List. In case of any discrepancies intimate to Executive/Head of QA or QC for necessary action.

5. Note down GRN date, material name, in-house batch no, quantity, vendor name, vendor batch no, date of manufacturing and date of expiry in the sampling record.

6. Open the packages carefully and observe the material for any abnormalities and record it on the Samplee's Remark Sheet.

7. Ensure that the surrounding area is clean while withdrawing the samples for testing.

8. The sampled materials are examined as per AQL against the approved standard specifications for general appearance, deviation from normal visual quality, color, text, etc. wherever applicable. The results are recorded in approved Visual Inspection Report for aluminum foil, PVC Foil, blister packs and labels.

9. After completion of sampling, the material packs are resealed with BOPP tape or tied with the help of cable tie.

10. Affix the 'SAMPLED BY QC' sticker label duly signed and mentioning the container number according to the sampling plan, on the outer container of the material from which sample was taken. Label the sampled packages with the 'sampled' labels duly signed. Mark the sampled packages as $N/1/n, N/2/n, ...,$ $N/S/n$, where N is the total number of containers, n is the number of containers sampled and S is the serial number of the sampled container.

11. Ensure that all the sampled rolls of labels and foils are affixed with 'under test' labels. On all other packaging materials at least two 'under test' labels shall be affixed on the bottom container/pack of each pallet.

12. Protect the samples from external contaminants like dust, water, and direct sunlight during sampling and testing operations.

13. In case of aluminum and PVC foils carry out the sampling under laminar air flow (LAF). The LAF shall be cleaned with wet mop followed by the dry mop.

14. For a sampling of glass bottles select at random 4 cases or boxes from the consignment. For visual examination sample all the bottles from the 4 cases.

15. For dimensions

    a. Neck finish and diameter: 20 bottles from each case sampled covering each cavity of the mould.

    b. Internal mould diameter and through bore diameter: all bottles from the top layer in each ease.

    c. Outer dimensions: 20 bottles from 4 cases.

    d. For overflow capacity: 3 bottles at random from each case.

16. Send the packaging material to the quality control department for testing as per the laid down specifications of the respective material.

17. All excess packaging materials after completion of testing and reporting shall be destroyed as per the laid down procedures.

Sampling of Intermediate, Bulk and Finished Products

The intermediate product is partly processed material which must undergo further processing (including packaging) before it becomes a bulk or finished product. Products that have completed all production stages but not packaging are called bulk products. Finished product is the products that have completed all the stages of manufacturing and packaging and is now ready for dispatch or market release. Pharmaceutical manufacturing process needs close monitoring and control of procedure to check out the occurrence of any variations in the characteristics of the final drug product. This is done by taking samples of in-process materials at intermediate stages of manufacturing and testing them for quality attributes to ensure that such attributes are under control. The important quality attributes are, i.e. adequacy ingredients mixing, uniformity, and homogeneity, tablet or capsule weight variation, the disintegration time of tablets and capsules, clarity and pH of solutions as in the in-process and intermediate stage.

Sampling of bulk and intermediate products: The frequency and extent of sampling of intermediate and bulk products are determined from pilot stage standards on acceptable process average and process variability estimated by application of appropriate statistical procedures. Where such information is not available, the sampling may be done by following the simple rule 'square root of N plus one' for determining sample sizes to be inspected from a given number of containers (N) in the batch. The square root of the lot size plus one is considered as a general rule to determine the number of units to be inspected.

Sampling of finished products: Sampling and testing of finished products batches are of high importance to ensure the market release of quality products. When the bulk products enter in the final packaging round,

as a general rule, samples must be taken at least at the beginning and the end of the batch packing operations. Preferably the samples must be drawn at frequent intervals, throughout the operations. Sampling of a balk, intermediate and finished products are carried out by QC laboratory staff following the finished product specification and test report:

1. QA persons receive in-process status or delivery report form and note all the details in bulk protocol data sheet and perform sampling arrangement based on the product details:
   a. Production unit
   b. Product name
   c. Type of bulk
   d. Batch No.
   e. Sampling date

   Before stating of packaging operation, visual assessment of all packaging materials received is done to check for quarantine or ongoing process labels. If any unconformity is observed in the bulk material, the quarantine warehouse section is informed to countercheck for any improper storing condition.

2. Sampling procedure: Finished product sampling is done based on the type of product, AQL, specification and testing schedule by QC persons. Sample labels are filled suitable to a number of the sample container and attached on sampling container or self-sealing polythene bags. The quantity of finished product required to be sampled from a batch depends on test control requirements and AQL sampling plan. Otherwise, commonly employed plan can be:
   a. 20 packs per batch randomly for powder product
   b. 10 strips of capsules randomly for capsules product
   c. 10 packs of pills per batch randomly for pills product

d. 20 tubes per batch randomly for cream product
e. 20 packs per batch randomly for liquids, syrup, emulsion, and suspension product
f. 150 ml per batch randomly for bulk liquid product
g. 30 packs per batch randomly for the pouch

Finally, all data and information set out in the sample label, and sampling memo is checked intermediately.

Retention Samples

After QC testing all remaining products can be stored as *Retention samples*. Finished goods sampling is required for *retention samples*, *test/reference samples*, *Stability samples* and *after-packing samples* other than the routine QC testing purpose. These samples are mostly retained to provide sample for analytical testing and as specimen of the final finished product.

Retention samples are a representative sample of a final finished packaged unit from a batch of finished product stored for identification purposes, i.e. presentation, packaging, labeling, patient information leaflet, batch number, and expiry date as need arises during the shelf life of the batch concerned as per label recommended storage conditions of the product.

Reference samples are the samples taken from a batch of starting material, packaging material or finished product which is stored as per label recommended storage conditions of the product. These samples are analyzed when required during the shelf life of the batch concerned.

For finished products, in most instances, the reference and retention samples are identical, i.e. as fully packaged units, and so such circumstances, reference and retention samples are regarded as interchangeable.

Stability samples are the samples of final finished products as in intact marketed packs which are stored for accelerated and long-term stability studies in quantity sufficient to perform stability indicating assay and tests to ascertain shelf life of the batch concerned. For each new products, stability samples are being collected form first three consecutive batches for stability study under accelerated temperature and humidity conditions. For all product categories manufactured in a facility, at least one batch per year should be sampled and kept under long-term stability test conditions.

After-packing samples or retail package samples are taken in an appropriate number of packs, bottles, bags or injections as a sample as an unopened intact pack. Fewer samples are required as all the pharmaceutical consignment are always homogeneous. In principle, this minimum amount/weight of identical final samples are required to be kept by the QC laboratory.

Retention and/or Reference and Stability Sampling

1. All retention and/or reference samples must be representative of the sealable product.
2. The samples must be logged into retention and/or reference sample logbook by production stuff and verified by QA personnel.
3. Retention and/or reference sample must be a representative from the start, middle and final stage of manufacturing.
4. Retention and/or reference samples are evaluated by QA staff.
5. Stability samples must be labeled with stability card. The quantity required for stability should be indicated in the SOP. The quantity indicated in the stability SOP is to be taken only from the batches with Packed Batch Document. These samples are taken in addition to samples normally required for testing, retention, and reference.

The reference and/or retention samples serve as a control record of a batch of starting material and finished product. These samples can be assessed and tested in the event of dosage form quality complaint, query related to compliance of marketing authorization, labeling/packaging query or for pharmacovigilance reports.

Duration of Storage

Reference and retention samples from all batches of finished products are to be retained for at least one year added to the expiry date. The reference sample should be contained in its finished primary packaging or in packaging composed of the same material as the primary container in which the product is marketed. Samples of starting materials (other than solvents, gases or water used in the manufacturing process) are usually retained for at least two years after the release of the product unless longer period is mentioned under the law. That period may be shortened if the period of stability of the material, as indicated in the relevant specification, is shorter. The reserve sample of an active ingredient in a drug product is retained for 1 year added to the expiration date of the last batch of the drug product containing this active ingredient. Packaging material samples are retained for the duration of the shelf life of the finished product concerned.

Quantity of Reference and Retention Samples

Reference samples are needed to be stored in sufficient quantity to carry out the full range of the analytical control tests of the batch at least for twice in accordance with the 'finished product specification and testing report' which has been approved by the relevant competent authorities. Unopened packs are used for carrying out each set of analytical controls, wherever necessary. Reference samples are the representatives of the starting material, intermediate product or finished product of the batch from which they are withdrawn. Where a batch is packaged in two, or more, distinct packaging operations, at least one retention sample should be taken from each packaging operation.

Storage Conditions

The reference samples of finished products and active substances are stored in conditions following the current version of the guidance on storage conditions for medicinal products and active substances. Storage conditions must comply with the licensing/marketing authorization requirements (e.g. refrigerated storage where relevant).

SAMPLING ACCESSORIES

Sampling Containers

Pharmaceutical containers hold, contains and protects the drug products and are or may be in direct contact with it along with the closure which is a part of the container. The container and closure must not interact physically or chemically with the drug substance in any way that could alter its quality. Specifically, the sampling containers are used for storing and transporting the samples collected. Based on the permeability characteristics the containers are categorized as:

Well-closed containers protect the drug contents from extraneous exposure or loss of the substance under the expected normal conditions of handling, shipment or storage.

Tightly closed containers must protect the contents from extraneous matter, from loss of the substance, and from efflorescence, deliquescence or evaporation under normal conditions of handling, shipment or storage.

Hermetically closed containers are impervious to air or any other gas under normal conditions of handling, shipment or storage.

The type of container to be used for a sample is determined by the physical and chemical properties of the substances and the storage and transport requirements. It is important to use the correct type of storage container for the pharmaceutical samples. After withdrawal of sample the container closure like cork plugs, crown caps, plastic or metal screw caps is reinforced to ensure better sealing. Cork plugs are wrapped in polyethylene before closure, and use of rubber plugs is prohibited.

The container used for containing samples must meet the following requirements:

·The containers and stoppers must not be susceptible to chemical attack by the samples and must not interact with or contaminate them:

- Containers are designed and manufactured in a way that allow leak-proof or air-tight closure;
- Containers must be strong enough to withstand transport and storage;
- Containers are such designed to ensure proper sealing and preclude unauthorized handling.
- The stoppers and caps used for closing the sample container/bottles must ensure a tight seal to prevent any leakage or evaporation of the samples.
- For solids side-mouthed, amber or color bottles closed by screw-caps with insert wads are most suitable. For hygroscopic material, tight filling polythene sheets may be used before the screw caps are fitted. For liquid materials, narrow-mouthed bottles, amber or colorless with suitable stoppers may be used. For volatile liquids, tight-fitting stoppers are used.

The most commonly used sample containers are polypropylene bottles, polyethyl entere phtalate bottles, glass bottles and vials, metal canisters, polyethylene, and polypropylene bags, metal gas cylinders, etc. along with screw caps, lids, stoppers, seals, desiccants, fillers. Light and/or moisture proof contains are used for substances requiring protection from light and/or moisture that are made up of light-resistant material or coated.

The bottle is a container with a more or less pronounced neck and usually a flat bottom.

The vial is a small container for parenteral medicinal products, with a stopper and over seal; the contents are removed after piercing the stopper. Both single-dose and multi-dose types exist.

The bag consists of surfaces, whether or not with a flat bottom, made of flexible material, closed at the bottom and the sides by sealing. The top of a bag may be closed by fusion of the material, depending on the intended use.

Sampling Devices

Different types of specially designed sampling devices are used for sampling of solid, liquid and solvents as per requirement. Sampling devices, tools, and implements must be used following the manufacturer's instructions for the use. Sampling tools must meet these general requirements:

- Robust enough to withstand handling operations;
- Easy to clean;
- Made of materials resistant to the effects of the substances being sampled and the cleaning agents;
- Must conform to safety requirements.
- Cleaning and maintenance of sampling devices must be ensured as per SOP.
- Some specific plastic and stainless steel devices are the most suitable.
- Proper cleaning and drying should be done of such equipment before use.
- Separate storage facility should be given to sampling equipment.

Sampling tools like scoops, spoons, spatula, spears, rods, thumb tube pipettes, dip tubes, thieves, dipping vessels or weighted disc containers mostly made up of stainless steel and rarely of glass is used. Scoops, spoons, spatula, spears, rods are used for sampling of solids received in small containers. Thieves and dipping vessels are used for solid material received in deep large containers or drum. Sack samplers are used for solid material received in bags or sacks, that is a specially designed device to withdraw samples through the side of the sack or bag. The powder trier sampler is ideal for taking a large volume, cross-sectional sample from a container and is suitable for sampling free-flowing powders, granules and even slightly cohesive powders. Powder lance is ideal for taking a cross-sectional sample through a bulk powder, and the slot sampler is ideal for taking a multilevel, cross-sectional sample from powders and granules.

Scoops, thumb tube pipettes, and dip tubes are normally used for sampling of liquids in a small container. Stainless steel drum samplers and dipping vessels are used for solvents and liquids received in large drums. Though conventionally thieves were used for sampling solid material now it has become highly versatile sampler with Visco thief for sampling of viscous materials such as oils, creams, shampoo. Liquid thief are used for less viscous liquids, micro thief and unit dose sample thief are used for taking multiple samples at multiple heights within the product. The tweezers (forceps) are ideal for picking up items up to 25 mm wide which is specially designed to pick up both small and large items. Other versatile tools useful for sampling in special cases are knives, stainless steel axes, scissors, tongs, cleaning brushes, etc. The sampling tools intended for the sampling of petroleum products, organic solvents, and other flammable liquids and gases are made of electro-conductive materials to prevent static electricity being generated. They must not create sparks when in contact with another metal object. The sampling tools used for taking samples from liquids from depth are tied to a cord, rope or chain long enough to take samples from the desired level.

Sampler

1. Sampler must be properly trained for performing sampling operation of different category of materials.
2. The sampler should strictly follow standard sampling procedure approved by QC personnel.
3. Sampler must be well versed with regular precautions to be taken while performing the sampling operation.
4. The person should be meticulous, observant and have adequate knowledge of materials to be handled.
5. Sampling person should know the precaution to be taken while handling hazardous and sensitive materials.
6. The person should know procedures for dealing with spillages.
7. The person needs to wear protective clothing and dress should not have any pockets.
8. The sampler should follow standard sampling procedure as approved by QC personnel.
9. Sampling person should work under the direction of QA manager.

SAMPLING PRECAUTIONS

The following are few recommended sampling precautions to be practiced for better quality compliance:

1. All solid and liquid items should be sampled inside the sampling booth except solvents.
2. The sampler must carefully read the sampling instructions given on the material specification and test report before sampling a material.
3. The label of the container should be thoroughly read. Before doing the sampling, sampler should ensure that sample containers are correctly showing the name of the material being sampled, the batch number of the material, the

reference number of the consignment and the container identifying number from which the sample is taken.

4. Container from which sample to be withdrawn should be thoroughly checked. All material containers are needed to be examined for damage before sampling, and any damage should be reported to the store manager immediately.

5. Material at the top and if possible in the bottom should be examined for contamination with foreign matter, variation in color in different portions of the materials, abnormal odor, infestation, extraneous matter.

6. In liquid suspended matter or sediment, different layers should be checked.

7. None of the materials are allowed to touch with bare hands, use of appropriate sampling tools are mandatory. Sampler needs to wear a mask, cap, hand gloves, and shoe covers. For sampling of hazardous materials protective clothing must be worn. Proper instructions for handling such materials must be documented and followed by the sampling staff.

8. Clean and dry sampling device kept in clean poly bags is to be used.

9. Material for microbiological testing is to be sampled with sterilized tools and into sterilized jars/bottles. Sampling device is mopped with 70% isopropyl alcohol for collecting samples for microbiological limit test. The sampling of items for microbiological testing and sterile raw material must be done under laminar airflow. Ensure the manometer reading of laminar airflow unit between 7 and 15 mm before sampling.

10. Sterile materials must be sampled in a way, which maintains the sterility of the bulk. All sterile material containers are taken to sampling booth maintained within the sterile area, containers are open under sterile conditions and sampled using sterile sampling kit.

11. Cleaning status room label should be checked before starting of sampling operation. Samplers should follow all clean room practice concerning abstinence for using watches, rings, nail polish, and other cosmetics while on duty.

12. Room temperature and humidity setting in the store and the sampling booth should not be disturbed or altered in any way.

13. Materials from one consignment shall be sampled at a time.

12. All containers to be sampled is cleaned with a damp cloth or vacuumed depending on the packing type immediately prior sampling.

14. Sampling of light-sensitive hygroscopic material is required to be performed in the sampling booth fitted with sodium lamp and dehumidifier. Sodium lamp should be switched on 5 minutes before sampling of the light-sensitive material.

15. While sampling all excess packaging are to be removed except the primary pack outside the sampling booth.

16. All the suppliers' RELEASED/PASSED labels attached to the received raw material and components should not be removed during the sampling process.

17. Before opening of a primary package or the immediate container, it is to be marked with a numerical order on the outer container. This is required for future identification of the container number from which the sample has been taken.

18. Containers must be opened carefully and re-sealed effectively after sampling. Care should be taken to protect the sample from contamination at all stages. Bags sampled with a spear or by cutting open must have the sampling area swabbed with 70% IPA before and after the operation.

19. In case of sampling of sterile products, all sampling tools should be prior sterilized, stored in sampling room and open inside the LAF only. They are to be rested only on sterile cloths throughout the sampling process to prevent contamination.

20. First Aid box should be available at the place of sampling with necessary medicines.

21. Due to expansion properties, volatile samples should not be filled to more than 70% of the capacity.

22. Spillages from sampling should be cleared immediately and disposed of safely. Any spillage of material on sampler skin should be washed off immediately.

23. All the sampling tools and clothing are disposed after sampling for cleaning and not to be reused in any case without cleaning and sterilization as required.

WHO GUIDELINES FOR SAMPLING OF PHARMACEUTICAL PRODUCTS AND RELATED MATERIALS

World Health Organization, WHO Technical Report Series, No. 929, 2005

(Courtesy: http://apps.who.int/medicinedocs/documents/s21440en/s21440en.pdf)

1. Introduction
   1.1 General considerations
   1.2 Glossary
   1.3 Purpose of sampling
   1.4 Classes and types of pharmaceutical products and related materials
   1.5 Sampling facilities
   1.6 Responsibilities for sampling
   1.7 Health and safety
2. Sampling process
   2.1 Preparation for sampling
   2.2 Sampling operation and precautions
   2.3 Storage and retention
3. Regulatory issues
   3.1 Pharmaceutical inspections
   3.2 Surveillance programmes
4. Sampling on the receipt (for acceptance)
   4.1 Starting materials

4.2 Intermediates in the manufacturing process and bulk pharmaceutical products
4.3 Finished products
4.4 Packaging materials (primary and secondary)
5. Sampling plans for starting materials, packaging materials and finished products
   5.1 Starting materials
   5.2 Packaging materials
   5.3 Finished products
Bibliography
Appendix 1: Types of sampling tools
Appendix 2: Sample collection form
Appendix 3: Steps to be considered for inclusion in a standard operating procedure
Appendix 4: Examples of types of containers used to store samples of starting materials and bulk products
Appendix 5: Examples of the use of sampling plans n, p and r

1. INTRODUCTION

These guidelines are primarily intended for the use of government organizations, such as drug regulatory authorities (inspectorates), quality control laboratories and customs and police officials, but the general principles are also appropriate for application by procurement agencies, manufacturers and customers. These guidelines are useful when surveying the national markets for the quality of drug products in accordance with national drug quality surveillance programmes for marketed products, whether registered for sale or compounded in pharmacies. The choice of a sampling plan should always take into consideration, the specific objectives of the sampling and the risks and consequences associated with inherent decision errors.

1.1 General Considerations

Sampling is the operation designed for the selection of a portion of a product for a defined purpose. The sampling procedure is to be developed appropriate to the purpose of sampling, type of controls intended to be applied and the material to be sampled described in writing. All operations related to sampling are to be performed with care, using proper equipment and tools. Any contamination of the sample by dust or other foreign material is liable to jeopardize the validity of the subsequent analyses.

1.2 Glossary

Available sample: Whatever the total quantity of sample materials is available.

Batch: A quantity of any drug produced during a given cycle of manufacture. If the manufacturing process is continuous, the batch originates in a defined period during which the manufacturing conditions are stable and have not been modified.

Combined sample: Sample resulting from combining all or parts of two or more samples of the material.

Consignment: The quantity of a bulk starting material, or a drug product, made by one manufacturer or supplied by an agent, and supplied at one time in response to a particular request or order. A consignment may comprise one or more batch identified packages or containers and may include material belonging to more than one batch identified batch.

Final sample: Sample ready for the application of the test procedure.

Homogeneity: A material is regarded as homogeneous when it is all of the same origins (e.g. from the same batch) and as non-homogeneous when it is of differing origins.

Original sample: Sample collected directly from the material.

Pharmaceutical product: Any material or product intended for human or veterinary use presented in its finished dosage form or as a starting material for use in such a dosage form that is subject to control by pharmaceutical legislation in the exporting state and/or the importing state.

Prequalification: The activities undertaken in defining a product or service need, seeking expressions of interest from enterprises to supply the product or service, and examining the product or service offered against the specification and the facility where the product or service is prepared against common standards of GMP.

The examination of the product or service and the facility where it is manufactured is performed by trained and qualified inspectors against common standards. Once the product is approved, and the facility is approved for the delivery of the specified product or service, other procurement agencies are informed of the approval. Prequalificationis required for all pharmaceutical products regardless of their composition and place of manufacture or registration, but the amount and type of information requested from the supplier for use in the assessment by the procurement agency may differ.

Production: All operations involved in the preparation of a pharmaceutical product, from receipt of materials, through processing, packaging and repackaging, labeling and relabeling, to completion of the finished product.

Random sample: In which the different fractions of the material have an equal probability of being represented.

Representative sample: Sample obtained according to a sampling procedure designed to ensure that the different parts of a batch or the different properties of a uniform material are proportionately represented.

Retention sample: Sample collected as part of the original sampling process and reserved for future testing. The size of a retention sample should be sufficient to allow for at least two confirmatory analyses. In some cases, statutory regulations may require one or more retention samples, each of which should be separately identified, packaged and sealed.

Sample: A portion of a material collected according to a defined sampling procedure. The size of any sample should be sufficient to allow all anticipated test procedures to be carried out, including all repetitions and retention samples. If the quantity of material available is not sufficient for the intended analyses and the retention samples, the inspector should record that the sampled material is the only available sample and the evaluation of the results should take into account of the limitations that arise from the insufficient sample size.

Sampler: Person responsible for performing the sampling operations.

Sampling method: That part of the sampling procedure dealing with the method prescribed for withdrawing samples.

Sampling plan: Description of the location, number of units and/or quantity of material that should be collected, and associated acceptance criteria.

Sampling procedure: The complete sampling operation is to be performed on a defined material for a specific purpose. A detailed written description of the sampling procedure is provided in the *sampling protocol*.

Sampling record: Written record of the sampling operations carried out on a particular material for a defined purpose. The sampling record should contain the batch number, date, and place of sampling, reference to the sampling protocol used, a description of the containers and the materials sampled, notes on possible abnormalities, together with any other relevant observations, and the name and signature of the inspector.

Sampling unit: Discrete part of a consignment such as an individual package, drum or container.

Selected sample: Sample obtained according to a sampling procedure designed to select a fraction of the material that is likely to have special properties. A selected sample that is likely to contain deteriorated, contaminated, adulterated or otherwise unacceptable material is known as an extreme *sample*.

Uniformity: A starting material may be considered uniform when samples drawn from different layers do not show significant differences in the quality control tests which would result in non-conformity with specifications. The following materials may be considered uniform unless there are signs to the contrary, i.e. organic and inorganic chemicals, purified natural products, various processed natural products such as fatty oils and essential oils; and plant extracts. The assumption of uniformity is strengthened by homogeneity, i.e. when the consignment is derived from a single batch.

1.3 Purpose of Sampling

Sampling of materials is required for different purposes, such as prequalification, acceptance of consignments, batch release testing, in-process control, special controls, inspection for customs clearance, deterioration or adulteration, or for obtaining a retention sample, the tests that are applied to the sample material includes the purpose of:

- Verifying the identity;
- Performing complete pharmacopoeial or analogous testing; and
- Performing special or specific tests.

1.4 Classes and Types of Pharmaceutical Products and Related Materials

The materials sampled in the pharmaceutical industry mostly belong to the following classes:

- Starting materials for use in the manufacture of finished pharmaceutical products;
- Intermediates in the manufacturing process (e.g. bulk granule);
- Pharmaceutical products (in-process as well as before and after packaging);
- Primary and secondary packaging materials; and
- Cleaning and sanitizing agents, comprising of gases and other processing agents.

1.5 Sampling Facilities

Sampling facilities are designed especially with the purpose of:

- Prevent contamination of the opened container, the materials, and the operator;
- Prevent cross-contamination by other materials, products, and the environment; and
- Protect the individual staff who withdraw samples (sampler) during the sampling procedure.

In pharmaceuticals, sampling is performed in a designated area or booth designed for and dedicated to this purpose, although this is not possible where samples are required to be taken from a production line (e.g. in-process control samples). In such cases, the area from where samples were taken are recorded in the sampling record, and a sequential log is to be kept of all materials sampled in each area. Sampling of materials from large containers of starting material or bulk products create difficulties. This type of sampling is mostly carried out in a separate, closed cubicle within the warehouse, to reduce the risk of contamination (e.g. by dust) of either the sample or the materials remaining in the container or of cross-contamination. Some materials are needed to be sampled in special or dedicated environments as contamination with dirt or particles from the environment are to be avoided, i.e. such as aerosol valves, hormones, and penicillin). While taking samples of the original sales pack as a sample from a pharmacy or hospital sampling area requirements need not be followed. However, the Drug Inspector should ensure that the quantity of the sample taken is sufficient for the intended analyses and retention samples. All units sampled should preferably be derived from the same batch and the same location except for special cases.

1.6 Responsibilities for Sampling

The persons generally responsible for following the defined sampling procedures are:

- *Governmental organizations*, as drug control authorities such as inspectors, quality control laboratories persons, customs and police authorities who are responsible for the clearance of drug products held in quarantine after manufacture or importation in suspect of being deteriorated, contaminated, adulterated or counterfeited are in need to sample products.
- *Customers,* like patients, private and public organizations can acquire drug products for complaint and research purpose.
- *Manufacturers* are mandatorily involved in sampling for compliance of good manufacturing practices (GMP), research and development purpose.

In the pharmaceutical manufacturing units, samplers are adequately trained in the practical aspects of sampling. They should be qualified to perform the sampling operation and should have sufficient knowledge of pharmaceutical substances to execute work effectively and safely. Given that the sampling technique itself can introduce bias, it is important that personnel carrying out the sampling are suitably trained in the techniques and procedures employed. Regular training is conducted and performance documented in the individual's training records.

Sampling records should indicate the date of sampling, the sampled container and the identity of the person who sampled the batch. A conscientious approach, with meticulous attention to detail and cleanliness, is essential. The sampler must remain alert to any signs of contamination, deterioration or tampering of the sampled containers. Any suspicious signs are to be recorded in detail in the sampling record and reported. When the government agencies need to sample a sterile bulk pharmaceutical product at the manufacturing site, it is best to have the manufacturer's personnel collect the sample following their procedures in the presence of the inspector.

The inspector should observe the procedure in a way not to increase the chance of contamination preferably through the glass window outside the aseptic sampling area.

1.7 Health and Safety

It is the responsibility of the sampler to read the relevant health and safety information (e.g. the safety data sheet for a pharmaceutical product and related materials) before sampling the material. The information should include necessary safety precautions and requirements for both the operator and the environment. The sampler needs to wear appropriate protective clothing for a specific sampling task that requires safety precautions such as the use of respiratory equipment and should be properly trained in its use. The sample storage areas should have adequate light and ventilation and should be arranged to satisfy the requirements for safety as well as any special requirement arising from the characteristics of the material being sampled. Care should be taken to guard against collapse of stacked containers of solids in bulk.

2. SAMPLING PROCESS

2.1 Preparation for Sampling

For the sampling of products, the responsible person needs to have at his or her disposal all the tools needed to open the containers (e.g. packages, barrels and others). Tools may include knives, pliers, saws, hammers, wrenches, implements to remove dust (preferably a vacuum cleaner), and material to reclose the packages (such as sealing tape), as well as self-adhesive labels to indicate that some of the contents have been removed from a package or container. Containers due to be sampled are cleaned before sampling. Sampling of uniform starting materials does not require complicated tools. A variety of pipettes fitted with suction bulbs, cups or beakers, dippers, and funnels are needed for liquids of low viscosity. The use of glass is preferably avoided. A suitable inert rod can be used for highly viscous liquid, and spatulas or scoops are needed for powdered and granular solids. Sterile pharmaceutical products are sampled with sterile tools under aseptic conditions to avoid the risk of loss of sterility. The tools for sampling non-uniform materials are more complicated and more difficult to clean. For example, a sampling tube with a shutter at the lower end may be used to sample liquids in drums or other large containers, and a slotted tube with a pointed end may be used for sampling of solids.

All sampling tools and implements should be made of inert materials and kept scrupulously clean. After use or before reuse, they should be thoroughly washed, rinsed with water or a suitable solvent, dried and stored in clean conditions. Adequate washing facilities are to be provided near the sampling area else the sampler is required to bring separate clean sets of implements for sampling of each product. The cleaning procedure used for all sampling tools and instruments is documented and recorded. The adequacy of the cleaning procedure for different types of material made sampling tools are to be demonstrated. The use of disposable sampling materials has distinct advantages. Examples of sampling tools suitable for each type of material are given in Appendix 1.

2.2 Sampling Operation and Precautions

Sampling procedures are maintained as written records describing the sampling operation, health and safety aspects of sampling. Samples are taken in sufficient quantities adequate for testing in accordance with the specifications. Closures and labels should preferably be such that it can detect unauthorized opening. Once sampled it should never be returned to the bulk in case excess or unused. Appendix 2 describes the details to be furnished in the sample collection form.

The sampling procedure should be designed in such a way that can detect non-uniformity of material. During the sampling operation, attention is paid to detect any signs of nonconformity of the material. Signs of non-uniformity include differences in shape, size or color of particles in crystalline, granular or powdered solid substances; moist crusts on hygroscopic substances; deposits of a solid pharmaceutical product in liquid or semi-liquid products and stratification of liquid products. These types of changes may readily be reversible and in some cases can occur during prolonged storage or exposure to extreme temperatures during transportation. Heterogeneous portions of the material or bulk as mentioned above should be sampled and tested separately from the rest of the material that has a normal appearance.

Pooling of the samples from the different portions are avoided, as this can mask contamination, low potency or other quality problems. Labeling of the sampled container at the time of sampling should provide appropriate details, including the batch number and the container number from which the sample was taken, amount taken and for what purpose. The container used to store the samples is also properly labeled with appropriate details such as sample type, the name of the material, identification code, batch/batch number, code, quantity, date of sampling, storage conditions, handling precautions and container number.

For finished drug products decision of sampling quantity required to be withdrawn take account of the official and non-official tests performed on an individual dosage form (e.g., tablets or parenteral preparations). The sampling procedure also takes account of experience with the pharmaceutical product or related material and with the supplier, and the number of sampling units in the consignment. In accordance with national legislation during on going investigations of legal cases related to counterfeit pharmaceutical products, samples may require to be taken in the absence of consignee. When a container is sampled by breaking the tamper-proof seal to obtain a sample outside the control of the consignee of the product, then the container is resealed with an appropriate tamper-proof seal, and the consignee of the product informed of its type and identification. If a container bag has been punctured to take a sample by an authorized sampler, then the sampling hole is appropriately closed and identified. Sampled containers are identified with a number, as they may not contain the quantity of product stated on the label. Sampling steps for sampling different category of substances are given in Appendix 3.

2.3 Storage and Retention

The container used to store a sample must not interact with the sampled material or allow any contamination. The container should also protect the sample from extremes of light, air, and moisture as per recommended storage directions for the pharmaceutical product or related material sampled. Samples of bulk solid or liquid materials are placed in one or more clean containers and sealed preferably with tamper-evident means. Liquid samples are transported in suitable bottles closed by screw tops with inert liners that provide a good moisture-proof seal for the contents. Suitable inert screw-top jars can also be used for solid or semi-solid pharmaceutical products. Light-sensitive materials are protected by using amber glass containers or by wrapping colorless glass containers in foil or dark-colored paper. Head space should be kept to a minimum to minimize any possible degradation. Any special procedures like nitrogen gassing are discussed with the consignee of the material and carried out as appropriate. Solid dosage forms such as tablets or granules are protected during transit, either by totally filling the container with the product or by filling any residual space with a suitable filling material. All containers are sealed, labeled, packaged adequately and transported in such a way as to avoid breakage and contamination during transport.

For all containers that come apart (e.g. screw-capped jars or metal tins with separate lids) precautions should be taken to avoid any mix up when they are opened for examination, such as by labeling all parts of each container whenever possible. If one sample is divided into several sample containers, they should be transported in a suitably sealed box, which should be labeled with the identity of the product, the consignment from which the sample was drawn, the size of the sample, the date and place of sampling, and the name of the sampler. Security and adequate storage conditions should be ensured for the areas where the samples are stored. Samples should be stored in accordance with the storage conditions as specified for the respective active pharmaceutical ingredient (API), excipient or drug product. Packaging materials similar to those in which the bulk is supplied should be used for long-term storage. The types of containers used to store samples of starting materials and bulk products are given in Appendix 4.

3. REGULATORY ISSUES

Sampling for regulatory purposes require additional samples to be taken apart from regulatory testing for other verification purposes (e.g. for duplicate testing and parallel testing by different regulatory laboratories and if demanded by the consignee of the product). The consignee of the product is informed regarding samples acquired, and if the consignee wishes to conduct his/her testing on the sample acquired by the regulatory purposes, authorities should provide a part of the sample to the consignee. Sampling of products for prequalification purposes also follows similar tracks.

3.1 Pharmaceutical Inspections

Drugs inspectors may take samples from retailers, wholesalers or hospital pharmacies and manufactured formulations or bulk from manufacturing units for a variety of reasons, such as:

- Routine monitoring and control;
- Following the suspicion or discovery of products that show signs of possible deterioration, contamination, adulteration or counterfeiting; and
- When a particular product is suspected of being either ineffective or responsible for adverse clinical reactions.

For deteriorated dosage forms, the sample should consist of one or more retail containers of the product that shows visual signs of deterioration. When sampling is done concerning a complaint on a drug product, the samples should include the original container and one or more unopened containers containing the same product, bearing the same batch number. Communication between the regulatory authority and the consignee of the goods is initiate concerning the findings and any necessary corrective action.

3.2 Surveillance Programmes

National drug regulatory authorities are responsible for monitoring the quality of all drug products marketed in their country and as defined by legislation. The extent of routine surveillance undertaken, unlike the assessment of suspect products depends upon factors, such as:

- The capacity of the national quality control laboratory;
- The extent to which the quality of the product has been assessed before registration;
- The extent to which the requirements for GMP are implemented; and
- The number of products that are imported from abroad.

The regulatory authority should ensure systematic implementation of drug quality surveillance programme for all the registered marketed products. Each product should be assessed regularly (e.g. every 2–3 years) for inclusion in the surveillance programme, but particular attention is accorded to products that are of prime importance to public health programmes or the ones that are potentially dangerous, unstable or difficult to formulate correctly. The responsible laboratory draws up the sampling programme, under the guidance of the drug regulatory authority on a yearly or half-yearly basis. This programme not only lists the products to be sampled during a given period but also to specify the sampling procedures and size of the samples to be collected taking into account the need for retention samples. The programme states level and extent of sampling of each brand of a given product and the local authority or inspector responsible for each sampling operation. It also indicates the laboratory (if more than one exists) where a sample should be sent for testing.

4. SAMPLING RECEIPT OR ACCEPTANCE

4.1 Starting Materials

The sample can be taken from any part of the consignment when the starting material consignment of a product is regarded as uniform. When the material is not physically uniform, special sampling tools may be required to withdraw a cross-sectional portion of the material. Alternatively, where applicable, a validated procedure can be followed to restore the uniformity of the material before sampling, based on information concerning the subsequent handling and manufacturing steps. A stratified liquid can be stirred, or a solid deposit in a liquid may be dissolved by gentle warming and stirring, but such interventions must not be attempted without adequate knowledge of the properties of the contents and appropriate communication with

the consignee of the goods. All partially processed natural products, both animal, herbal (dried plants and their parts) and mineral, are treated as intrinsically non-uniform. Special procedures requiring considerable practice are needed to prepare representative samples from such consignments. Details of appropriate procedures are available with the relevant International Organization for Standardization (ISO) documents.

4.2 Intermediates in the Manufacturing Process and Bulk Pharmaceutical Products

Pharmaceutical intermediates and bulk products are like, liquids and semi-solid pharmaceutical products, powdered solids or granulates transported in large containers intended either for further processing or direct packaging into final marketed containers, and unit dosage forms (tablets, capsules) supplied in bulk which is intended for repackaging into smaller containers. There is a risk of segregation of bulk materials during transportation should be taken into account when drawing up the sampling plan. Products of this kind may be assumed to be uniform with a validated transportation process and provided that they:

- Are labeled with the name of the manufacturer and batch number;
- Have been produced in accordance with GMP; and
- Are supplied with a certificate, issued in the country of origin, according to the WHO Certification Scheme on the quality of pharmaceutical products moving in international commerce. In these circumstances collection of a single sample is sufficient for the intended analyses.

4.3 Finished Products

The quality of finished pharmaceutical products frequently needs to be verified at the time of release and importation. The necessary sampling is performed using an appropriate method with regard to the presumed uniformity. A single consignment of a product from a single manufacturer and labeled with a single batch number is assumed to be uniform. The minimum size of the samples is determined as per the requirements of the analytical procedure used to test the product. Testing of unit dosage forms for uniformity of weight, volume or content requires a considerable number of units as well as tests for sterility. Depending upon the type of material, the size of the consignment and the way in which the material is packed, a unit to be sampled is regarded as the transport container, e.g. 20 packs shrink-wrapped or boxed together, rather than an individual container. The required number of unit dosage forms is then withdrawn from any individual container from a selected transit container. If a consignment consists of one very large batch or if little experience has been recorded with the product to be sampled, it may be prudent to carry out two independent analyses. Two independent final samples are then be taken from different sampling units. Conversely, when a consignment is composed of two or three batches from the same manufacturer, a single sample taken from each batch may suffice, provided that favorable documented experience existed with the product and the manufacturer, and it is evident from the expiry date and other information that the batches were produced at approximately the same time.

4.4 Packaging Materials (Primary and Secondary)

There is a potential chance of mixing up of printed packaging materials during the sampling operations and, therefore, only one material is recommended to be handled at a time. **Samples of packaging materials should never be returned to the consignment.**

Adequate protection of packaging material integrity (e.g. collapsible metal tubes) and identification is required for the packaging material samples to avoid damage and mixing. Primary packaging materials further need adequate protection during sampling operation to avoid environmental contamination. Appropriate sampling protection is practiced considering the final use of the packaging (e.g. parenteral ampoules). Based on several reasons, a consignment of packaging materials may not be considered homogenous, such as:

- Materials manufactured on different days or equipment line.
- Materials manufactured on one machine line but different stations (e.g. 16 printing dye stations and 12 molding stations).
- Packaging material manufactured with different source materials (e.g. polyethylene from two different sources).
- Change in quality occurred during the process (e.g. container wall thickness, color variation, text legibility or change of printing plate).

5. SAMPLING PLANS FOR STARTING MATERIALS, PACKAGING MATERIALS AND FINISHED PRODUCTS

The choice of the sampling plan should always take into consideration the specific objectives of the sampling and the risks and consequences associated with inherent decision errors. Ideally, each sampling unit should be examined to ensure that it is intact and also checked for possible damage to the container. The contents should be inspected for uniformity and appropriately tested for identity. Uniformity should be tested on selected layer samples at different points in the material without previous intermixing. However, if in case the ideal procedure is not possible to follow or justified by the purpose of sampling, the number of sampling units is randomly selected. It is not prudent to open all containers of products, which are liable to deteriorate under the influence of moisture or oxygen when held in a transit warehouse. However, materials in damaged containers or those found to be non-uniform should either be rejected or individually sampled for complete quality control. Unlabeled sampling units should be rejected.

For random sampling, whenever possible, each sampling unit should be consecutively numbered, and the required number of random sampling units are selected using tables of random numbers. The number of units to be sampled depends on different assumptions and three possible plans are shown in Table 7.8. It is important to recognize that the "n-plan" is not statistically based thus be used only as a guiding principle.

5.1 Starting materials

While sampling of starting materials proper consideration has to be given to decide on a sampling plan.

5.1.1 The n plan

The 'n plan' is used with great caution and only when the material to be sampled is considered uniform and is supplied by a recognized source. Samples can be withdrawn from any part of the container (usually from the top layer). The *n plan* is based on the formula $n = 1 + \sqrt{N}$, where N is the number of sampling units in the consignment. When the minimum number of containers needed to be sampled (N) is less than or equal to 4, then every container is sampled. According to this plan, n samples are taken from N sampling units selected at random, and these are subsequently placed in separate sample containers. The control laboratory inspects the appearance of the material and tests the identity of each original sample according to the relevant specification. If the results are concordant, the original samples are combined into a final composite sample from which ananalytical sample is prepared, the remainder being kept as a retention sample. The *n* plan is not recommended for use by control laboratories of manufacturers who are

Table 7.8: Values of *n*, *p* or *r* for the *N* sampling units

Values of	Values of N		
n, p or *r*	*n* plan	*p* plan	*r* plan
2	up to 3	up to 25	up to 2
3	4–6	26–56	3–4
4	7–13	57–100	5–7
5	14–20	101–156	8–11
6	21–30	157–225	12–16
7	31–42	–	17–22
8	43–56	–	23–28
9	57–72	–	29–36
10	73–90	–	37–44

required to analyze and release or reject each received consignment of the starting materials used to produce a drug product.

5.1.2 The p plan

The 'p plan' is used when the material is uniform, received from a recognized source and the main purpose is to test for identity. The p plan is based on the formula $p = 0.4\sqrt{N}$, where N is the number of sampling units. The figures for p are obtained by rounding up to the next highest integer. According to this plan, samples are taken from each of the N sampling units of the consignment and placed in separate sample containers. These original samples are transferred to the control laboratory, visually inspected and tested for identity. If the results are concordant, p final samples are formed by appropriate pooling of the original samples.

5.1.3 The r plan

The 'r plan' is used when the material is suspected to be non-uniform and/or is received from a source that is not well known. The *r* planis also used for herbal medicinal products used as starting materials. This plan is based on the formula $r = 1.5\sqrt{N}$, where N is the number of sampling units. The figures for r are obtained by rounding up to the next highest integer. Samples are taken from each of the N sampling units of the consignment and placed in separate sample containers. These original samples are transferred to the control laboratory and tested for identity. If the results are concordant, r samples are randomly selected and individually subjected to testing. If these results are concordant, the r samples are combined for the retention sample.

5.2 Packaging Materials

Sampling plans for packaging materials should be based on defined sampling standards, for example, British Standard BS 6001-1, ISO2859 or ANSI/ASQCZ1.4-1993. The objective is to ensure that there is a low probability of accepting material that does not comply with the predefined acceptance level.

5.3 Finished Products

As for packaging materials, sampling plans for finished products should also be based on defined sampling standards. For physical and chemical testing, the sampling units should consist of whole packs, and individual packs should not be broken open for sampling.

APPENDIXES

APPENDIX 1: TYPES OF SAMPLING TOOLS

Scoops

Spatula or scoops are most commonly used for sampling of solid materials. Figure 7.13 shows the recommended designs of scoops, which should preferably be rounded.

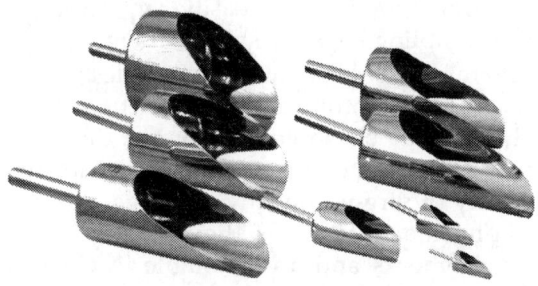

Fig. 7.13: Sampling scoops for solids

Using a perfect size scoop is essential for correct sampling practice. If the scoop is too small for the sizes of the particle being sampled, large particles will roll off, and testing bias may be introduced. If the scoop is too big, it may unnecessarily obtain a large sample size for a given number of increments. A scoopful of the sample should be taken in a single movement and transferred to the sample container. Avoid tapping the scoop to remove the product as this is likely to cause segregation for the sample.

Dip Tubes

Dip tubes made up of polypropylene or stainless steel are used for sampling of liquid and topical products. A typical dip tube is shown in Fig. 7.14.

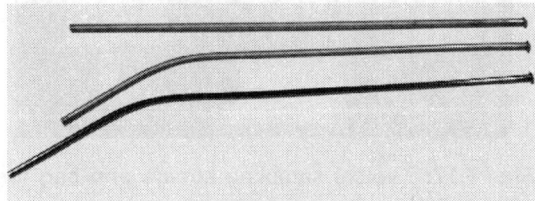

Fig. 7.14: Typical dip tubes for liquids

Dipping Vessels or Weighted Containers

Containers in weighted carriers are used for taking samples from large tanks and storage vessels. These containers are designed in such a way that they can be opened at a required depth. Marks on the cord used for lowering the container is used to determine the correct sampling depth. A typical weighted container is shown in Fig. 7.15.

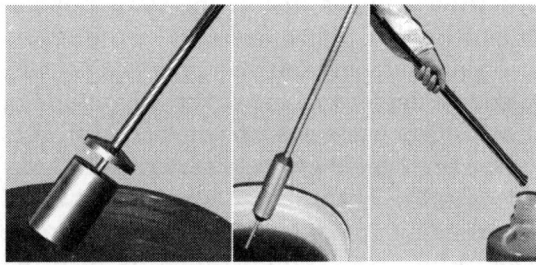

Fig. 7.15: Typical dipping vessels used for collecting liquid or solid samples from a variable depth of large containers

Thieves

Sample thieves are used for taking samples from deep containers of solids, that is also sometimes referred to as "double-tube spears". Typical thieves are shown in Fig. 7.16.

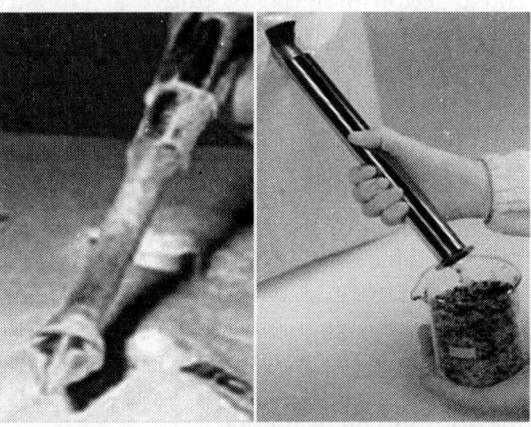

Fig. 7.16: Sample thieves

A plug thieve consists of a hollow tube with an inner rod that has a tip on the end to allow the thieve to enter the powder bed inclosed position. The geometry of this tip can influence the sample taken as the pointed tips to cause less distortion of the powder bed than the blunt-tipped probes, thereby reducing sampling error.

Chamber thieve consists of two concentric tubes, in which the inner tube is solid except the sample collection chambers. The outer tube is hollow with openings that can be aligned with the inner tube chambers. Following insertion a thieve distort the static powder blend bed of pharmaceutical product by carrying material from the upper layers of the blend to the lower layers. The magnitude of this distortion depends on whether the thieves are inserted into the blend with a smooth, jerky or twisting action. The angle of thieves insertion into the powder bed can also create sampling error. When thieve is inserted vertically, it can extract samples of different particle size in contrast obtained while inserting the same thieve at an acute angle. Also, the position of a chamber thieve while in the powder bed (i.e. whether the chamber is at the top, the bottom or in the middle of the thief) can also influence the sampling error. A well-designed thieve have a sharp end to minimize disruption to the powder bed. The construction material of thieve are mostly stainless steel or poly propylene. Sampling error can be affected by construction material and also bed depth as the static pressure of the bulk blend forces the material into the sample chamber(s). This pressure is far greater at the bottom of a large container than it is in the middle or at the top. It is quite possible that the same thieve could extract samples of different particle size from the top or bottom of a static powder blend. It is essential to define the correct sampling procedure for using thieves, and the staff is to be trained for the appropriate technique.

Sample Bag and Sampling Spears

Sampling spears are the most commonly used instruments for taking samples from bags because they are relatively cheap, simple and quick. Sampling spears have a maximum external diameter of about 12 mm, but can be up to 25 mm. The spear should be 40–45 cm in length to obtain a good cross-sectional sample. The tapered type sampling spears penetrate container bags easily. Typical spears and sampling bags are shown in Fig. 7.17.

Sampling bags are made of flexible material closed at the bottom and the sides by sealing. The top may be closed by fusion of the material, depending on the intended use. Mostly a variety of virgin polyethylene bags are used in pharmaceuticals as they meet all FDA requirements and are available in clear or light-sensitive amber color with an open end or zip. Other specialty designed bags are also available as per specific need for sampling, pharmaceutical and lab applications including self-adhesive bags, anti-static bags, biohazard bags, hazmat bags and custom pre-printed bags indifferent sizes. Polyethylene bags are advantageous as they are unbreakable, collapsible, light as well as very economical.

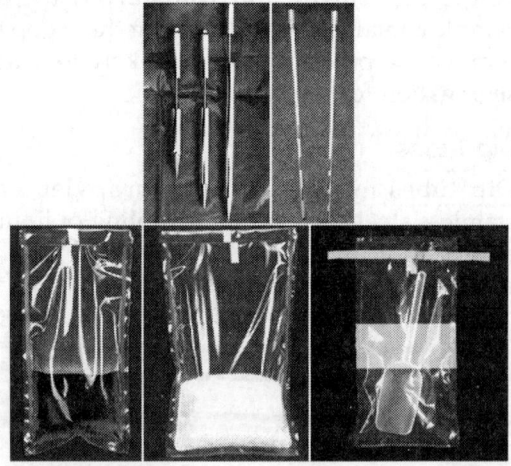

Fig. 7.17: Typical sampling spears and bag for solid sample

APPENDIX 2: FORMS

Sample Collection Form

Product name of the sample: ....

Name of (active) starting material (INN, generic or scientific name) with dosage strength:
....

Dosage form (tablet, capsule, etc.): ....

Batch number: ....

Date of manufacture:........................... Expiry date: ....

Registration or license number (if applicable): ....

Date of sampling: ....

Name of the manufacturer: ....

Name of location/place where sample was taken: Serial number: ....

....

Address (with telephone and fax number, if applicable):

....

A number of sample unit taken (tablet, capsule, etc.: At least 20 but not more than 30 units):

....

A brief physical/visual description of sample:

....

Names of person who took samples:

1. ....

2. ....

Signature of person(s) taking samples   Signature of the representative
where the sample(s) was taken (optional)   of the establishment

1. ....

2. ....

Sampling Label

Material Code ....

Material Description ....

....

Laboratory Batch Number ....

Manufacturer's Batch Number ....

Number of Samples ....

Sample Quantity ....

Date ....

Container no: .... of ....

	Name	Signature
Sampled by:		
Authorized by:		
Supervised by:		
Submitted to:		

APPENDIX 3: STEPS TO BE CONSIDERED FOR INCLUSION WHILE PREPARING SAMPLING STANDARD OPERATING PROCEDURE (SOP)

These steps of a sampling SOP described below are based on purely theoretical basis and are required to be rectified and refined for particular use.

Bulk Liquid Products Sampling Steps

1. Read and understand the precautions to be observed for the safe handling of the material.
2. Gather all the required sampling equipments (sampling tube or weighted sampling can, sample bottles and labels) and check that all are properly cleaned.
3. Locate the batch.
4. Examine the container(s) for signs of contamination and record faults if any.
5. Examine the labels for obvious differences and signs of changes including obliterations and mislabeling, and record faults, if any.
6. Investigate and clarify the sources and reasons for any observed faults before proceeding for sampling.
7. Based on the viscosity of the liquid choose a suitable size and orifice liquid-sampling tube.
8. Sample the liquid, suspension or emulsion (well stirred, if appropriate) by slowly pushing the open sampling tube vertically downwards through the liquid so that material is collected from each layer.
9. Seal the tube, withdraw it from the bulk liquid. Transfer all the contents of the tube to a clean, labeled sample bottle.
10. Repeat steps 8 and 9 until sufficient samples for analytical and retention purposes have been obtained.
11. Seal the sample bottles.
12. Reseal the sampled container and label as 'sampled'.

13. Clean and dry the sampling tube, observing the relevant safety precautions.
14. Sample other required containers in the same manner following steps 8–12 above.
15. Clean the sampling tube using the recommended cleaning procedure.
16. Deliver the analytical samples to the laboratory and the reserve samples to the retention sample store. Report any aspects of the sampling that should be brought to the attention of the analyst or the inspector.
17. Check supplier certificate versus the specifications, if applicable.

Powdered Starting Material

The steps to be considered in sampling a powdered starting material are as follows.

1. Read and understand the precautions to be observed for the safe handling of the material.
2. Gather together the required sampling equipment (sampling spear, sample bottles, and labels) and check that all items are clean.
3. Locate the consignment and count the number of containers. Record this number.
4. Examine all the containers for obvious differences and signs of damage. Record any faults.
5. Examine all the labels for obvious differences and signs of changes, including obliterations and mislabeling. Record any faults.
6. Segregate any damaged containers and those with suspected spoiled contents for separate examination. These should then be referred *to or rejected* and dealt with accordingly.
7. Segregate any containers with different batch numbers and treat these separately.

8. Number the remaining containers.

9. Choose the appropriate sampling plan (n, p or r).

10. Choose the containers to be sampled in accordance with the requirements of the chosen plan (by the use of random number tables, by drawing batches or by the use of a random number generator if applicable).

11. Open the containers one at a time and inspect the contents. Record any differences.

12. Choose a suitable, clean sampling spear and plunge this (gates closed) into the powder so that the point of the spear reaches the bottom of the container.

13. Open the gates to allow the powder to enter the spear cavities, then reclose them.

14. Withdraw the spear from the container and transfer the spear contents to a labeled sample bottle.

15. Repeat steps 12–14 until sufficient material has been collected for analytical and retention requirements.

16. Seal the sample bottle.

17. Reseal the container from which the samples were withdrawn and label as "sampled."

18. Wipe clean the sampling spear if required, observing the safety precautions, before sampling the other chosen containers.

19. Repeat steps 12–18 for each chosen container.

20. Clean the sampling spear using the recommended cleaning procedure.

21. Deliver the analytical samples to the laboratory and the reserve samples to the retention sample store. Report any aspects of the sampling that should be brought to the attention of the analyst or inspector.

22. Check the supplier certificate versus the specifications, if applicable.

Packaging Materials

The steps to be considered in sampling of packaging materials are as follows.

1. Check the consignment against any associated documentation.

2. Check transit containers for the following and report any deviations as necessary:
   a. correct identification;
   b. integrity of the seal, if appropriate; and
   c. absence of physical damage.

3. Obtain the required sample from the required number of containers.

4. Place the sample units into identified appropriate sample containers.

5. Identify the consignment containers that have been sampled.

6. Note any special situations found during the sampling process (e.g. rogue items or component damage). Report any such observations as necessary.

7. Remove all sampled material pallets or containers from the sampling area together with all documentation.

8. Check supplier certificate against the specifications, if applicable.

Finished Products

The following steps should be considered when sampling finished products.

1. Determine the number of pallets per batch in the consignment.

2. Work out as per ISO 2859–1 table level II, the number of pallets to be checked visually.
   a. Check condition of pallet and packaging for the integrity of outer packaging material.
   b. Check outside of goods on the pallets for general cleanliness.
   c. Check that the overall labeling of the pallets matches the packing list.
   d. Count, categorize and record the number of defects.

3. Count the total number of transport packs on the number of pallets present and verify the total against the packing list.

4. From the number of pallets work out the number of transport packs to be sampled using the ISO table.

    a. Check condition of boxes for the integrity of packaging material.

    b. Check for cleanliness of boxes.

    c. Check the labeling of the boxes for damage.

    d. Check the boxes for overall damage.

    e. Check the labels for spelling mistakes.

    f. Check the labels for manufacturing and expiry dates.

    g. Count, categorize and record the number of defects.

5. From the number of boxes selected work out the number of unit packs to be examined visually using the ISO table.

    a. Check condition of the containers for the integrity of packaging material.

    b. Check for cleanliness of containers.

    c. Check condition of containers for shape and color.

    d. Check the labeling of containers for damage.

    e. Check the containers for overall damage.

    f. Check the labels for spelling mistakes.

    g. Check the labels for manufacturing and expiry dates.

    h. Count, categorize and record the number of defects.

6. From the number of containers selected, determine the number of containers to be taken for physical and chemical testing and retention.

7. Check the supplier certificate against the specifications, if applicable.

APPENDIX 4: CONTAINERS USED TO STORE SAMPLES OF STARTING MATERIALS AND BULK PRODUCTS

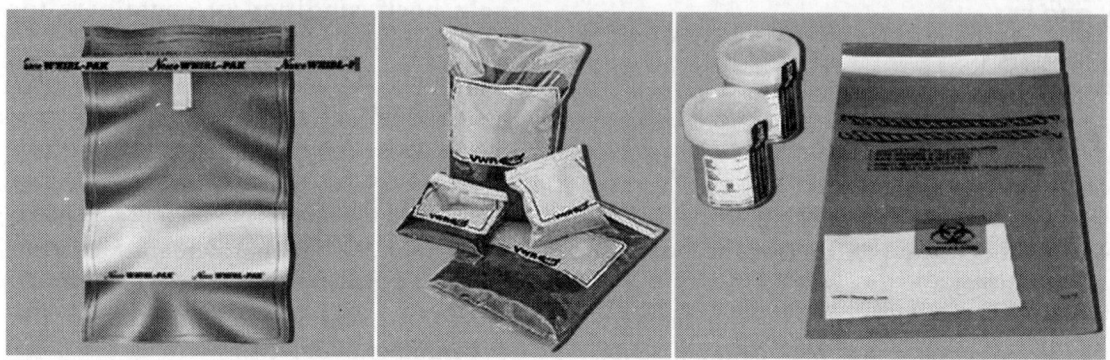

Fig. 7.18: Different types of sampling containers

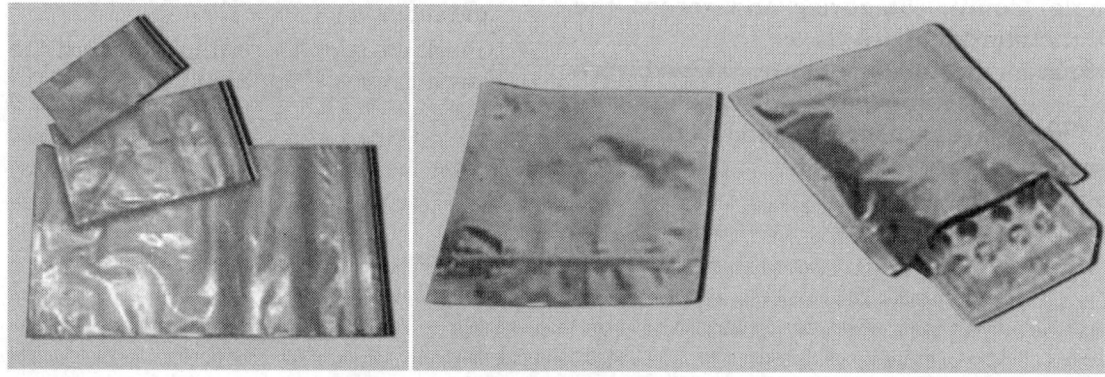

Fig. 7.19: Bag for storage of samples

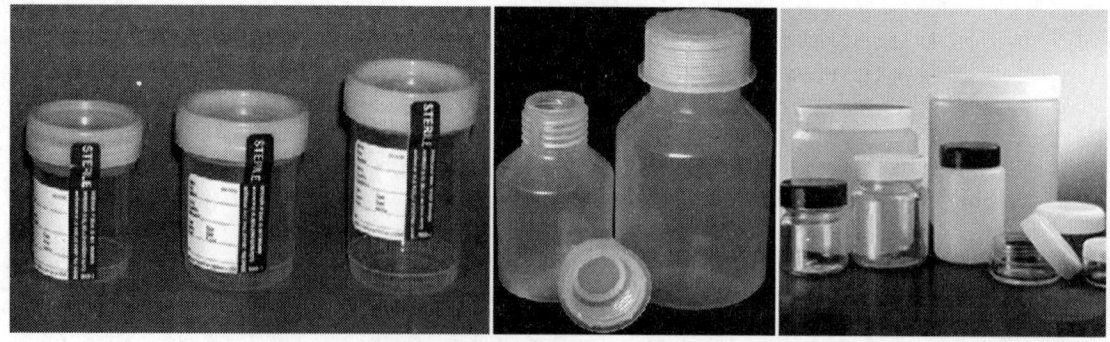

Fig. 7.20: Screw-top containers

APPENDIX 5: SAMPLING PLAN

Examples of the use of sampling plan n, p, and r

Consider a consignment of 40 containers of a starting material.

n Plan

Assuming a uniform material from a recognized source where there is a high degree of confidence in the source

While using the *n plan*, the $n = 1 + 6.32 = 7.32 \cong 7$. Samples are to be taken from seven containers selected at random. The appearance and identity of each of the seven samples are checked. If the results are concordant, all the seven samples are combined to produce a single, composite sample from which an analytical sample is prepared for full testing.

p Plan

Assuming a uniform material from a recognized source with the main purpose of checking the identity

Using the *p* plan, $p = 0.4\sqrt{N}$, $p = 0.4 \times 6.32 = 2.53 \cong 3$. Three samples would be taken from each container. The appearance and identity of each of these samples are checked. If the results are concordant, the samples are appropriately combined to form three final, composite samples to be used for retention (or full testing if required).

r Plan

Assuming the material is non-uniform and/or from a source that is not well known

Using the *r* plan, $r = 1.5\sqrt{N}$, $r = 1.5 \times 6.32 = 9.48 \cong 10$. Nine samples would be taken from each container. The appearance and identity of each of these samples are checked. If the results are concordant, 10 samples are selected at random and individually subjected to full testing.

BIBLIOGRAPHY

1. Acceptance sampling plans and procedures for the inspection of bulk materials. Geneva, International Organization for Standardization; 2000: ISO 10725.

2. American National Standards Institute/ American Society for Quality. Sampling procedures and tables for inspection by attributes. American Society for Quality, Washington, DC; 1993: ANSI/ASQCZ1. 4-1993.

3. European Commission Enterprise and Industry Directorate-General. Consumer goods Pharmaceuticals Brussels, 14 December 2005 EudraLex The Rules Governing Medicinal Products in the European Union Volume 4 EU Guidelines to Good Manufacturing Practice Medicinal Products for Human and Veterinary Use Annex 19 Reference and Retention Samples.

4. Good practices for national pharmaceutical control laboratories. WHO Expert Committee on Specifications for Pharmaceutical Preparations. 36th report, Geneva, World Health Organization; 2002: WHO Technical Report Series, No. 902, Annex 3.

5. Guidelines on packaging for pharmaceutical products. WHO Expert Committee on Specifications for Pharmaceutical Preparations. 36th report, Geneva, World Health Organization; 2002: WHO Technical Report Series, No. 902, Annex 9.

6. Gy P. Sampling of particulate materials - theory and practice.2nd Ed, Elsevier, New York; 1979.

7. Koratochvil B, Taylor JK. Sampling for chemical analysis.Analytical Chemistry, 53; 1981: 925A.

8. Methods for sampling chemical products. Introduction and general principles. British Standard BS 5309-1.British Standards Publishing, London; 1976.

9. Methods for sampling chemical products. Sampling of liquids.British StandardBS 5309-3.British Standards Publishing, London; 1976.

10. Methods for sampling chemical products. Sampling of solids.British StandardBS 5309-4. British Standards Publishing, London; 1976.

11. Oakland JS. Management tools in the manufacture of chemicals: statisticalquality control. Chemistry and Industry 16; 1981: 562–567.

12. Quality assurance of pharmaceuticals.A compendium of guidelines and related materials. 2ndVol, Updated Ed, Good manufacturing practices,and inspection.Geneva, World Health Organization; 2004.

13. Sampling procedures for inspection by attributes. Procedures for assessment ofstated quality levels. British Standard BS 6001-5:2000. Geneva, International Organization for Standardization; 1999: ISO 2859-4.

14. Sampling procedures for inspection by attributes. Sampling schemes indexedby acceptance quality limit for lot-by-lot inspection. British Standard BS6001-1. Geneva, International Organization for Standardization; 1999: ISO2859-1.

15. Sampling procedures for inspection by variables. Specification for singlesampling plans indexed by acceptable quality level (AQL) for lot-by-lotinspection. British Standard BS 6002-1. Geneva, International Organizationfor Standardization; 1993: ISO 3951:1989.

16. Sommer K. Sampling of powders and bulk materials.Springer-Verlag, Heidelberg; 1986.

17. WHO Expert Committee on Specifications for Pharmaceutical Preparations. 39th report, Geneva, World Health Organization; 2005: WHO Technical Report Series, No. 929, Annex 2.

8

Supply Chain Management

CHAPTER OVERVIEW

- Importance of supply chain management
- Evolution of supply chain management
- Significance of logistics management in pharmaceuticals
- Indian pharmaceutical supply chain
- Challenges of adopting SCM practices
- Physical distribution of pharmaceutical products
- Cold chain supply (Drug Tracing System)

- Critical issues in understanding the pharmaceutical supply chain management
- Importation supply chain management
- Advantages of adopting SCM practices
- European Medicines Verification System (EMVS)
- Current perspectives
- Bibliography

KEY POINTS

- The pharmaceutical supply chain is the crucial aspect of distribution logistics for speedy and on time delivery of finished products to the end level customer. Beyond near management of transportation and logistics, the pharmaceutical supply chain has matured into the integration of planning, collaboration, quality transportation, documentation, and legal aspects management.
- Pharmaceutical product distribution activities are highly controlled due to the maintenance of quality and safety aspects and liability of time-bound supply. Most of the pharmaceutical products need temperature controlled storage and distribution under strict regulatory control to keep pace with developed countries. The Indian pharmaceutical supply chain is witnessing biggest reform imminent with the implementation of GST changing the market scenario.
- Pharmaceutical companies are now implementing a supply chain management technique to improve the functional process of quality controlled drug delivery. Shipping of temperature-sensitive drug products is required to be done in thermally controlled shipping condition. Cold chain supply vehicles are used for biologicals, injectable and thermolabile products applying refrigerants like dry ice and/or wet ice.
- Understanding product characteristics and typical environmental conditions the distribution stability programs are developed for performance measurement of the supply chain. The combined data of in-house stability study and transportation data is utilized to develop product-specific shipping criteria. When the need arises for product recall reverse logistics play an important role which collects all products distributed through the entire supply chain operation and sends back to the manufacturer.
- Seal control transit programmes are nowadays practiced with shipment issue in a tracked and sequential manner. The integrity of seals are monitored, and approved procedures are followed to deal with the situations of suspected or found to be counterfeit pharmaceutical products. The manufacturer is required to provide a batch certificate, no objection certificate and certificate of origin from drug controller for each imported consignment of a pharmaceutical product as recommended by the WHO Certification Scheme. The currently implemented EMVS system of EU is enabled with a Data Matrix Unique Identifier code on the medicine pack for online tracking of consignment all over the supply chain till dispensing to the patients preventing entry of falsified medicines in the legal supply chain

IMPORTANCE OF SUPPLY CHAIN MANAGEMENT

Logistics is the branch of science relating to procuring, maintaining and transporting material, personnel, and facilities. The term logistics comes from the Greek logos, originally used to describe the science of movement, supply, and maintenance of military forces in the field. Later on, it was used to describe the management of materials flows through an organization, from the raw materials stage to finished goods. Logistics is the management of goods flow from the point of origin to the destination ensuring maintenance of customers and legal requirements.

Regarding human resources management, logistics means giving inputs, i.e. "recruiting manpower", which ultimately work for the final consumer or to delivery. Logistics involves the integration of information on material handling, packaging, transportation, inventory, warehousing with material security. Logistics is a channel of the supply that adds the value of time and place utility. Logistics aspect of the supply chain plans, implements and controls the forward and reverses movement and storage of goods, services and related information between the point of origin and the point of consumption.

Logistics management subdivided into the following:

- Materials management
- Channel management
- Distribution (or physical distribution)
- Business or logistics management
- Supply chain management (SCM)

Currently, the supply chain of products is built focusing on flexibility, responsibility, and reliability, shifting the supply paradigm from a stock-based system to an order-based model. Its characteristics are:

- Rapid commission and decommission of new products in the markets following the application of current techniques.
- Implementation of alternate supply methods to match the technological shift in the sales models, e.g. direct delivery to the consumer rather than through a wholesaler channel.
- Advanced product design and packaging system for better customer satisfaction and intellectual property right protection
- Application of new inventory tracking tools to eliminate counterfeiting and parallel-importing risks.

The primary task of distribution logistics is speedy and on time delivery of finished products to the customer coordinating the steps like order processing, warehousing, delivery packaging, and transportation. Distribution logistics has gain importance as the time, place, and quantity of production are correlated with the difference in the time, place and quantity of consumption. Organizations nowadays must collaborate and rely on effective supply chains or networks to compete in the global market and the online networked economic culture. Traditionally, the companies working in the field of supply network used to concentrate on the inputs and outputs to the processes, with little concern for the internal management level and employee level working. In the 21st century, expansion of business environment has developed supply chain networks beyond local boundaries. Multinational companies are proliferating nowadays through joint ventures, strategic alliances, and business partnerships. The companies are implementing the concepts of 'Just-In-Time', 'Lean Manufacturing' and 'Agile Manufacturing' practices. Revolution in information technology has also contributed significantly in product promotion and effortless transaction leading to easy going coordination among the manufacturer and supply chain network enabling fastest product delivery.

EVOLUTION OF SUPPLY CHAIN MANAGEMENT

A U.S. industry consultant first coined the initiation of supply chain management in the early 1980s. Though, the concept of supply chain management was of great importance long before the early 20th century with the introduction to assembly line in manufacturing technology. In the 1060s, development of Electronic Data Interchange (EDI) systems has helped in the integration of supply chain management which was further developed by the introduction of Enterprise Resource Planning (ERP) systems in the 1990s. This period had continued to develop until the 21st century when with the expansion of internet-based collaborative systems characterized both increases in value-addition and cost reductions through integration.

The era of globalization has driven the development of comprehensive worldwide systems of suppliers networking expanding the supply chains over national boundaries into other continents. Organizations have welcomed globalization of supply chain management with the goal of increasing their competitive advantage, value-adding and reducing costs through global sourcing. Supply chain management evolved as a specialized service with the inception of transportation brokerages, warehouse management, and non-asset-based carriers. Beyond mear transportation and logistics aspects, it has matured into the integration of planning, collaboration, execution and performance management. At the beginning of the nineties, industries have started shifting focus on 'core competencies' with an increasing tendency to outsource manufacturing and distribution, specialized models. With the adoption of contract manufacturing practices, it started managing bills of material with different part numbering schemes, for work-in-process visibility and vendor-managed inventory (VMI). Outsourced technology hosting for supply chain solutions had grown primarily in transportation and collaboration categories. The specialized model composes multiple steps of distribution networks for the individual supply chains specific to products and suppliers, who work together to distribute, market and sell a product. According to unique characteristics and demands of a given market, region or channel trading partner environment also proliferates. This variability had a significant effect on the supply chain infrastructure ranging from secure establishment and management of the electronic communication to the more complex configuration of processes and workflows that are essential to the management of the network between the trading partners.

SIGNIFICANCE OF LOGISTICS MANAGEMENT IN PHARMACEUTICALS

The pharmaceutical industry is facing unparalleled challenges impacting the business globalization, economical pricing policy, government controls over pricing and fast advancing technology. Logistics is a crucial part of pharmaceutical business as the pharmaceutical product distribution activities are highly sensitive to the maintenance of quality and safety aspects and also time-bound. Pharmaceutical products need a temperature controlled storage and distribution under strict regulatory control. The pharmaceutical industry in India is highly focused on quality products, and focusing this continual evolution of research and development are going to keep pace with developed countries. Over time, the Indian pharmaceutical industry has given importance to quality supply chain services for logistic activities for delivering products to the end customer at right time, right place, in a secure form and also at a competitive operational cost. Some of the critical factors affecting pharmaceutical supply chain in India are:

1. The notable contribution of the supply chain system in the pharmaceutical industry is inventory recycling and reduction of order cycle time. Operational performance is directly linked to logistics costs, while inventory recycling and the reduced order cycle time are related to on-time delivery.

2. Product liability refers to the legal liability that arises out of the design, manufacture, distribution, sale, and disposal of a product. The pharmaceutical industries are concerned about quality consistency throughout the lifetime of the product, defined by stability conditions. Stability is defined as the ability of a drug product to remain within established specifications, maintain its identity, strength, quality, and purity until the expiration date. Although the storage conditions in the production facility and the drug store are maintained relatively constant, the distribution environment can vary greatly while the drug product is shipped between various climatic zones in different countries challenging the quality and stability of a product.

3. Seasonal changes, mode of transportation and number of drop-off points varies within the pharmaceutical supply chain that can deviate the quality specification. Distribution of drug products requiring controlled-temperature storage conditions must be in a manner ensuring no adverse effect on product quality. It is virtually impossible to validate the quality consistency of a shipping method against all environmental conditions. So there is always a risk of quality deviation due to physical, chemical or microbiological instability in products during inland or abroad shipping.

   Stability testing recommends thermal cycling studies to validate the effects of temperature variation on drug products quality. Packaged drug products are stored in stimulated high-temperature conditions likely to be encountered while the drug product is in distribution or consumption phase. The products are cycled from high to low temperatures for several days and repeated several times. Distribution stability studies generate additional data on the effect of temperature excursion on product quality.

4. An effective and written procedure is required for the prompt recall of pharmaceutical products, with a designated person(s) responsible for recalls. The procedure should comply with the guidance issued by the national or regional regulatory authority. Recall information must be provided to the appropriate national or regional regulatory authority. In case recall of a genuine original product is necessary due to a complaint related to its counterfeited product which is not readily distinguishable from the original product, the manufacturer of the original product should inform the relevant health authority.

5. Pharmaceutical supply chains do not allow much flexibility relative to non-pharmaceutical supply chains. As pharmaceutical industries have fixed places of production and prices making it difficult to maintain logistic cost while dealing with issues of distances to markets and lead times of production and procurement. Pharmaceutical organizations mostly do not use the end-to-end supply chain model as used by non-pharmaceutical organizations as it has Carrying and Forwarding Agents (C&F), wholesalers and retailers as part of the supply chain.

INDIAN PHARMACEUTICAL SUPPLY CHAIN

The Indian pharmaceutical industry is ready to become globally competitive. The Indian healthcare sector is one of the fastest growing and is expected to cross $372 billion by 2022. Pharmaceutical product export value in 2017–18 stood at $17 billion and are expected to reach $20 billion by 2020. With the implementation of GST, the *Indian logistics market* is expected to reach above $200 billion in 2020. The pharma logistics market has an addressable size of $500 million in India, with an average annual growth rate of 4% whereas the global pharma logistics market is expected to grow at 5.5% rate by 2020. The logistics costs of the industry incurred towards packaging, ground transportation, marketing, cold chain supply, and storage, are been growing at a compound annual growth rate (CAGR) of 5–7% since 2002 onwards. The major logistics costs of pharmaceutical products are expensed for packaging and distribution. Logistics comprises 45–55% costs of the pharmaceutical product value chain. Pharmaceutical companies worldwide have started using supply chain management technique to improve the entire functional process. Supply chain management has helped pharma companies to enhance their efficiency in managing resources and improving relationships. Cold chain supply is a complicated and challenging affair in India with the coexistence of six different *climates* zones from hot, dry, humid, to cold and cloudy. India is a big country with the presence of more than 55,000 retail pharmacies spread across the states. The supply chain management interacts with challenges while transporting temperature sensitive drugs such as vaccines, biologicals, and injections of life saving drugs to the far-flung areas also affecting the cost factor.

The Indian pharmaceutical supply chain is witnessing a paradigm shift in the distribution cycle with the introduction of single shoot GST (Goods and Services Tax) taxation, consolidation of pharma companies, the emergence of pharma retail store chains and government-initiated Jan Aushadhi stores. The introduction of value added tax (VAT) in 2005 replac-

ing general sales tax along with increasing government pressure to constrain retail drug prices has squeezed domestic margins. The biggest reform of the Indian pharmaceutical supply chain is imminent again with the implementation of GST in 2016-17 changing market functions. GST came with a great deal of ambiguity concerning its impact on the pharmaceutical industry, creating a lot of uncertainty in the supply chain also. With GST applicable many raw materials, salts, compounds, and APIs in 5% VAT bracket has moved to 12% GST bracket. The pharmaceutical companies have to spend more in manufacturing as the material cost has gone up urging to change the MRP of the product to absorb that impact. GST replaced the multistage taxation in the pharmaceuticals industry, i.e. central excise duty on manufacturing, central sales tax or VAT on sale of goods, customs duty on imports, Service tax on provision of services and levies such as entry tax, cess by the State or municipalities with a single tax rate rationalizing the tax structure and helping in reducing cost on transportation, warehousing and inventory holding.

CHALLENGES OF ADOPTING SCM PRACTICES

Transportation of pharmaceutical products are done following precaution to maintain:
- Product identity
- Package integrity
- Product should not get contaminated
- Adequate precautions should be taken against spillage, breakage, misappropriation, and theft.
- Appropriate environmental conditions should be maintained, especially while transporting thermolabile products.

The complex quality issues related to the pharmaceutical supply chain can be apprehended with a full understanding of interdependency between the transportation process and product characteristics. Pharmaceutical products should not get adversely affected by environmental conditions while in shipment. Pharmaceutical products are to be sold and/or distributed by persons or entities authorized to acquire such products as per the regulations of applicable national, regional and international legislation. All the distribution channel involved in dealing pharmaceutical products supply must obtain requisite authority permission prior distribution of products. An extensive regulatory requirement leads to inflexibility and inability to react quickly to changes and facilities that are either capacity constrained or underutilized.

Production: Selection of a specific manufacturing site for particular product tactical factors such as compliance, profitability, labor skill, costs, and age of equipment are key factors in making strategic decisions. For winning, market strategy pharmaceutical companies should recognize the need for competence in global siting and production network rationalization. Nowadays manufacturing plants are typically designed for a specific drug, formulation or therapeutic class. Therefore optimum asset utilization and fulfilling supply of high-demand products are systemic problems. High inventory overdue, low turns, and late deliveries have plagued many pharmaceutical manufacturers over the years. Nowadays competition has increased in the pharma sector due to shorter exclusivity periods, the boom in the generic market, availability of more drugs with a locked-out patent period. Pharmaceutical companies need repositioning to respond more accurately towards changing customer demand assuring real-time business performance.

Distribution: Distribution is the most important part of the integrated supply-chain management of pharmaceutical products. Mostly different agencies are responsible for handling, storage, and distribution of pharmaceutical products in the supply chain, however, in some cases, a single agency can also be involved for the entire elements of the distribution process. "WHO Good Distribution Practices for Pharmaceutical Products" guideline provides a details description of all aspects of the pharmaceutical products distribution process ensuring the quality and identity of drugs during supply. These aspects include but not limited to, procurement, purchasing, storage, distribution, transportation, repackaging, relabelling, documentation and record-keeping practices. Good Distribution Practices help in the integration and coordination of Indian and international businesses.

Goods and inventory management: Pharmaceutical products shipment containers are designed to maintain product quality providing adequate protection from external influences and contamination. Various companies, institutions, as well as individuals are involved in pharmaceutical products distribution, storage, sale provided with licensing from the FDAs. Guidelines and documentation assist in proper fulfillment of the different aspects of the distribution process in the supply chain to avoid the introduction of counterfeits into the market place.

Traceability: "Electronic track and trace" technology is used by the pharmaceutical manufacturers, and also by supply chain intermediaries like distributors, traders, and wholesalers, which is necessary for the compliance of recall. The person or entity responsible for the transportation of the pharmaceutical products should be aware of the pharmaceutical products distribution requirements and complies with the appropriate storage and transport conditions. The dispatch and transportation of pharmaceutical products are initiated only after receipt of a valid delivery order. Dispatch records must contain enough information to enable traceability of the product batch all along its distribution channel to facilitate recall of a batch, if necessary, and also for any investigation related to counterfeit pharmaceutical products matching the original one.

Recall and return: A product recall is a request based return of an entire marketed batch of a product, usually due to complaint related to safety issues. Management of successful product recall is one of the most critical challenges for the pharmaceutical company. The regulatory guidelines of the FDAs are evolving and becoming increasingly stringent for product recall requirement. Handling product recall related issues can seriously impact on the daily operations of the organization. Automated software solutions can be used for both forward and backward lot traceability and serial number tracking and mock recall testing. Establishment of recall-specific contacts for suppliers, storing of pre-defined documents, press releases associated with potential recalls and the ability to e-mail these documents directly to the intended recipients helps in the management of effective recall.

Reverse supply chain: Reverse logistics also called as 'Aftermarket Customer Services' is the process of managing the return of marketed products from each and every point of distribution. As logistics is the movement of goods from suppliers to customers, *reverse logistics* is movement in the opposite direction. When the need arises for product recall reverse logistics play an important role which has become an integral part of today's supply chain operations. Reverse logistics strategy is mostly based on supply chain transparency enabling tracking of product using the lot and/or batch number, identifying product shipping locations, receivers contact details and successfully recapturing the product to be returned to the manufacturer immediately.

PHYSICAL DISTRIBUTION OF PHARMACEUTICAL PRODUCTS

The manufacturing units produce and supply products to the distribution channels based on past forecasts. Activities are related to planning, scheduling and supporting manufacturing operations, such as work-in-process storage, handling, transportation and time phasing of components, inventory management and maximum flexibility in the coordination of geographic and final assemblies controlling the physical distribution of products. Physical distribution is the movement of a finished product/service to the customer or the final destination of the marketing channel. On time availability of the product/service is a vital part of the success of each marketing channel effort. Pharmaceutical companies are increasing inclining towards the practice of production and services outsourcing that traditionally have been provided in-house. This trend is particularly evident in logistics where the provision for transport, warehousing, and inventory control is subcontracted to specialist logistics partners. Management and control of this type of network having external partners and suppliers require a blend of both central and local management level involvement. Strategic decisions are always taken by the central management of the company with a plan to monitor and control suppliers performance and day-to-day liaisoning with logistics partners at a local level.

Understanding product characteristics, typical environmental conditions and anticipating environmental extremes the protocols for the distribution stability programs are developed for performance measurement. Stability experts and distribution personnel must share information for a collaborative approach for adopting efficient transportation conditions. The combined data of in house stability study and transportation data provide the information necessary to develop product-specific shipping criteria. Shipping and distribution control strategy document complements the overall robustness of a distribution program. Special storage and environmental conditions (e.g. temperature and/or relative humidity) required for transportation of pharmaceutical products must be standardised, monitored and recorded. Records regarding transportation condition data monitoring are needed to be kept for a minimum of the shelf-life of the product distributed plus one year, or as required by national legislation. Monitoring data is made available for inspection of the regulatory or other oversight bodies when required.

Methods of transportation, including suitable vehicles to be used for ground transport, is selected with care considering local conditions of climate and seasonal variations experienced. Delivery of products requiring controlled temperatures should be in accordance with the applicable storage and transport conditions. Shipping containers must bear labels specifying information on handling and storage conditions and precautions to be exercised ensuring the products are properly handled and secure at all times. Internationally and/or nationally accepted abbreviations, names or codes are used while labeling of shipment containers enabling identification of the containers' content and source. Special care must be exercised while using dry ice in shipment containers as it may have an adverse effect on the quality of the product if cames in contact with the pharmaceutical product. Damaged and/or broken shipment containers are handled as per written procedures. Vehicles and containers are needed to be loaded carefully and systematically, as it helps in unloading on first-out/last-in basis saving time and prevent physical damage.

Particular attention should be paid while transporting potentially toxic and hazardous products such as toxic, radioactive materials, and other dangerous pharmaceutical products presenting special risks of abuse, fire or explosion (e.g. combustible/flammable liquids, solids, and pressurized gases). Loading and unloading of boxes of hazardous products require special care. Pharmaceutical products containing hazardous substances should be stored and transported in safe, dedicated and secure areas, and vehicles marked outside with special precaution. Products containing toxic and/or flammable substances are transported in suitably designed dedicated containers in compliance with applicable international and national legislation. Products containing narcotics and other dependence-producing substances should be transported in safe and secure containers and vehicles to prevent any attempted theft or misuse. Special attention should be given to the designing, cleaning, and maintenance of all equipment used for the handling of vehicles used for transportation of hazardous pharmaceutical products. Equipment and cleaning agents used for the cleaning of vehicles should be chosen and used so as not to constitute a source of contamination. Special provision should be available for segregation of rejected, recalled and returned pharmaceutical products as well as those suspected to counterfeit during transit. These type of products are securely packaged and labeled and transported accompanied with appropriate documentation. Measures should be in place to prevent unauthorized persons from entering and/or tampering with vehicles and/or equipment engaged with pharmaceutical product transport.

Distributors receive and process pharmaceutical product returns or exchanges under the terms and conditions of the agreement between the distributor and the recipient. Both distributors and such respective parties are accountable for the return process administration ensuring that operation is secure and do not permit the entry of counterfeit product. The rejected and returned products are transported following the appropriate process in accordance with the relevant storage and other provision requirements.

COLD CHAIN SUPPLY (DRUG TRACING SYSTEM)

The pharmaceutical supply chain is becoming increasingly complex, involving a number of storage and transit locations including airports and docks. Pharmaceutical product distribution is widely variable and depends upon a range of factors:

- Points of origin and destination
- Products sensitivity to temperature
- Transit mode, ground, air, sea or combination
- Time, weather and season
- Carrier vehicle type

Shipping of temperature-sensitive articles requiring thermally controlled shipping presents particular challenges. Thermal hazards tend to be unique regarding its product degradation capabilities compared to shock, vibration, and other physical hazards. Label indication of storage temperature is not at all indicative of the allowable temperature tolerances during shipping, i.e. parenteral products labeled with storage conditions between 2 and 8°C may vary widely in their stability characteristics for short-term exposure of heat and cold.

Temperature cycling study data gives a clear indication of drugs got affected by multiple, short-term excursions beyond the storage temperature limits. Wholesalers and retailers of those drug products must exercise special handling practices during particular climate conditions. The commonly used refrigerants are dry ice (frozen carbon dioxide gas) and wet ice (frozen water). These refrigerants come as crushed ice or in various sized refrigerant packs containing water mixtures with specific freezing points and also as special phase-change materials for specialized needs. Refrigerant packs are cooled to the correct freezing point to get the proper surface temperature before use. An insulating barrier is placed between the refrigerant and the product with some special packaging material for the products liable to get damaged by accidental freezing. Commonly available insulating materials are foil laminates, bubble pack, corrugated, fabricated, and molded expanded polystyrene (EPS) cartons, and fabricated or molded urethane foam cartons, with or without additional interior components. Dry ice is placed in such a manner that the drug product and the primary package does not get adversely affected while in transportation. Validated temperature-controlled vehicles are an expensive investment for the transport service provider. It is imperative that the safety of the pharmaceutical products must not be compromised by placing consignments of other articles in the vehicle. Exclusive and special condition transportation requirements of pharmaceutical products make the distribution costs higher. A solution can be packaging the thermolabile pharmaceutical products in thermostable packing which is again not very cost-effective as these types of thermal resistant packaging is expensive enough.

Drug traceability during the whole course of transportation has become increasingly important not only to detect and deter entry of counterfeit drugs but also to track and trace biological products like vaccines, antisera, blood components, and hormonal products having high sensitivity to transportation environment variations. Drug tracing system provides integrated end-to-end management and control on drugs movement from the manufacturer to the distributors, through intermediate wholesalers, to the healthcare institutions and medical stores involved in the retail sale of drugs, and ultimately to the patients who receive the prescription drugs. The ability to identify the individual product by barcode or microchip identification tags is a unique approach to implement for product traceability. Microchip-based tags are generally more effective as they can store substantial amounts of data and also permit additional data to be added in the course of progress in distribution route, if necessary. Microchips are affected by liquid, metal, noise, magnetic and electroconductive substances.

Microchip tags vary in size and functional capabilities, therefore are selected as per the specific requirements like shape, content, and purpose to fit for the drug product packs to be traced. Quality of some specific drug products can only be ensured if the product does not spend longer than a specified length of time under certain temperature conditions during the transportation process. The drug manufacturers are implementing sensor-based tracking devices in the lot unit level packing in order to comply with new mandatory history control requirements for biological products. The quality of such products is ensured by using sensors or an active tag as periodic collection, recording, and monitoring of transit temperature, vibration, and other pertinent condition related data is not possible to review while in transit from one point to another. The sensors can be mounted over the batch or lot unit pack or in close proximity to the drug product storage shelves to measure actual environmental conditions.

CRITICAL ISSUES IN UNDERSTANDING THE PHARMACEUTICAL SUPPLY CHAIN MANAGEMENT

The core elements of supply chain management are gathering, monitoring, measuring, simulating, notifying and managing product across the supply chain processes, viz. internal organizations and external trading communities. The objective is to create smooth-running operations by seamlessly notifying the right people at the right time when action or intervention may be necessary. Regulations aim to foster safe, transparent, and secure distribution system by establishing measures to ensure that pharmaceutical products are supplied with proper documentation permitting traceability of the products throughout distribution channels from the manufacturer/importer to the entity responsible for selling or supplying the product to the patient. Distribution records including the labeling details

on expiry dates and batch records are an integral part of secure distribution documentation enabling traceability. The significant critical issues concerning pharmaceutical supply chain management are:

1. The pharmaceutical supply chain dislikes any other supply chain, is not only bringing products from the manufacturers to the retailer but also guarantee product integrity. The pharmaceutical supply chain is also inherently different in its organization as the pricing for a particular product may be different for each end user. A hospital can get a drug at lower rates than does a patient from a corner pharmacy. There are programs like Medicare, Medicaid, Red Cross and Jan Aushadhi where the procurement prices for the generic drugs are different from a corner pharmacy.

2. Authorized procurement and release procedures are followed for all administrative and technical operations performed in the supply process to ensure procurement of appropriate pharmaceutical products from approved suppliers and distributed by approved entities under the approval of competent regulatory authority of the individual country.

3. An adequate number of competent personnel are involved in all stages of the distribution of pharmaceutical products in order to ensure product quality and legal obligation compliance. All personnel involved in distribution activities are to be qualified and trained as per the requirements of Good Distribution Practices. Training module mostly includes aspects of product identification, safety, security, environmental condition maintenance and the detection and control of counterfeits entering into the supply chain. Personnel dealing transportation of hazardous pharmaceutical products (bioactive drugs, radioactive

materials, narcotics, and other hazardous, environmentally sensitive products and/or products presenting special risks of abuse, fire or explosion) need specific training.

4. Appropriate measures are adopted to ensure the integrity of the pharmaceutical products in transit. Seal control transit programmes are practiced for shipment issued in a tracked and sequential manner. The integrity of seals are monitored and numbers verified during transit and upon receipt. Approved procedures are followed to deal with the situations of suspected or found to be counterfeit pharmaceutical products.

5. Transit risk assessments studies are conducted by the distributors frequently to assess potential risks to the quality and integrity of pharmaceutical products. Control systems are developed and implemented to address any potential risks identified. The quality system is reviewed and revised periodically to address new risks identified during risk assessment.

6. Product traceability must be ensured throughout the supply chain as a shared responsibility among all the parties involved in the supply chain. Documented traceability for products received and distributed are ensured along with the identity of all parties involved in the supply chain to facilitate product recalls. "Electronic track and trace system" is implemented following the national policies and legislation depending on the type of product as it is beneficial in the long run for the pharmaceutical companies as well as the ultimate end users. Only the authorized persons are entitled to perform all electronic communication and transactions related to the distribution of pharmaceutical products.

7. Pedigree documentation review along with the visual and/or analytical identification enables to trace entry of potentially counterfeit products in the supply chain. The distributor must notify the marketing authorization holder, the labeled entity as if marketed by other company (if different from manufacturer), the appropriate national and/or international regulatory bodies, as well as other relevant competent authorities when a potential counterfeit pharmaceutical product is identified. Counterfeit products found in the distribution chain are kept apart clearly labeled as not for sale from other pharmaceutical products to avoid any confusion.

8. Internationally applicable product coding and identification system are applied in consultation and collaboration with the various parties involved in the supply chain for the export pharmaceutical product. A differentiated approach is necessary for different products and regions, pedigree and/or track-and-trace technologies provide possible options to ensure traceability.

9. Vehicles and equipment used to distribute pharmaceutical products are to be suitable to prevent contamination and prevent exposure of the products to environmental conditions adversely affecting stability and package integrity. The design and use of vehicles and equipment must aim to minimize the risk of errors and/or contamination. Effective cleaning is done to make the vehicle free of dust or dirt that may have an adverse effect on the quality of pharmaceutical products being distributed. Vehicles and containers should have sufficient capacity and space to allow orderly storage of the various categories of pharmaceutical products during transportation. Overloading of vehicles carrying pharmaceutical products is not allowed. Equipment planted in the vehicles and containers for monitoring

temperature and humidity are calibrated at regular intervals. Where non-dedicated vehicles and equipment are used, appropriate cleaning is performed, checked and recorded, to ensure that the quality of the pharmaceutical product has not been compromised.

10. In case of third-party carriers, written agreements are being made between distributors and carriers in line with national and regional regulatory requirements to ensure that appropriate measures are taken to safeguard pharmaceutical products, including maintaining appropriate documentation and records. Delegation of any activity related to the distribution of a pharmaceutical product to another person or entity is done only with the parties appropriately authorized for that function in accordance with the terms of a written contract which is agreed upon by the contract giver and the contract acceptor. The contract should define the responsibilities of each party including observance and compliance of the principles of GDP and relevant warranty clauses. It should also include the responsibilities of the contractor to adopt measures to avoid the entrance of counterfeit medicines into the distribution chain and is audited periodically.

11. In the case of recall requirement, all wholesalers and retailers distributed with particular pharmaceutical product and the competent regulatory authorities is promptly informed. All distribution records must be readily available to the designated person(s) responsible for recalls. These records contain sufficient information on products supplied to customers including exported products. The progress of the recall process is recorded, and a final report is issued describing reconciliation between delivered and recovered quantity, recall reason, investigation of compliant, test results of recalled products and action taken on the product. The effectiveness of the arrangements for recalls should be evaluated at regular intervals. All recalled pharmaceutical products should be stored in a secure, segregated area pending appropriate action.

IMPORTATION SUPPLY CHAIN MANAGEMENT

Pharmaceutical products are exported outside India following "WHO guidelines on import procedures for pharmaceutical products." Customs, enforcement agencies and regulatory agencies are responsible for the supervision of pharmaceutical products export activities. These agencies establish cooperation and information exchange in order to prevent the importation of counterfeit pharmaceutical products. Requirements to import pharmaceutical products are country-specific although most of the procedures and formalities are similar for all countries after globalization of trade by General Agreement on Tariff and Trade (GATT). For World Trade Organization (WTO) countries more trade liberalization is expected in the near future through Trade Facilitation Agreement (TFA).

In most of the countries, registration in foreign trade agency is required to become an importer. In India, IEC (Import Export Code) Number is obtained from the office of Director General of Foreign Trade. Nowadays, the information about registration for importer–exporter is linked with customs location and reserve bank, making it online digitalized. Some common requirements to import Pharmaceutical products in major countries are:

The manufacturer provides a warranty or batch certificate for each imported consignment of a pharmaceutical product as recommended by the WHO Certification Scheme.

No objection certificate from Drug controller of importing country is required to import some of the special items under pharmaceutical products, drugs, medicines, cosmetics, etc.

The Certificate of origin issued by drug control authority for imported Pharmaceutical products is required in almost all countries. This certificate helps to determine the origin of imported goods to avail exemption on import duties and taxes as per different unilateral, multilateral and bilateral agreement between countries.

The number of ports of entry for imported pharmaceutical products enforced with formalities of appropriate legislation is limited in every country. The port most appropriately located and best equipped to handle imported pharmaceutical products are chosen as the port(s) of entry in a country for the imported products. The importer is responsible for undertaking all requisite steps to ensure that products are not mishandled or exposed to adverse storage conditions at wharves or airports. Persons having training on the handling of pharmaceutical products are involved with the customs procedures and be readily contactable.

Legal responsibilities: Pharmaceutical products are imported in conformance with the national drugs act or other relevant legislation enforced by the national drug regulatory authority of India and the country of import. All transactions relating to the importation of pharmaceutical products consignments are to be conducted either through the governmental drug procurement agency or through independent wholesale dealers specifically designated and licensed by the national drug regulatory authority for this purpose. The customs authorities have the discretionary powers to request for technical advice and opinions from other appropriately qualified persons, if particular circumstances warrant this. The WHO Certification Scheme on the "Quality of Pharmaceutical Products Moving in International Commerce" are

followed to provide data regarding the quality assessment of imported pharmaceutical products.

In countries where no formal system of product licensing being imposed, for importation of products the national drug regulatory authority formalizes the process by issuing permits in the name of the authorized importing agency or agent. The national drug regulatory authority compiles a comprehensive and frequently updated list of licensed products and authorized importing agents, and issue notifications of any product licenses withdrawn on the grounds of safety. Efficient and confidential channels for communicating information on counterfeit products and other illicit activities are established between all interested official bodies.

Customs clearance: Customs clear the duly licensed pharmaceutical products supported by appropriate documentation for marketing within the importing country. All customs posts designated to handle consignments of pharmaceutical products are consequently provided with secure storage facilities, including refrigerated compartments for thermolabile products. At the port of entry, consignments of pharmaceutical products are to be stored under suitable conditions for as short period as possible. The National Drug Regulatory Agency of a particular country is responsible for inspecting the facilities periodically to ensure that all equipment and facility is in good working condition. The importing agency or agent should alert the customs authorities in advance of the anticipated arrival of consignments for a speedy transfer from the international carrier to the designated storage facility with the minimum of delay and, as for appropriate cases, without breaking the cold chain. Consignments of pharmaceutical products and pharmaceutical starting materials are accorded high priority for clearance through customs.

ADVANTAGES OF ADOPTING SUPPLY CHAIN MANAGEMENT PRACTICES

Healthy relationship when exists between the largest arcs of supplier and customer, integration can generate maximum market share and profitability. Taking advantage of supplier capabilities and emphasizing on customer relationships a firm can excel in performance aiming long-term supply chain perspective.

Customer targeting: Customer-based diversification primarily from wholesalers and group purchasing organizations (GPOs) to retailers, service providers, and consumers provide opportunities for manufacturers to gain visibility with a real-time demand based delivery but may increase the overall supply chain costs. The GPOs helps the healthcare providers such as hospitals, nursing homes and home health service providing agencies to cut down medical and supply costs while ensuring supply of necessary medical equipments and medicines on time. The GPOs do aggregated purchasing in high volume and uses this leverage to negotiate discounts with manufacturers, distributors and other vendors. A cost-management-based sales approach by disease/indication and segment-based marketing and sales channel management can reduce the cost to a great extent.

Inventory cost: Over the past decade, improvement of the efficiency of purchasing activities has become an essential and strategic part of the goals of most organizations as an increase in profitability can be equally accomplished by spending less. The practice of supply chain management fundamental in daily working can reduce materials inventory from 40 percent to 25 percent, which is much lower than the industry's normal average.

Raw material supply: Supply chain management practices enable the industry to procure materials from a reasonable number of suppliers to reduce the risk factors, and the company can get shifted to a single window system. In the pharmaceutical industry, e-procurement has been massively embraced because of its association with lower transaction costs, reduced unit price and a drive toward contract compliance. E-procurement may lower the costs when supported by strategic sourcing or supplier management, so that cost structures and productivity are also enhanced downstream. The benefits of strategic sourcing not only reduce total costs for buyer and supplier, but also ensure higher quality, low working capital, ongoing reduction in lead times, and welcoming to productive partnerships.

Cost reduction: Successful adoption of supply chain management practices allows companies to gain bargaining power and reduce sales prices by five to ten percent. Efficiency of supply chain structure, when positioned in best, reduces the cost by increasing market share. In the coming years, pharmaceutical companies that do not adapt to optimized cost and business effective supply structures will risk market survival. Drug utilization review shows a potential shift in customers from efficacy to cost efficiency.

Service quality: Efficient supply chain management not only helps in reducing the number of transporters but also reduce the delivery time. When a new product is developed, the cycle for commercializing of that product and rolling it out become a much tighter job. Intelligent synchronization between production, marketing, and channel networking can enable faster rollouts. Information and feedback on the effectiveness of reverse logistics functionality are needed to be considered parallel to demand generation and fulfillment processes.

Customer Service: Innovations are now being implemented by the pharmaceutical business world to improve and implement a value added supply chain. Nearly half of the health-insured population in the United States now receives medical care from Pharmaceutical Benefits Managers. As a consequence, the mail order channel has grown dramatically, with a unique supply chain requirements differing from those of the hospital or retail store channel. Drug manufacturers and health care providers are implementing Disease Management Programs that provide specialized services for a specific disease to a particular patient directly, i.e. diabetic control, cancer care centers, etc. These programs allow drug manufacturers to get much closer to the consumer and better control of manufacturing starting from the inventory levels correlated with demand planning. It needs undoubted adoption of SCM practices, to bypass multileveled supply chain. Following these practices enable the companies to outsource facilities in the supply chain extending from research and marketing, sales and distribution, and call center functions. Evolution of new comprehensive supply chain dissolving the intermediation of wholesalers and distributors reduce the cost for the customer by developing the lower-cost-service channel.

Security: Software for supply management provides a web-based solution with an integrated database. This also provides multiple level security and user level access control for authorized persons for each operation. All the functions of logistics can be controlled from a single assess point stating from purchase to supply chain, inventory, warehouse, distribution, and sales. Internet access provides with flexible operational philosophy. Tight controls on Master data and Multi-layer Security have a limited risk of information pilferage.

Productivity measures: The pharmaceutical companies are experiencing a decline in market share and margins due to increased competition from generics market with a greater impact on profitability. Price pressures, shortened new drug exclusivity periods, mergers, acquisitions, consolidation, and escalating R&D costs also play a significant role. Consumers are becoming more knowledgeable about medicines due to mass communications (including advertising),

websites and information centers. Buying decision power continues to change with a shift in treatment strategies requiring more agile, tiered marketing at the same time handling the nonrevenue products. Sales processes that have traditionally focused on educating and building awareness within the medical care provider community, now need to anticipate and accommodate power shifts due to the entry of mass communications based marketing. More recently, large pharmaceutical companies have started mass marketing to US consumers.

Asset management: The time frame for the sales and marketing department to place a product, generate demand and influence market is shrinking due to increased generics competition and shortening exclusivity periods. Shrinking time frame and price pressures require adopting innovative sales distribution methods for marketing. Drug manufacturers are now marketing directly to consumers—via television and via the internet worldwide, but this particular mode of sales and marketing channel are only appropriate for certain products. Direct-to-consumer (DTC) advertising produces mixed results, and may also increase budgets significantly. Although DTC generates extra cost, these direct channels also present new opportunities to build loyalty and get closer to real-time demand. Identification and evaluation of the efficacy of these evolving sales channels should become integral to the commercialization process.

Channel management: New channel opportunities paired with the increasing role of Pharmaceutical Benefits Managers and disease management programs could present a ripe-for-picking time to address channel costs and performance for both nonrevenue and revenue business streams. To deal with the nonrevenue side, pharmaceutical companies are now exploring the value of alternative distribution possibilities, like distributing direct to disease management programs or leveraging the role of retail pharmacies. This strategy may provide opportunities to strengthen retail relationships and gather more accurate demand information on the real market.

On the other hand, revenue side can be dealt with shifting to cost- and performance-based channel management leading to cost savings. More reliable distribution and improved demand visibility can be achieved through e-marketplaces such as the Worldwide Retail Exchange and Global Healthcare Exchange. The drug manufacturers can now sell directly to retailers and health care providers. Additionally, as Pharmaceutical Benefits Managers and disease management programs continue to evolve and mature, drug makers should anticipate their technology and information needs in order to seek ways to integrate with their customer management, and financial processes.

EUROPEAN MEDICINES VERIFICATION SYSTEM (EMVS)

The EMVS is a new system of end-to-end verification of medicines designed to ensure patient safety by preventing falsified medicines from entering the legal supply chain of EU. The EMVS covers mainly prescription medicines for human use. According to the legislation, pharmaceutical manufacturers and parallel importers are required to print an embedded two-dimensional Data Matrix code on the medicine pack. The code incorporates a Unique Identifier (UI) along with an anti-tampering device to the outer packaging for each individual sales package. The Data Matrix includes information about the batch number, expiry date, and the UI that consists of a random serial number unique to each pack and a product code. The UI is then uploaded to the European hub EVMS by the manufacturer. The UI is checked at various points during the supply chain. Using specifically designed software, the distributors carry out verification checks of the UI in data matrix on the outer packaging. It verifies the authenticity as the product travels through the supply chain. The medicines are scanned at the point of dispense and verified for authenticity against a national (or supranational) repository. When the UI on the pack matches the UI in the repository, the pack is decommissioned from the EMVS by the pharmacist and dispensed to the patient. In case there is a warning related to this pack, the system will highlight this as an exceptional event following an investigation to determine whether the pack has tampered. Medicines packages without UI is no longer produced from 9th February 2019 and will, over time, permanently leave the supply chain. The EMVS has entered into its operational phase on 9th February 2019 in 28 European countries participating all in the European Economic Area (EEA). Italy and Greece will make use of a longer implementation period. This system aims to provide a final safety measure to ensure the endpoint verification of the medicines authenticity.

CURRENT PERSPECTIVES

Logistics in the pharma industry play a very critical role in providing the right medicine to the right place, at the right time, and most importantly at the right price. Pharmaceutical business has become highly competitive today, and success largely depends upon the efficiency of the supply chain. The supply chain is very important as it maintains the complex network relationship between the organizations (drug manufacturers), trading partners to source raw materials, product partners, delivery, retailers and hospitals. With the growing competition among major pharmaceutical players in the country, inventory control plays a significant role in the value maintenance of the pharma supply chain. In today's business environment, out of stock situation is unacceptable. The end retailer and customers must be supplied with the requisite amount of products as assured. Research and development require a huge investment to bring a successful product into the the market when it finally arrives, shortfall due to supply related issues is unbearable. As the value margins on pharma products are very high, different channels of distribution share around 30 percent of profit. Pharmaceutical companies agreeably spend a lot to improve the efficiency of supply chains. Consideration is given for adding feasible technology, such as global positioning system (GPS) electronic tracking devices and engine kill buttons to vehicles enhancing the security of pharmaceutical products while in the vehicle. Dedicated vehicles and equipment are used by the logistic facility providers while handling pharmaceutical products.

In the coming years, logistics and supply chain management are expected to play a significant role in the Indian pharma industry and could contribute to the enhancement of productivity as well as the growth of the industry. Supply chain specialization enables companies to improve their overall competencies in the same way what the manufacturing and distribution outsourcing has done before. It allows to focus on core competencies and assemble networks of specific, best-in-class partners to contribute to the overall value chain itself, thereby enhancing performance and efficiency. The ability to quickly supply products to its destined places maintaining the unique and complex competency is the leading reason for supply chain management popularity. Logistics competency becomes a more significant factor in creating and maintaining a competitive advantage. Logistic management becomes increasingly important as the difference between profitable and unprofitable operations are becoming narrower. Pharmaceutical companies are no longer satisfied with dictating the temperature-controlled agenda but are looking to partners who can maintain product safety, efficacy and

visibility across the supply chain globally. Logistics suppliers are under increasing pressure to raise their standards to the level of leading pharmaceutical companies. Companies are also rationalizing and consolidating supply chain operations and are looking to supply chain provider who can ensure end-to-end temperature control across the local, regional and global scale. Pricing pressures along with the adoption of new trends have already forced the profit margins down where any inefficiency in the pharmaceutical products supply chain could put the organization at risk. Pharmaceutical companies thriving to be well positioned for the future can achieve excellence despite the growing hardships and complexity for compliance with regulatory guidelines by focusing on distribution aspects through efficient supply chain management.

BIBLIOGRAPHY

1. Agarwal S, Desai S, Holcomb MM, Oberoi A. Unlocking the Value in Big Pharma. McKinsey Quarterly. http://www.mckinseyquarterly.com.
2. Bhandari M, Garg R, Glassman R, Philip CMa, Rodney WZ. A genetic revolution in healthcare. The McKinsey Quarterly. http://www.mckinsey-quarterly.com.
3. Cooper MC, Lambert DM, Pagh J. Supply Chain Management: More Than a New Name for Logistics. The International Journal of Logistics Management 1997; 8(1): 1–14.
4. Food and Drug Administration. Draft Guidance for Industry: Stability Testing of Drug Substances and Drug Products. Rockville, MD. 1998.
5. Good trade and distribution practices for pharmaceutical starting materials. In: WHO Expert Committee on Specifications for Pharmaceutical Preparations. Thirty-eighth report. Geneva, World Health Organization, WHO Technical Report Series. 2004.
6. Guidelines for implementation of the WHO Certification Scheme on the quality of pharmaceutical products moving in international commerce. WHO Expert Committee on Specifications for Pharmaceutical Preparations. Thirty-fourth report. Geneva, World Health Organi-

zation, WHO Technical Report Series, No. 863, Annex 10. 1996.

7. Guidelines on import procedures for pharmaceutical products. In: WHO Expert Committee on Specifications for Pharmaceutical Preparations. Thirty-fourth report. Geneva, World Health Organization, WHO Technical Report Series, No. 863, Annex 12. 1996.

8. Halldorsson A, Kotzab H, Mikkola JH, Skjoett-Larsen T. Complementary theories to supply chain management. Supply Chain Management: An International Journal 2007; 12(4): 284–296.

9. Harland CM. Supply Chain Management, Purchasing and Supply Management, Logistics, Vertical Integration, Materials Management and Supply Chain Dynamics. In: Slack, N edn. Blackwell Encyclopedic Dictionary of Operations Management. UK, Blackwell. 1996.

10. Hines T. Supply chain strategies: Customer driven and customer focused. Oxford: Elsevier press; 2004.

11. Ketchen JrG, Hult TM. Bridging organization theory and supply chain management: The case of best value supply chains. Journal of Operations Management 2006; 25(2): 573–580.

12. Kouvelis P, Chambers C, Wang H. Supply Chain Management Research and Production and Operations Management: Review, Trends, and Opportunities. Production and Operations Management 2006; 15(3): 449–469.

13. Mentzer JT, DeWitt W, Keebler JS, Min S, Nix NW, Smith CD, Zacharia ZG. Defining Supply Chain Management. Journal of Business Logistics 2001; 22(2): 1–25.

14. Murray A, Frazier H. A Prescription for Direct Drug Marketing. McKinsey Quarterly. http://www.mckinseyquarterly.com. 2000.

15. Otoshi K, Tomita H, Kaneko T. RFID Solutions for the Medical and Pharmaceutical Industries. Hitachi Review 2007; 56: 83–87.

16. Pear R. Drug Industry is told to stop gifts to doctors New York times. http://www.ny-\times.com.

17. Pharmaceutical Research and Manufacturers of America (PhRMA). Industry Profile, Washington, DC. http://www.phrma.org.

18. Simchi-Levi D, Kaminsky P, Simchi-levi E. Designing and Managing the Supply Chain, 3rd ed., New York: Mcgraw Hill; 2007.

19. Storage, temperature and humidity. USP27–NF 22, US Pharmacopeial Convention. General Notices _26_, Rockville, MD. 2004.

20. Taylor J. Good Shipping and Distribution Practices: paper presented at the United Kingdom Medicines and Healthcare Products Regulatory Agency, USP Packaging, Storage, and Distribution Open Conference. Washington, DC. 2003.

21. The European Medicines Verification System (EMVS) explained: The European Medicines Verification Organisation (EMVO). Brussels, Belgium. https://emvo-medicines.eu/new/wp-content/uploads/The-European-Medicines-Verification-System-explained-2.pdf.

Index